Whole Body Computerized Tomography

Practical image analysis
by
Otto Henning Wegener

Supplemented by films
contributed by
Detlev Behrendt
Claus Claussen
Thomas Grumme
Michael Haertel
Bernd Lochner
Detlev Rehnitz
Klaus Sartor
Burckhard Trempenau
Christian Utesch

English translation
by
Joseph H. Long

Berlex Imaging
Division of
Berlex Laboratories, Inc.

A publication
in the medico-scientific book series.
The book-shop edition is published by
S. Karger Basel – München – Paris – London – New York – Sydney.
A translation of
Ganzkörper-Computertomographie

All rights reserved.
No part of this publication may be translated into other languages, reproduced or utilized in any form or by any means, electronic or mechanical, including photocopying, recording, microcopying, or by any information storage and retrieval system, without permission in writing from the publisher.
© Copyright 1983 by Schering AG West Germany
Printed in Germany
Design: Werbestudio of
Schering AG West Germany
with the
collaboration of Urte von Bremen
Anatomical drawings: Klaus Bohm
Lithography:
Walter Bohm GmbH & Co KG, Berlin;
Carl Schütte & C. Behling, Berlin
Composition: Hellmich KG, Berlin
Printing: Oraniendruck GmbH, Berlin
ISBN 3-8055-2773-X

Schering AG West Germany
is not associated with Schering Corp.,
Kenilworth, N.J., USA.

To my academic tutor,
Prof. Dr. Heinz Oeser

Addresses

Dr. med. Detlev Behrendt
Abteilung für Röntgendiagnostik
(Chefarzt: Prof. Dr. H. Witt)
Rudolf-Virchow-Krankenhaus
1000 Berlin 65

Dr. med. Claus D. Claussen
Oberarzt und Ass. Prof. an der
Strahlenklinik und Poliklinik
(Direktor: Prof. Dr. R. Felix)
Klinikum Charlottenburg der
Freien Universität Berlin
1000 Berlin 19

Prof. Dr. med. Thomas Grumme
Oberarzt an der
Neurochirurgischen Abteilung
(Leiter: Prof. Dr. E. Katzner)
der Neurochirurgischen-
Neurologischen Klinik
und Poliklinik im
Klinikum Charlottenburg der
Freien Universität Berlin
1000 Berlin 19

Prof. Dr. med. Michael Haertel
Chefarzt des Instituts für
Diagnostische Radiologie am
Kantonsspital St. Gallen
CH-9000 St. Gallen

Dr. med. Bernd Lochner
Strahlenklinik und Poliklinik
(Direktor: Prof. Dr. R. Felix)
Klinikum Charlottenburg der
Freien Universität Berlin
1000 Berlin 19

Dr. med. Detlev Rehnitz
Oberarzt der Röntgenabteilung
(Chefarzt: Priv.-Doz. Dr. Jürgen Treichel)
Kreiskrankenhaus Ludwigsburg
7140 Ludwigsburg

Dr. med. Klaus Sartor
Oberarzt an der
Strahlendiagnostischen Abteilung
(Leiter: Prof. Dr. H. Schmidt)
des Allgemeinen Krankenhauses
Hamburg-Altona
2000 Hamburg

Dr. med. Burckhard Trempenau
Oberarzt an der Abteilung für
Röntgen-Diagnostik
(Chefarzt: Prof. Dr. H. Witt)
des Rudolf-Virchow-Krankenhauses
1000 Berlin 65

Dr. med. Christian Utesch
Röntgen- und Strahlenabteilung
(Chefarzt: Prof. Dr. P. Schaefer)
im Krankenhaus Neukölln
1000 Berlin 47

Priv.-Doz. Dr. med. O. H. Wegener
Oberarzt an der Röntgenabteilung
(Kommiss. Leiter: Prof. Dr. R. Felix)
im Klinikum Steglitz
der Freien Universität Berlin
Hindenburgdamm 30
1000 Berlin 45

Preface

When Professor Heinz Oeser asked me to write a short appreciation of the English translation of Dr. Wegener's book on Whole Body Computerized Tomography I accepted with great pleasure.

I had already been aware of the German text and was very impressed by the excellent overview of the wide and extensive field of computer tomography presented by the author and his colleagues. It is a very authoritative, well balanced, well illustrated account of the present state of the art. The student and more experienced radiologist is provided with all the necessary information required to master most problems which require computerized tomographic examinations.

The excellent anatomical diagrams and their correlations with CT scans will be most valuable to those learning the technique. Many clinical examples of various types of pathology and indications for CT examinations, established by personal experience gained from a large number of patient studies over several years by Dr. Wegener, will be most helpful to radiologists.

I am convinced that this English edition will be a very welcome book to doctors working in the field when technical and diagnostic decisions have to be made about CT investigations. The layout of the book is excellent and the text very readable. This new English edition will establish it as an eminently suitable handbook to be found in all departments of radiology where computerized tomography is being practised.

London, January 1983   R. E. Steiner

Preface

The introduction of computerized tomography is, without any doubt, the greatest technological breakthrough in the diagnostic sector of clinical radiology of recent decades. It has opened up a brand new field of diagnostic activity for clinical radiologists, challenging them to update and perfect their diagnostic knowledge and to keep up with changes.

Whole body computerized tomography has now been in clinical use long enough to justify an attempt at a systematic text book which goes beyond individual case reports. The different radiological journals have published a multitude of papers in recent years and it is frequently very difficult — particularly for the would-be specialist — to overlook, evaluate and assimilate the results of this literature.

To find a way through this maze Dr. Wegener has undertaken the highly laudable task of compiling the accumulated knowledge from the literature and his own experience in our clinic within the covers of a single textbook. With its systematic layout, the book attempts to be a pillar of support to the student and a reference work for daily practice to the experienced radiologist. The author's own experience spans five intensive years.

At the same time the book tries to show the limits of the method, which are often set too high in individual problems because of the great progress made. Attention to this aspect of the book could save unnecessary and, above all, expensive examinations. In this context the book is naturally also directed at the doctor establishing the indication for computerized tomography and referring the patient for this examination. By referring to the chapters on the individual organs he can see for himself what is possible and what is not.

In addition to typical films, the book also contains a number of assiduously drawn diagrams to facilitate understanding.

I wish the book the rapid and widespread distribution it deserves.

Berlin, November 1981   R. Felix

Acknowledgements for the English edition

Thanks are also extended to Joseph H. Long for the excellent translation of this book and to Dr. Janet Husband for her kind and friendly assistance.

Berlin, October 1982   O. H. Wegener

Foreword

Analysis of the computed tomogram demands new knowledge from the radiologist. In addition to the operation of a technically complicated evaluation unit, the unaccustomed anatomy in transverse sections and the correct estimation of the density value, knowledge of the pathological anatomy of diseases in particular enters into the process of diagnosis. The matching of computed tomogram and specimen proves just how much the new, non-invasive imaging procedure has succeeded in approaching the macroscopic pathological anatomy. The radiologist will still find many of the visualized structures familiar, since the computed tomogram is still an X-ray picture. Established radiological criteria still apply in the analysis of the image, but their value has shifted within the spectrum of new signs.

The present book is intended both as an introduction to whole body computerized tomography and as an aid to radiologists already working with scanners. Its aim is to show how the individual clinical pictures appear in the computed tomogram. The first chapter deals briefly with the technique of computerized tomography. The CT terminology is explained at the end of the book. A great deal of space has been devoted to the normal anatomy to make the new form of representation in transverse sections with its advantages – but also its limitations – more understandable to the reader. The individual clinical pictures are described in separate chapters to facilitate reference in daily practice. The orbit and the spinal canal as neuroradiological border regions have been given appropriate space, since they are also demonstrable in the transverse section. Alternative imaging procedures have been listed briefly in an indication table without consideration of their content.

Since December 1976, more than 12,000 patients have been examined with a 20-second scanner at the Klinikum Steglitz. Only a little of the copious film material is reproduced in this book, since films of better quality made with faster scanners have become available in the meantime.

My particular thanks are extended to my colleagues Dr. D. Behrendt, Dr. C. D. Claussen, Professor Dr. Th. Grumme, Professor Dr. M. Haertel, Dr. B. Lochner, Dr. D. Rehnitz, Dr. K. Sartor, Dr. B. Trempenau and Dr. Chr. Utesch, who provided me unreservedly with a large number of case examples.

The generous layout of the book was made possible by Schering AG West Germany. I am particularly indebted to Dr. F. Masberg for his friendly support. The graphic concept of the book was developed in close cooperation with members of the company, and I should like to thank Dr. K. Friebel, Miss A. Schneider and H. Würfel of the Medical Publications Department and W. Miethke, H. Grünert, Mrs. U. von Bremen, and K. Bohm of the Werbestudio for their patient and creative cooperation.

Many colleagues, friends and acquaintances have contributed indirectly to the completion of this book, and thanks are also due to them: Mrs. U. Conner, Mrs. M. Laqua, Dr. D. Apitzsch, D. Conner, Farouk Mouhammed, Mrs. M. Heinrich, Dr. T. Ikonomidis, Dr. A. Kaernbach, Miss K. Klüter, Prof. P. Koeppe, Dr. Chr. Koch, Prof. W. Oelkers, Priv. Doz. Dr. A. Rost, Mrs. G. Schaefer, Mrs. H. Schlick, Dr. R. Schupp, Dr. R. Souchon, Miss B. Steinert, Dr. M. Vowinckel, Dr. R. Wolf and Miss G. Weiskopf.

Since the development of computerized tomography is not yet concluded, it can be assumed that some of the information in this book will be superseded in the course of time. So that the necessary deeper knowledge can be gained, an extensive bibliography broken down into organ regions has been provided. Particular attention is drawn to the recently appeared CT monographies (98-00).

My fervent hope is that the book will prove to be a valuable, practical aid.

Berlin, May 1981   O. H. Wegener

Contents

Technique of computerized tomography	**1-00**
Mathematical principles	1-10
Technical realization	1-20
The volume element	1-30
The density value	1-40
The partial volume effect	1-50
Anatomical outline	**2-00**
Density measurement	**3-00**
Evaluation	3-10
Falsification of density values	3-20
Density scale	3-30
Terminology	3-40
Pathomorphological substrate	3-50
Cystic contents, transudate, exudate	3-51
Blood – haematomas	3-52
Abscesses	3-53
Solid tissue	3-54
Regressive change	3-55
Contrast media	**4-00**
Forms of opacification	4-10
Intracavitary contrast media	4-20
Retrograde cystography	4-21
Bowel opacification	4-22
Modes of administration	4-23
Peritoneography	4-24
Myelography	4-25
Renal contrast media	4-30
Pharmacokinetics	4-31
Guided bolus injection	4-32
Controlled bolus injection	4-33
Reduced bolus injection	4-34
Infusions	4-35
Forms of administration	4-36
Biliary contrast media	4-40
Pathophysiological correlate	4-50
Indications for whole body computerized tomography	**5-00**
Cranium, neck	**50-00**
Orbit	**51-00**
Anatomy and imaging	51-10
Examination technique	51-20
Tumours of the orbit	51-30
Intraconal tumours	51-40
Haemangiomas	51-41
Tumours of the optic nerve	51-42
Neurinomas	51-43
Malignant lymphomas	51-44
Other malignant intraconal tumours	51-45
Retinoblastoma, melanoma	51-46
Extraconal tumours	51-50
Meningeomas	51-51
Tumours of the lacrimal gland	51-52
Periorbital malignant tumours	51-53
Dermoid cysts	51-54
Fibromas	51-55
Neurofibromas	51-56
Inflammations	51-60
Acute inflammations of the retrobulbar space	51-61
Granulomatous changes	51-62
Dacryoadenitis	51-63
(Idiopathic) pseudotumours	51-64
Endocrine ophthalmopathy	51-65
Retrobulbar neuritis	51-66
Mucocele, pyocele	51-67
Vascular processes	51-70
Arteriovenous malformations	51-71
Trauma	51-72
Foreign bodies	51-73
Visceral cranium	**52-00**
Anatomy and imaging	52-10
Examination technique	52-20
Tumours of the paranasal sinuses	52-30
Cystic forms	52-31
Benign solid tumours	52-32
Malignant tumours	52-33
Inflammations of the paranasal sinuses	52-40
Mucoceles, pyoceles	52-41
Mucocele vs tumour	52-42
Tumours of the nasopharynx	52-50
Benign tumours	52-51
Malignant tumours of the epipharynx	52-52
Tumours of the oro- and mesopharynx	52-60
Thyroid	**53-00**
Anatomy and imaging	53-10
Examination technique	53-20
Diffuse diseases of the thyroid	53-30
Focal disease of the thyroid	53-40
Thorax	**60-00**
Mediastinum	**61-00**
Anatomy and imaging	61-10
The mediastinal spaces	61-11

The mediastinal vessels	61-12
Trachea, oesophagus	61-13
Fasciae	61-14
Lymph nodes	61-15
Examination technique	61-20
Lymph node enlargements	61-30
Malignant lymphomas	61-31
Lymph node metastases	61-32
Primary tumours of the anterior mediastinum	61-40
Mesenchymal tumours	61-41
Thymomas	61-42
Teratoid blastomas	61-43
Endothoracic goitre	61-44
Parathyroid tumours	61-45
Primary tumours of the middle mediastinum	61-50
Tumours of the trachea	61-51
Bronchogenic cysts	61-52
Pleuropericardial (mesothelial) cysts	61-53
Primary tumours of the posterior mediastinum	61-60
Solid neurogenic tumours	61-61
Cystic masses	61-62
Tumours of the oesophagus	61-63
Vascular processes	61-70
Aorta	61-71
Aneurysms of the thoracic aorta	61-72
Brachiocephalic trunk	61-73
Azygous vein	61-74
Inflammations of the mediastinum	61-80
Acute mediastinitis	61-81
Chronic mediastinitis	61-82
Injuries of the mediastinum	61-90
Pneumomediastinum (mediastinal emphysema)	61-91
Mediastinal haematomas	61-92

Heart – pericardium	**62-00**
Anatomy and imaging	62-10
Examination technique	62-20
Functional conditions of the heart	62-30
Volume load	62-31
Pressure load	62-32
Cardiomyopathy	62-40
Coronary diseases	62-50
Valvular defects	62-60
Intracavitary masses	62-70
Pericardium	62-80
Anatomy and imaging	62-81
Examination technique	62-82
Pericardial accumulations of fluid	62-83
Chronic constrictive pericarditis	62-84
Tumours	62-85

Lung – pleura	**63-00**
Anatomy and imaging	63-10
Pulmonary structure	63-11
Pulmonary nodules	63-12
Density of the lung	63-13
Examination technique	63-20
Emphysema	63-30
Bronchopulmonary malformations, bronchiectasis	63-40
Inflammations of the lung	63-50
Exudative processes	63-51
Granulomatous inflammations (sarcoidosis)	63-52
Fibroses	63-53
Granulomas	63-54
Neoplasias of the lung	63-60
Benign tumours	63-61
Bronchial carcinoma	63-62
Multiple circumscribed lesions (metastases)	63-63
Vascular lesions	63-70
Pleura	63-80
Anatomy and imaging	63-81
Examination technique	63-82
Pleural effusion	63-83
Pleural thickening	63-84
Asbestosis, talcosis	63-85
Primary neoplasias of the pleura	63-86
Diffuse mesothelioma	63-87
Secondary tumours of the pleura	63-88

The chest wall	**64-00**
Anatomy and imaging	64-10
Examination technique	64-20
Tumours	64-30
Inflammations	64-40
Trauma	64-50

Abdomen, peritoneal space	**70-00**
Liver	**71-00**
Anatomy and imaging	71-10
Examination technique	71-20
Cystic diseases of the liver	71-30
Dysontogenetic cysts	71-31
Solitary hepatic cysts	71-32
Echinococcus granulosus	71-33
Echinococcus alveolaris	71-34
Solid tumours of the liver	71-40
Adenomas and focal nodular hyperplasia	71-41
Mesenchymal hamartomas	71-42
Haemangioma	71-43
Benign mesodermal tumours	71-44

Hepatocellular carcinoma	71-45
Cholangiocarcinoma	71-46
Secondary tumours of the liver (liver metastases)	71-47
Inflammatory changes of the liver	71-50
Fatty degeneration of the liver	71-51
Hepatitis	71-52
Cirrhosis	71-53
Haemochromatosis	71-54
Abscesses	71-55
Trauma	71-60

Biliary system	**72-00**
Anatomy and imaging	72-10
Examination technique	72-20
Cholecystomegaly	72-30
Inflammatory changes of the gallbladder	72-40
Cholecystitis	72-41
Cholelithiasis	72-42
Hydrops and empyema of the gallbladder	72-43
Tumours of the gallbladder (including hyperplastic cholecystoses)	72-50
Inflammations of the biliary tract	72-60
Tumours of the biliary tract	72-70
Choledochal cyst	72-71
Caroli syndrome	72-72

Pancreas	**73-00**
Anatomy and imaging	73-10
Examination technique	73-20
Cystic diseases of the pancreas	73-30
Dysontogenetic cysts	73-31
Retention and pseudocysts	73-32
Solid tumours of the pancreas	73-40
Cystadenoma	73-41
Adenocarcinoma (including anaplastic carcinoma)	73-42
Cystadenocarcinoma	73-43
Islet cell tumours	73-44
Secondary tumours	73-45
Pancreatitis	73-50
Acute pancreatitis	73-51
Chronic pancreatitis	73-52
Pancreatic abscess	73-53
Trauma of the pancreas	73-60
Lipomatosis and atrophy	73-70

Gastrointestinal tract	**74-00**
Anatomy and imaging	74-10
Examination technique	74-20
Gastrointestinal tract	74-30
Recurrence following proctectomy	74-31

Peritoneal cavity	**75-00**
Anatomy and imaging	75-10
Examination technique	75-20
Ascites	75-30
Peritoneal metastases	75-40
Intraperitoneal abscesses	75-50
Intraperitoneal haemorrhage	75-60

Spleen	**76-00**
Anatomy and imaging	76-10
Examination technique	76-20
Splenic cysts	76-30
Solid tumours of the spleen	76-40
Inflammatory diseases of the spleen	76-50
Trauma	76-60
Splenic haematoma	76-61
Vascular lesions	76-70
Splenic infarction	76-71
Thrombosis of the splenic vein	76-72
Splenic anomalies	76-80

Urogenital tract, retroperitoneal space	**80-00**

Kidney	**81-00**
Anatomy and imaging	81-10
Examination technique	81-20
Cystic diseases of the kidney	81-30
Solitary cysts	81-31
Polycystic diseases of the kidney	81-32
Other cystic masses	81-33
Solid parenchymal tumours	81-40
Hypernephroid carcinomas	81-41
Adenoma and cystadenoma	81-42
Angiomyolipoma	81-43
Mesenchymal tumours	81-44
Wilms' tumour (nephroblastoma)	81-45
Tumours of the renal pelvis	81-46
Secondary tumours of the kidney	81-47
Inflammations	81-50
Local bacterial nephritis, abscesses, carbuncles	81-51
Xanthogranulomatous pyelonephritis	81-52
Chronic pyelonephritis	81-53
Renal tuberculosis	81-54
Transplanted kidney	81-55
Fibrolipomatosis	81-56
Renal trauma	81-60
Renal haematoma	81-61
Obstructive uropathy	81-70
Hydronephrosis (congestion kidney)	81-71
Pyonephrosis	81-72
Urolithiasis	81-73
Vascular processes	81-80

Renal infarct	81-81
Variants, anomalies	81-90

Adrenals 82-00

Anatomy and imaging	82-10
Examination technique	82-20
Hyperplasia and adrenocortical tumours	82-30
Adrenocortical hyperplasia	82-31
Adrenocortical adenomas	82-32
Adrenocortical carcinomas	82-33
Adrenomedullary tumours	82-40
Myelolipomas	82-41
Phaeochromocytoma	82-42
Phaeochromoblastoma	82-43
Neuroblastoma	82-44
Metastases	82-45
Adrenal cysts	82-50
Haemorrhage	82-60
Inflammation, atrophy	82-70
Inflammation	82-71
Hypoplasia, atrophy	82-72

Urinary bladder 83-00

Anatomy and imaging	83-10
Examination technique	83-20
Changes of position	83-30
Inflammations of the urinary bladder	83-40
Tumours of the urinary bladder	83-50
Papillomas, carcinomas	83-51
Mesenchymal tumours	83-52

Prostate 84-00

Anatomy and imaging	84-10
Examination technique	84-20
Adenoma and carcinoma of the prostate	84-30
Inflammations of the prostate	84-40

Female genital organs 85-00

Anatomy and imaging	85-10
Examination technique	85-20
Tumours of the uterus	85-30
Myoma (uterine leiomyoma)	85-31
Cervical carcinoma	85-32
Uterine carcinoma	85-33
Recurrence of malignant uterine tumours	85-34
Ovarian tumours	85-40
Cysts	85-41
Dermoid cysts	85-42
Malignant and hormone-producing tumours of the ovary	85-43
Inflammations	85-50
Inflammations of the uterus	85-51
Inflammations of the adnexa	85-52
Inflammations of the parametrium	85-53

Retroperitoneal cavity 86-00

Anatomy and imaging	86-10
Retroperitoneal vessels	86-11
The retrocrural space	86-12
The diaphragm	86-13
Fascial spaces of the retroperitoneum	86-14
Lymph nodes	86-15
Examination technique	86-20
Perirenal and pararenal lesions	86-30
Exudative haemorrhagic lesions of the perirenal space	86-31
Urinomas (perirenal pseudocysts)	86-32
Perirenal haematoma	86-33
Solid perirenal lesions	86-34
Lesions in the anterior pararenal space	86-35
Lesions in the posterior pararenal space	86-36
Iliopsoas muscle	86-37
Lesions in the subperitoneal space	86-38
Retroperitoneal fibrosis	86-40
Secondary retroperitoneal fibrosis	86-41
Pelvic fibrolipomatosis	86-42
Lymph node diseases	86-50
Malignant lymphomas	86-51
Lymph node metastases	86-52
Benign lymphadenopathies	86-53
Primary retroperitoneal tumours	86-60
Vascular lesions	86-70
Aneurysms	86-71
Aneurysms of the abdominal aorta	86-72
Trauma of the aorta	86-73
Anomalies of the inferior vena cava	86-74
Thrombosis of the inferior vena cava (including pelvic veins)	86-75

Skeleton and soft tissues 90-00

Soft-tissue tumours (of the extremities) 91-00

Pathology of soft-tissue tumours	91-10
Examination technique	91-20
CT of soft-tissue tumours	91-30

Muscle tissue 92-00

Examination technique	92-10
Atrophy	92-20
Progressive muscular dystrophy	92-30
Inflammatory muscle changes	92-40
Purulent myositis (muscular abscess)	92-41
Sarcoidosis	92-42

Polymyositis	92-43
Muscle haematoma	92-50

Skeleton — **93-00**

Anatomy and imaging	93-10
Examination technique	93-20
Mineralization of bone	93-30
Bone tumours	93-40
Vertebral column and vertebral canal	93-50
Anatomy and imaging	93-51
Examination technique	93-52
(Lumbar) spinal stenosis	93-53
Disc herniation	93-54
Vertebragenic tumours and tumour-like lesions	93-55
Intraspinal masses	93-56
Trauma of the vertebral column	93-57
Inflammations of the vertebral column	93-58
Osseous pelvis	93-60
Anatomy and imaging	93-61
Osteogenic tumours	93-62
Bone injuries	93-63
The sacroiliac joints	93-64

CT terminology — **97-00**

Literature — **98-00**

Index — **99-00**

Technique of
computerized tomography (1-00)

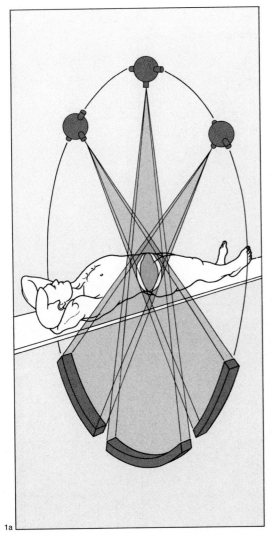

Technique of computerized tomography (1-00)

Tomography was introduced to radiology in the twenties. It splits up the summation image of the X-ray film by movement of the scanning system into parallel image layers arranged spatially behind each other. The application of new technologies to this entirely mechanical concept has led to the development of computerized tomography. With this technique, data (attenuation values) are collected from a body region from various directions (Fig. 1-1a) until the spatial arrangement of the absorbing structures can be determined. A matrix of attenuation values – the computed tomogram – creates a pictorial impression of the region scanned displayed in shades of grey. The method permits reproducible measurement of the tissue density, providing important diagnostic information.

Mathematical principles (1-10)

Fig. 1-1b shows an object of square cross-section broken down into 8 x 8 quadratic elements, each with different attenuation values. Determination of the attenuation values of row I_y and column I_x is not sufficient to establish the individual attenuation values unequivocally via a set of equations. Additional measurements are required from various angles up to a total number of n x n, in this case 8 x 8 projections. The following rule therefore applies to the technical conception of a scanner: the number of absorption measurements from different directions determines the number of picture elements, i. e. the spatial resolution, whereby the sequence of data acquisition can be chosen at will.

Fig. 1-1a: **Scanning.** Bundled X-rays penetrate the body from various directions vertical to the longitudinal axis of the body. The attenuation is recorded by a detector system.

Fig. 1-1b: **Mathematical principles** (cf. 1-10).

Technical realization (1-20)

The attenuation measurements are made with detectors arranged behind the X-ray tube and behind the patient. Four scanning principles have been developed:

● Single-detector rotation-translation scanners (1st generation scanners). A finely gated beam of X-rays with a detector chamber situated opposite the tube scans the object in 180 angular steps of 1°. A "linear" translation movement across the body is made after every angular step (Fig. 1-2a). The briefest scanning time amounts to several minutes.

● Multidetector rotation-translation scanners (2nd generation scanners). A detector system with 5–50 chambers is situated opposite the X-ray tube (Fig. 1-2b). A bundle of diverging X-rays or a fan-shaped beam reduces the number of angular steps, which are usually set at 10° and correlate with the angle of the fan beam. The briefest scanning time ranges from 20 to 6 seconds.

● Rotation scanners with a movable detector system (3rd generation scanners). A broad fan of X-rays covering the entire object angularly faces a detector field of 200–600 detectors which is moved around the body (Fig. 1-2c). The scanning time lies between one and four seconds.

● Rotation system with stationary detectors (4th generation scanners). A fan-shaped beam of X-rays covering the entire object angularly moves within or outside a fixed detector ring of 300–1,000 detectors (Fig. 1-2d). The briefest scanning time amounts to 3–8 seconds.

Brief scanning times are desirable for whole body computerized tomography to reduce to a minimum movement artifacts due to respiration, peristalsis and heart beats.

The attenuation values acquired in the individual projections are fed into a computer, where they represent the individual elements of a set of equations (see above). The computed tomogram is created by means of a complicated mathematical process of image reconstruction. This is a matrix with a limited number of picture elements, each of which has a numerical value corresponding to its absorption behaviour. Conversion of these numerical values into shades of grey gives rise to an image of the cross-sectional area scanned in which the structures can be recognized by virtue of their varying ability to absorb X-rays.

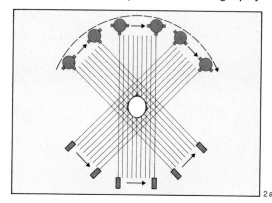
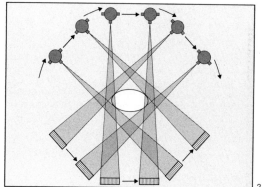
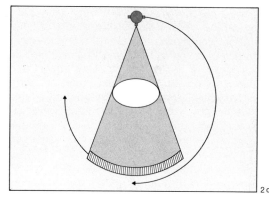
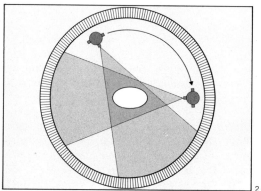

Fig. 1-2 a–d: **Scanning principles** of the various generations of scanner.

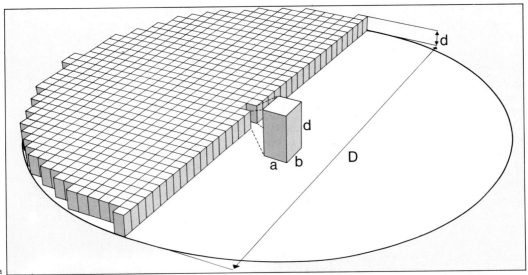

Fig. 1-3 a: **Volume of a volume element.** The area of the picture element and the slice thickness (d) determine the volume of a volume element. a = b = edge length of a picture element, D = diameter of the scanning field.

The volume element (1-30)

The smallest unit of the computed tomogram is the picture element (pixel) which, depending on the chosen size of the scanning field and picture matrix, represents a certain proportion of the cross-sectional area depicted. In conformity with the slice thickness used, the pixel also represents a tissue volume, the content of which is made up in a simple way by the slice thickness, the size of the matrix and the diameter of the scanning field (Fig. 1-3a). The term "volume element" is also used instead of "picture element". The introduction of this term highlights two features of computerized tomography: the limited spatial resolution and the provision of a density value.

The density value (1-40)

Each volume element has a numerical value – the density value – which represents the mean attenuation of the tissue contained within it. The density value stands in direct (linear) relationship to the linear attenuation coefficient. By means of internal calibration of the scanners, the density value of water is set at 0 and that of air at – 1,000. The absorption values of the other body tissues are expressed in relation to this scale (Fig. 3-3a), which was named after Hounsfield. The density value is therefore an arbitrary unit and represents a **relative linear absorption coefficient**.

The partial volume effect (1-50)

The density value is a mean value for the tissue contained in the volume element. When the volume element is filled with structures of varying density, the latter contribute to the density value in proportion to the extent to which they occupy the volume element. This partial volume effect is therefore a consequence of limited spatial resolution and is reduced by finely gridded image matrices and the use of small slice thicknesses, i. e. small volume elements.

In the evaluation of the image the partial volume effect manifests itself in two ways:

● **Quantitatively:** It falsifies the density value at the boundaries of structures (3-20).

● **Qualitatively:** the demonstration of structures running obliquely through the spatially orthogonal architecture of the volume elements is indefinite, i. e. in varying shades of grey. Fissures narrower than the edge length of a volume element can no longer be depicted directly, but at the most by a change in density of the volume element. Large slice thicknesses mask horizontal fissures, while large picture elements (coarse image matrices) mask vertical fissures (Fig. 1-5b).

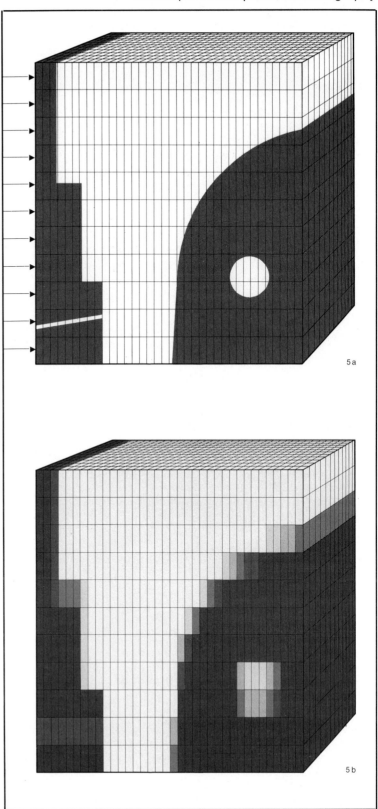

Fig. 1-5 a,b: **The partial volume effect.** An object comprised of two media of different density (a) produces a coarse image due to scanning in slices (→) and because of gridding in picture elements (b). Contours at the borders of the structure become distorted, fissures are masked and density values adulterated.

Anatomical outline (2-00)

Key

* = ramus

Arteriae*

A 1	Aorta abdominalis/ Aorta thoracica	
A 2	Truncus pulmonalis	
A 3	A. pulmonalis	
A 4	Truncus brachiocephalicus	
A 5	A. carotis communis	
A 6	A. subclavia	
A 7	A. axillaris	
A 8	A. vertebralis	
A 9	A. thoracica interna	
A 10	Truncus coeliacus	
A 11	A. hepatica	
A 12	A. lienalis	
A 13	A. gastrica sinistra	
A 14	A. mesenterica superior	
A 15	A. renalis	
A 16	A. lumbalis	
A 17	A. mesenterica inferior	
A 18	A. iliaca communis	
A 19	A. iliaca interna	
A 20	A. iliaca externa	
A 21	A. femoralis	
A 22	A. pudenda	
A 23	A. penis dorsalis	
A 24	A. obturatoria	

Venae*

V 1	V. cava inferior V. cava superior
V 2	V. thyreoidea ima
V 3	V. pulmonalis
V 4	V. brachiocephalica (anonyma)
V 5	V. jugularis interna
V 6	V. subclavia
V 7	V. axillaris
V 8	V. jugularis externa
V 9	V. thoracica interna
V 10	V. azygos
V 11	V. hemiazygos
V 12	V. lienalis
V 13	V. portae
V 14	V. mesenterica superior
V 15	V. renalis
V 16	V. lumbalis
V 17	V. vertebralis
V 18	V. iliaca communis
V 19	V. iliaca interna
V 20	V. iliaca externa
V 21	V. femoralis
V 22	V. pudenda
V 24	V. obturatoria

Musculi

M 1	M. trapezius
M 2	M. deltoideus
M 3	M. semispinalis capitis
	M. longissimus colli
M 4	M. splenius capitis
M 5	M. levator scapulae
M 6	M. rhomboideus (minor, major)
M 7	M. supraspinatus
M 8	M. infraspinatus
M 9	M. teres major
M 10	M. teres minor
M 11	M. subscapularis
M 12	M. latissimus dorsi
M 13	M. scalenus anterior
M 14	M. scalenus medius
M 15	M. scalenus posterior
M 16	Mm. sternohyoideus, omohyoideus, sternothyreoideus
M 17	M. sternocleidomastoideus
M 18	M. longus colli
M 19	M. pectoralis major
M 20	M. pectoralis minor
M 21	M. intercostalis (interior, intermedius, exterior)
M 22	M. serratus anterior
M 23	M. erector spinae
M 24	M. rectus abdominis
M 25	M. obliquus externus abdominis
M 26	M. obliquus internus abdominis
M 27	M. transversus abdominis
M 28	M. quadratus lumborum
M 29	M. psoas
M 30	M. iliacus
M 31	M. iliopsoas
M 32	M. erector trunci
M 33	M. iliocostalis
M 34	M. longissimus dorsi
M 35	M. multifidus
M 36	M. glutaeus maximus
M 37	M. glutaeus medius
M 38	M. glutaeus minimus
M 39	M. piriformis
M 40	M. obturatorius internus
M 41	M. gemellus (superior, inferior)
M 42	M. obturatorius externus
M 43	M. pectineus
M 44	M. adductor longus
M 45	M. gracilis
M 46	M. sartorius
M 47	M. rectus femoris
M 48	M. tensor fasciae latae
M 49	M. vastus lateralis
M 50	M. levator ani
M 51	Diaphragma
M 52	M. subclavius
M 53	M. pyramidalis
M 54	M. quadratus femoris
M 55	M. serratus posterior superior

Skeleton

S 1	**Vertebra**
S 11	Corpus vertebrae
S 12	Pediculus arcus vertebrae
S 13	Articulatio intervertebralis
S 14	Processus spinosus
S 15	Processus transversus
S 16	Processus articularis superior
S 17	Processus articularis inferior
S 18	Canalis vertebralis
S 19	Discus intervertebralis
S 2	**Costa (Corpus costae)**
S 21	Caput costae
S 22	Collum costae
S 23	Articulatio costotransversaria
S 24	Articulatio capitis costae
S 25	Sternum
S 26	Articulatio sternoclavicularis
S 27	Arcus costalis
S 28	Cartilago costalis
S 29	Clavicula
S 3	**Scapula**
S 31	Spina scapulae
S 32	Acromion
S 33	Processus coracoideus
S 34	Cavitas glenoidalis
S 4	**Os coxae**
S 41	Ala ossis ilium
S 42	Acetabulum
S 43	Tuber ossis ischii
S 44	Corpus ossis ischii
S 45	Ramus ossis ischii
S 46	Symphysis pubica
S 47	Ramus superior ossis pubis
S 48	Ramus inferior ossis pubis
S 5	**Femur**
S 51	Caput femoris
S 52	Collum femoris
S 53	Trochanter major
S 54	Articulatio coxae
S 6	**Os sacrum, Os coccygis**
S 61	Foramina sacralia pelvina
S 62	Crista sacralis
S 63	Canalis sacralis
S 64	Promontorium
S 65	Articulatio sacroiliaca
S 66	Os coccygis
S 7	**Humerus**
S 71	Caput humeri

Organa

O 1	**Cor**
O 11	Ventriculus sinister
O 12	Ventriculus dexter
O 13	Atrium sinistrum
O 14	Atrium dextrum
O 15	Septum interventriculare
O 16	Pericardium
O 2	**Pulmo**
O 21	Trachea
O 22	Bronchus principalis
O 23	Bronchus lobaris
O 24	Carina
O 25	Pleura
O 26	Sinus phrenicocostalis
O 3	**Hepar**
O 31	Lobus dexter
O 32	Lobus sinister
O 33	Lobus quadratus
O 34	Lobus caudatus
O 35	Ligamentum falciforme (Ligamentum teres hepatis)
O 36	Porta hepatis
O 37	Vesica fellea
O 38	Ductus hepaticus
O 39	Ductus choledochus
O 4	**Pancreas, Lien**
O 41	Caput pancreatis
O 42	Processus uncinatus
O 43	Corpus pancreatis
O 44	Cauda pancreatis
O 45	Lien
O 46	Hilus lienis

Organa (cont.)

O 5	**Organa uropoetica (ren)**
O 51	Hilus renalis
O 52	Sinus renalis
O 53	Pelvis renalis
O 54	Calices renales
O 55	Cortex, Medulla renalis
O 56	Ureter
O 57	Vesica urinaria
O 58	Urethra
O 6	**Organa genitalia masculina**
O 61	Prostata
O 62	Vesicula seminalis
O 63	Funiculus spermaticus (Ductus deferens + vasa)
O 7	**Canalis alimentarius**
O 71	Oesophagus
O 72	Gaster
O 73	Duodenum
O 74	Jejunum
O 75	Ileum
O 76	Colon
O 77	Flexura colica
O 78	Colon sigmoideum
O 79	Rectum
O 8	**Glandulae sine ductibus**
O 81	Glandula thyreoidea
O 82	Glandula suprarenalis

Cetera

C 1	N. ischiadicus
C 2	N. femoralis
C 3	N. pudendus
C 4	Plexus lumbosacralis
C 5	Fossa ischiorectalis

Cetera (cont.)

C 6	Sinus phrenicocostalis
C 7	Fascia renalis
C 8	Nodus lymphaticus
C 9	Linea alba
C 10	Radix nervi spinalis

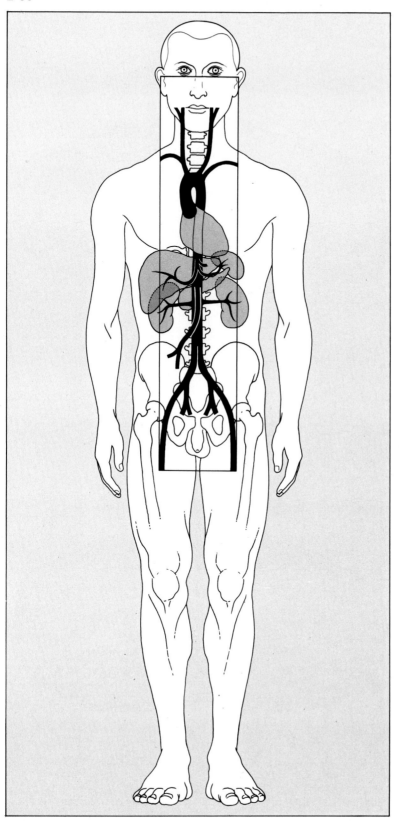
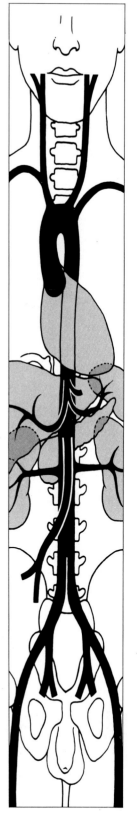

Anatomical outline

2-1/2

	1/2
A 5	A. carotis communis
A 7	A. axillaris
A 8	A. vertebralis
V 5	V. jugularis interna
V 7	V. axillaris
O 21	Trachea
O 71	Oesophagus
O 81	Glandula thyreoidea
M 1	M. trapezius
M 2	M. deltoideus
M 3	M. semispinalis capitis
	M. longissimus colli
M 4	M. splenius capitis
M 5	M. levator scapulae
M 6	M. rhomboideus (minor, major)
M 7	M. supraspinatus
M 8	M. infraspinatus
M 9	M. teres major
M 10	M. teres minor
M 11	M. subscapularis
M 12	M. latissimus dorsi
M 13	M. scalenus anterior
M 14	M. scalenus medius
M 15	M. scalenus posterior
M 16	Mm. sternohyoideus, omohyoideus, sternothyreoideus
M 17	M. sternocleido-mastoideus
M 19	M. pectoralis major
M 20	M. pectoralis minor
S 1	Vertebra
S 21	Caput costae
S 29	Clavicula
S 31	Spina scapulae
S 32	Acromion
S 33	Processus coracoideus
S 34	Cavitas glenoidalis
S 71	Caput humeri

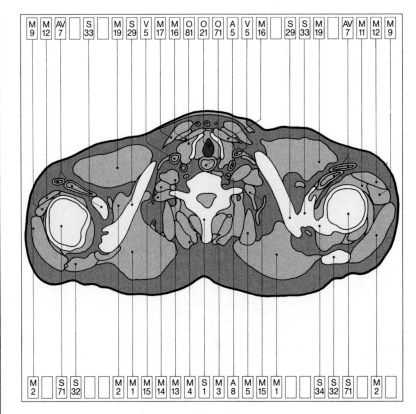

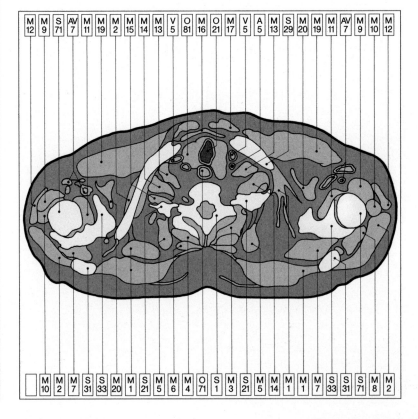

2-1/2

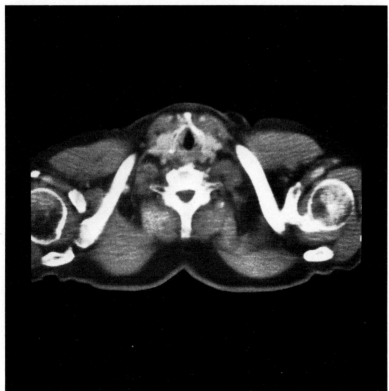

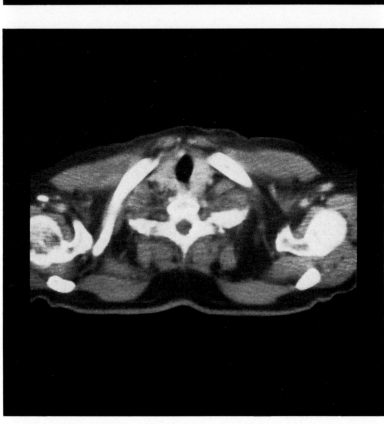

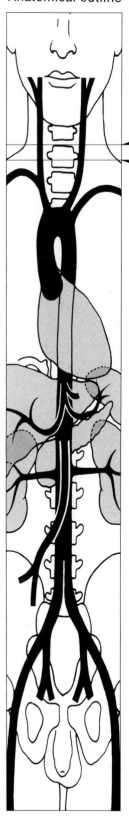

Anatomical outline

2-3/4

	3/4
A 4	Truncus brachio-cephalicus
A 5	A. carotis communis
A 6	A. subclavia
A 7	A. axillaris
V 2	V. thyreoidea ima
V 4	V. brachiocephalica (anonyma)
V 5	V. jugularis interna
V 6	V. subclavia
V 7	V. axillaris
O 2	Pulmo
O 21	Trachea
O 71	Oesophagus
O 81	Glandula thyreoidea
M 1	M. trapezius
M 2	M. deltoideus
M 3	M. semispinalis capitis
	M. longissimus colli
M 4	M. splenius capitis
M 5	M. levator scapulae
M 6	M. rhomboideus (minor, major)
M 7	M. supraspinatus
M 8	M. infraspinatus
M 9	M. teres major
M 10	M. teres minor
M 11	M. subscapularis
M 12	M. latissimus dorsi
M 19	M. pectoralis major
M 20	M. pectoralis minor
M 21	M. intercostalis (interior, intermedius, exterior)
M 55	M. serratus posterior superior
S 1	Vertebra
S 2	Costa (Corpus costae)
S 21	Caput costae
S 26	Articulatio sternoclavicularis
S 29	Clavicula
S 3	Scapula
S 31	Spina scapulae
S 32	Acromion

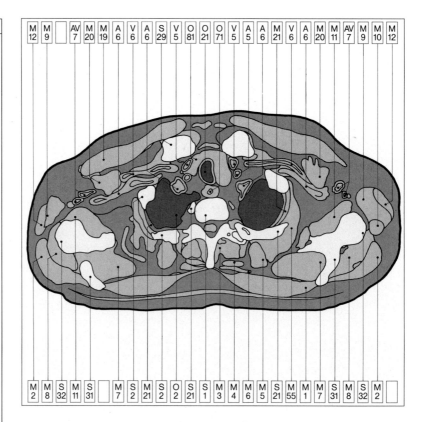

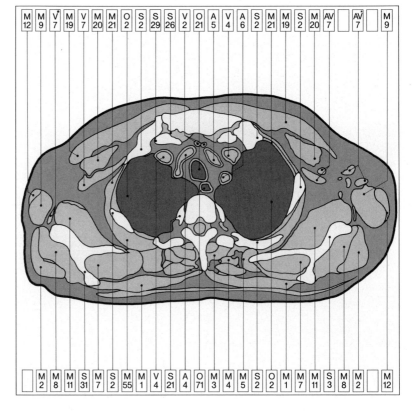

2-3/4

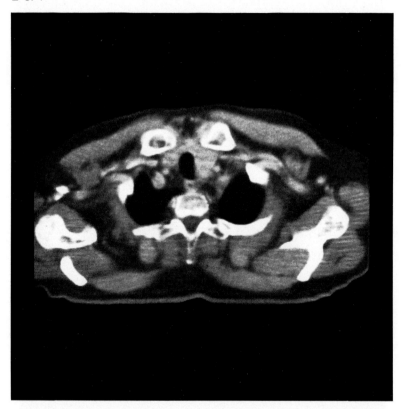

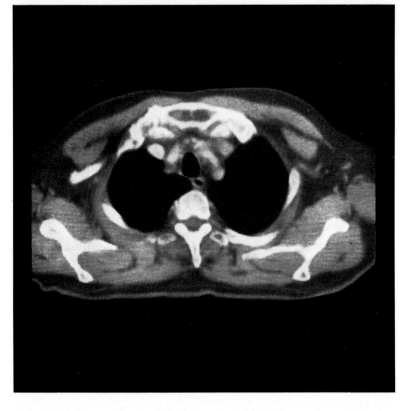

Anatomical outline

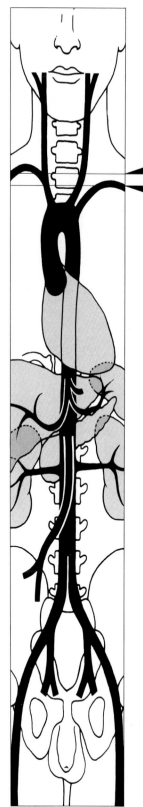

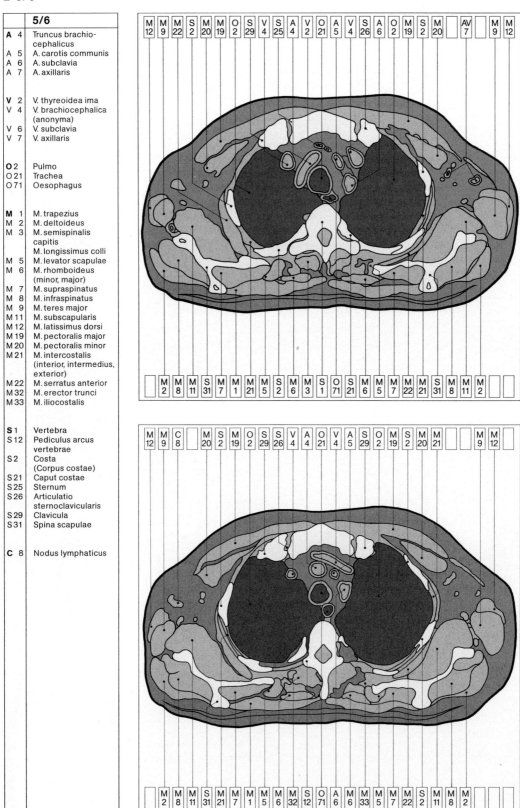

2-5/6

	5/6
A 4	Truncus brachiocephalicus
A 5	A. carotis communis
A 6	A. subclavia
A 7	A. axillaris
V 2	V. thyreoidea ima
V 4	V. brachiocephalica (anonyma)
V 6	V. subclavia
V 7	V. axillaris
O 2	Pulmo
O 21	Trachea
O 71	Oesophagus
M 1	M. trapezius
M 2	M. deltoideus
M 3	M. semispinalis capitis
	M. longissimus colli
M 5	M. levator scapulae
M 6	M. rhomboideus (minor, major)
M 7	M. supraspinatus
M 8	M. infraspinatus
M 9	M. teres major
M 11	M. subscapularis
M 12	M. latissimus dorsi
M 19	M. pectoralis major
M 20	M. pectoralis minor
M 21	M. intercostalis (interior, intermedius, exterior)
M 22	M. serratus anterior
M 32	M. erector trunci
M 33	M. iliocostalis
S 1	Vertebra
S 12	Pediculus arcus vertebrae
S 2	Costa (Corpus costae)
S 21	Caput costae
S 25	Sternum
S 26	Articulatio sternoclavicularis
S 29	Clavicula
S 31	Spina scapulae
C 8	Nodus lymphaticus

2-5/6

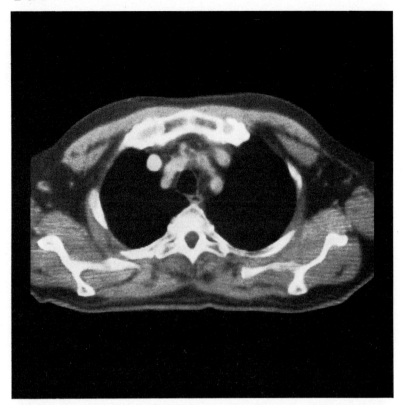

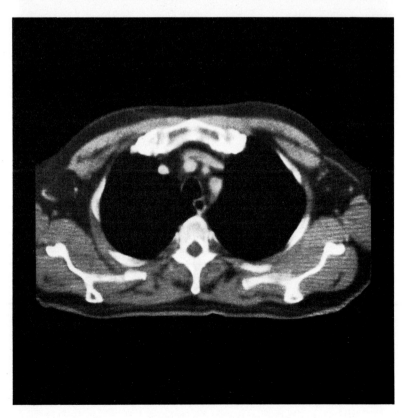

Anatomical outline

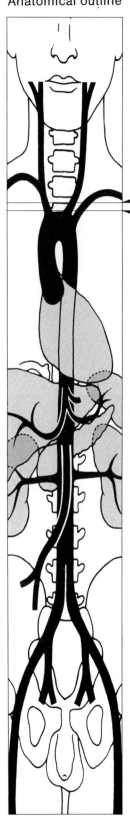

2-7/8

	7/8
A 1	Aorta thoracica
A 4	Truncus brachiocephalicus
A 5	A. carotis communis
A 7	A. axillaris
A 9	A. thoracica interna
V 1	V. cava superior
V 4	V. brachiocephalica (anonyma)
V 7	V. axillaris
V 9	V. thoracica interna
V 10	V. azygos
O 2	Pulmo
O 21	Trachea
O 71	Oesophagus
M 1	M. trapezius
M 2	M. deltoideus
M 5	M. levator scapulae
M 6	M. rhomboideus (minor, major)
M 7	M. supraspinatus
M 8	M. infraspinatus
M 9	M. teres major
M 10	M. teres minor
M 11	M. subscapularis
M 12	M. latissimus dorsi
M 19	M. pectoralis major
M 20	M. pectoralis minor
M 21	M. intercostalis (interior, intermedius, exterior)
M 22	M. serratus anterior
M 32	M. erector trunci
M 33	M. iliocostalis
S 1	Vertebra
S 2	Costa (Corpus costae)
S 23	Articulatio costotransversaria
S 25	Sternum
S 28	Cartilago costalis
S 3	Scapula
S 31	Spina scapulae
C 8	Nodus lymphaticus

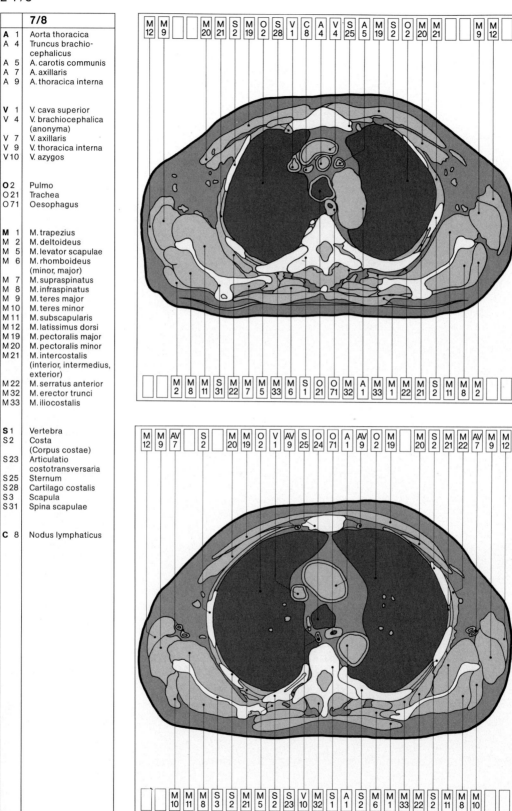

2-7/8

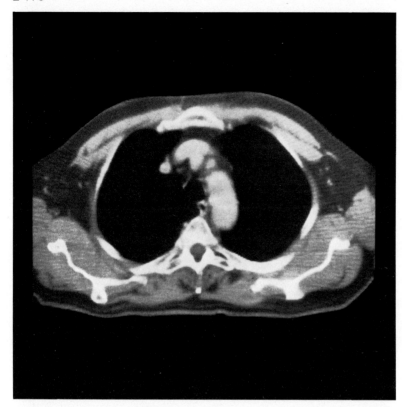

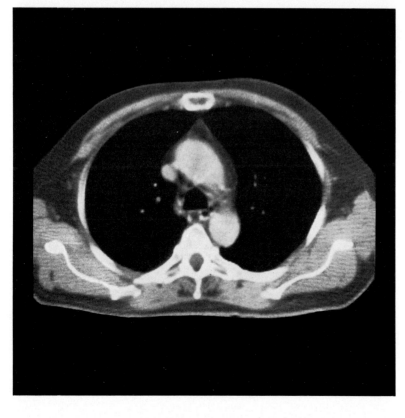

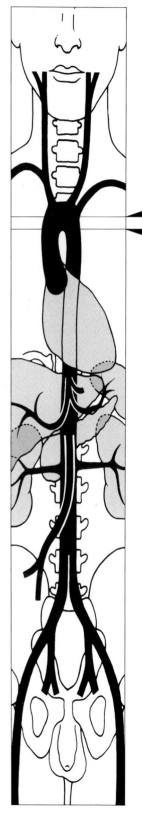

Anatomical outline

2-9/10

9/10

A	1	Aorta thoracica
A	3	A. pulmonalis
A	7	A. axillaris
A	9	A. thoracica interna
V	1	V. cava superior
V	7	V. axillaris
V	9	V. thoracica interna
V	10	V. azygos
O	2	Pulmo
O	21	Trachea
O	22	Bronchus principalis
O	71	Oesophagus
M	1	M. trapezius
M	6	M. rhomboideus (minor, major)
M	8	M. infraspinatus
M	9	M. teres major
M	10	M. teres minor
M	11	M. subscapularis
M	12	M. latissimus dorsi
M	19	M. pectoralis major
M	20	M. pectoralis minor
M	21	M. intercostalis (interior, intermedius, exterior)
M	22	M. serratus anterior
M	32	M. erector trunci
M	33	M. iliocostalis
S	1	Vertebra
S	2	Costa (Corpus costae)
S	25	Sternum
S	27	Arcus costalis
S	28	Cartilago costalis
S	3	Scapula

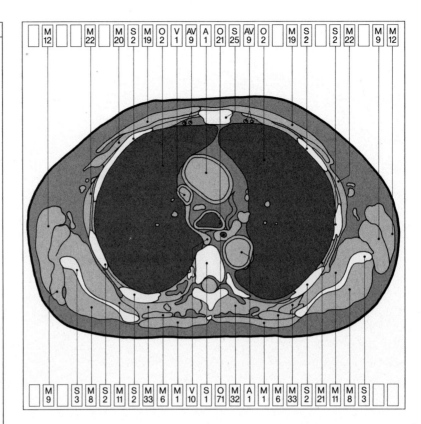

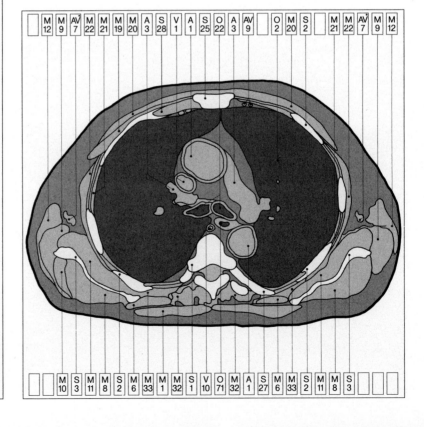

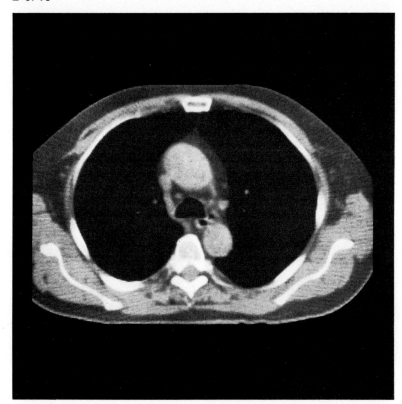
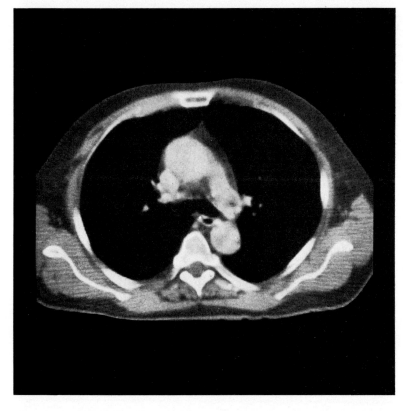
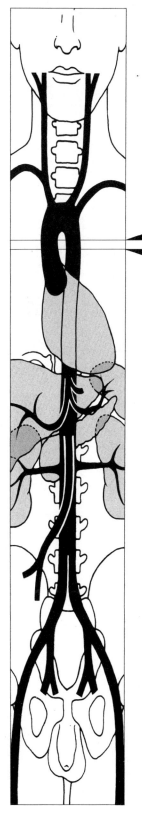

Anatomical outline

2-11/12

	11/12
A 1	Aorta thoracica
A 2	Truncus pulmonalis
A 3	A. pulmonalis
A 9	A. thoracica interna
V 1	V. cava superior
V 3	V. pulmonalis
V 9	V. thoracica interna
V 10	V. azygos
O 2	Pulmo
O 22	Bronchus principalis
O 71	Oesophagus
M 1	M. trapezius
M 6	M. rhomboideus (minor, major)
M 8	M. infraspinatus
M 9	M. teres major
M 11	M. subscapularis
M 12	M. latissimus dorsi
M 19	M. pectoralis major
M 21	M. intercostalis (interior, intermedius, exterior)
M 22	M. serratus anterior
M 32	M. erector trunci
M 33	M. iliocostalis
S 1	Vertebra
S 2	Costa (Corpus costae)
S 21	Caput costae
S 22	Collum costae
S 25	Sternum
S 28	Cartilago costalis
S 3	Scapula

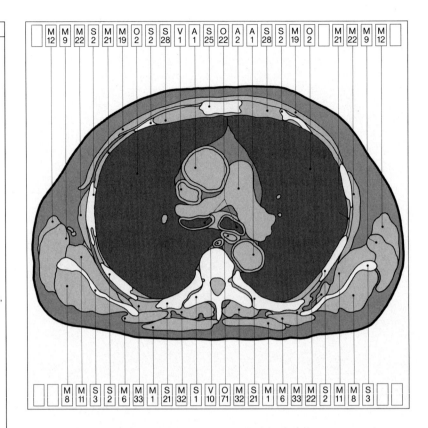

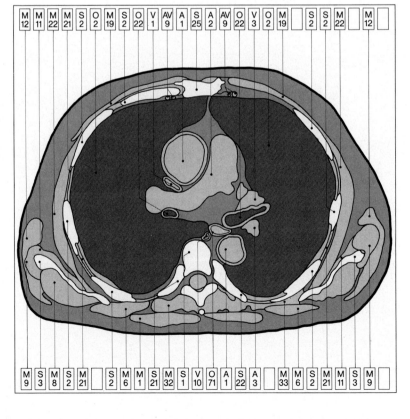

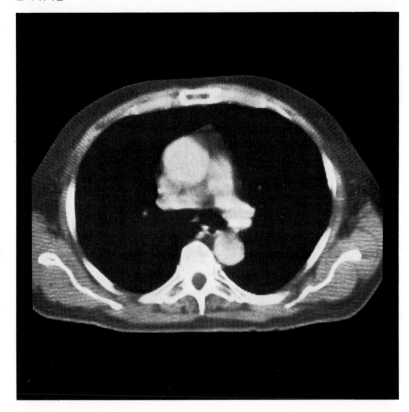
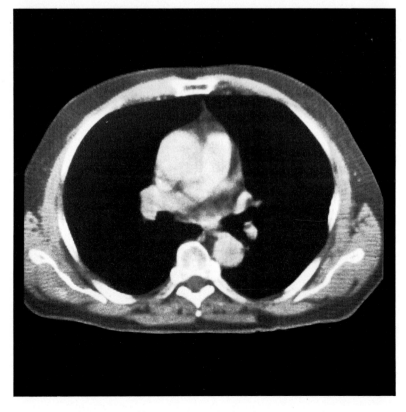
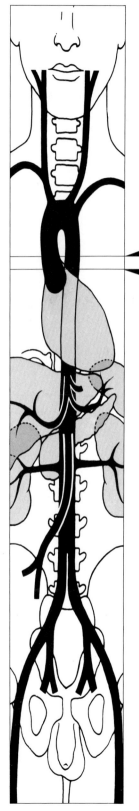

Anatomical outline

2-13/14

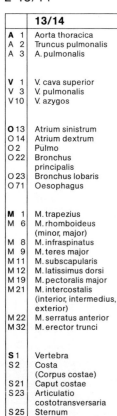

	13/14	
A	1	Aorta thoracica
A	2	Truncus pulmonalis
A	3	A. pulmonalis
V	1	V. cava superior
V	3	V. pulmonalis
V	10	V. azygos
O	13	Atrium sinistrum
O	14	Atrium dextrum
O	2	Pulmo
O	22	Bronchus principalis
O	23	Bronchus lobaris
O	71	Oesophagus
M	1	M. trapezius
M	6	M. rhomboideus (minor, major)
M	8	M. infraspinatus
M	9	M. teres major
M	11	M. subscapularis
M	12	M. latissimus dorsi
M	19	M. pectoralis major
M	21	M. intercostalis (interior, intermedius, exterior)
M	22	M. serratus anterior
M	32	M. erector trunci
S	1	Vertebra
S	2	Costa (Corpus costae)
S	21	Caput costae
S	23	Articulatio costotransversaria
S	25	Sternum
S	28	Cartilago costalis
S	3	Scapula

* = ramus

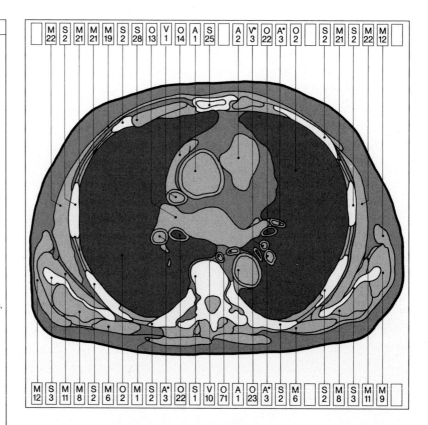

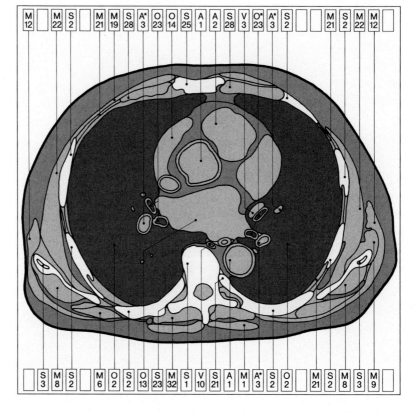

2-13/14

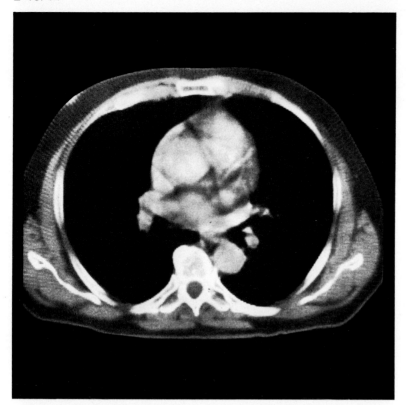

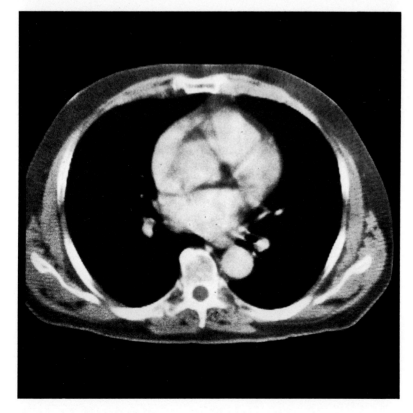

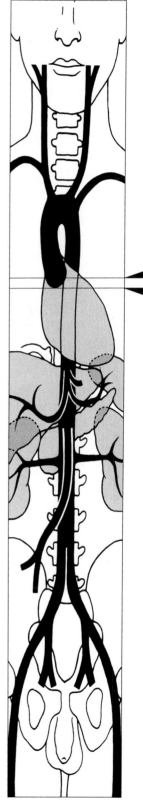

Anatomical outline

2-15/16

	15/16	
A	1	Aorta thoracica
A	2	Truncus pulmonalis
A	3	A. pulmonalis
A	9	A. thoracica interna
V	1	V. cava superior
V	3	V. pulmonalis
V	9	V. thoracica interna
V	10	V. azygos
O	11	Ventriculus sinister
O	12	Ventriculus dexter
O	13	Atrium sinistrum
O	14	Atrium dextrum
O	15	Septum interventriculare
O	16	Pericardium
O	2	Pulmo
O	23	Bronchus lobaris
O	71	Oesophagus
M	1	M. trapezius
M	6	M. rhomboideus (minor, major)
M	8	M. infraspinatus
M	9	M. teres major
M	12	M. latissimus dorsi
M	21	M. intercostalis (interior, intermedius, exterior)
M	22	M. serratus anterior
M	32	M. erector trunci
M	51	Diaphragma
S	1	Vertebra
S	14	Processus spinosus
S	2	Costa (Corpus costae)
S	21	Caput costae
S	22	Collum costae
S	25	Sternum
S	28	Cartilago costalis
		* = ramus

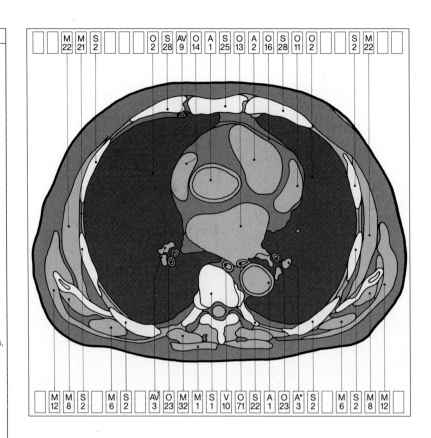

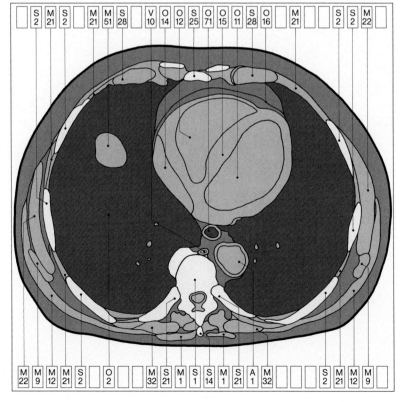

2-15/16

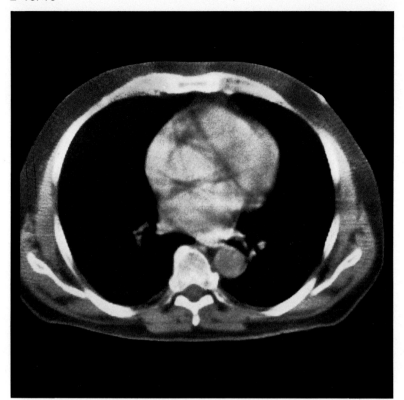

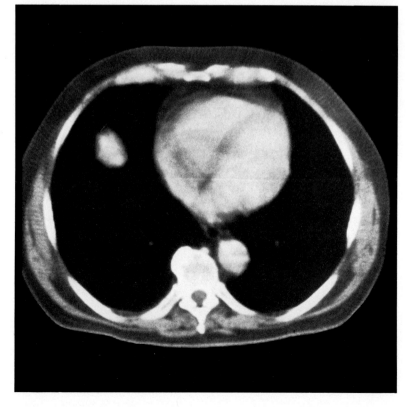

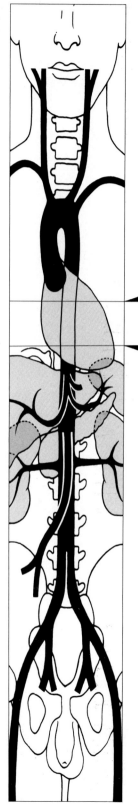

Anatomical outline

2-17/18

17/18

A 1	Aorta thoracica
A 12	A. lienalis
V 1	V. cava inferior
V 10	V. azygos
V 11	V. hemiazygos
O 26	Sinus phrenicocostalis
O 3	Hepar
O 45	Lien
O 72	Gaster
O 76	Colon
O 77	Flexura colica
M 1	M. trapezius
M 12	M. latissimus dorsi
M 21	M. intercostalis (interior, intermedius, exterior)
M 22	M. serratus anterior
M 24	M. rectus abdominis
M 25	M. obliquus externus abdominis
M 32	M. erector trunci
M 33	M. iliocostalis
M 51	Diaphragma
S 1	Vertebra
S 2	Costa (Corpus costae)
S 25	Sternum
S 26	Articulatio sternoclavicularis
S 27	Arcus costalis
S 28	Cartilago costalis

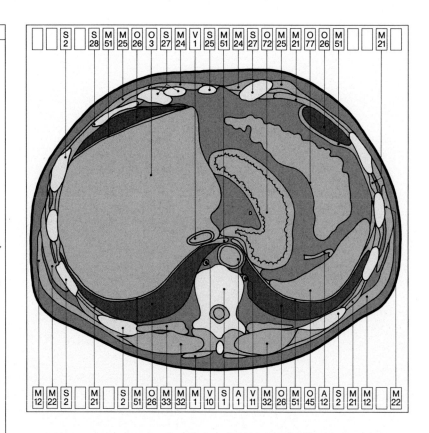

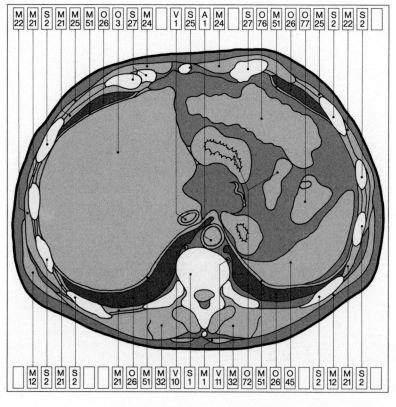

2-17/18

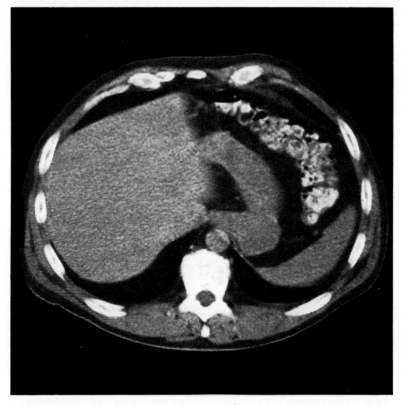

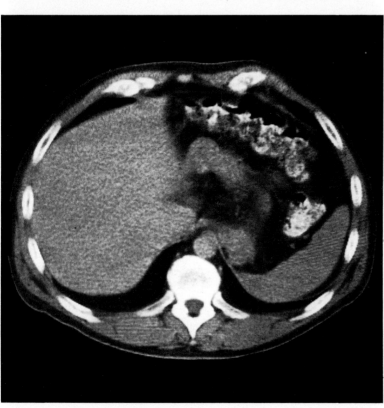

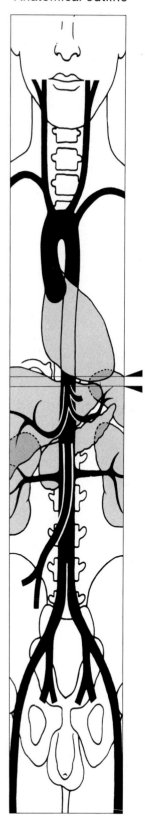

Anatomical outline

2-19/20

19/20

A 1	Aorta thoracica
A 12	A. lienalis
A 13	A. gastrica sinistra
V 1	V. cava inferior
V 10	V. azygos
V 11	V. hemiazygos
V 12	V. lienalis
O 26	Sinus phrenicocostalis
O 3	Hepar
O 34	Lobus caudatus
O 36	Porta hepatis
O 43	Corpus pancreatis**
O 44	Cauda pancreatis**
O 45	Lien
O 46	Hilus lienis
O 72	Gaster
O 74	Jejunum
O 76	Colon
O 77	Flexura colica
M 12	M. latissimus dorsi
M 21	M. intercostalis (interior, intermedius, exterior)
M 22	M. serratus anterior
M 24	M. rectus abdominis
M 25	M. obliquus externus abdominis
M 27	M. transversus abdominis
M 32	M. erector trunci
M 51	Diaphragma
S 1	Vertebra
S 2	Costa (Corpus costae)
S 22	Collum costae
S 26	Articulatio sternoclavicularis
S 27	Arcus costalis

** = lipomatosis pancreatis

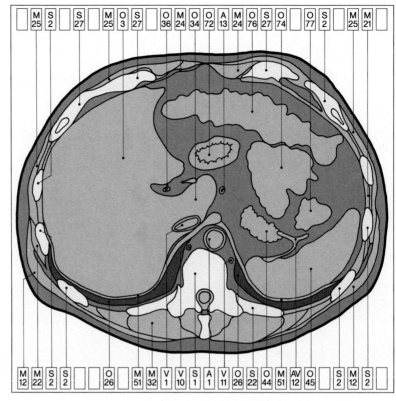

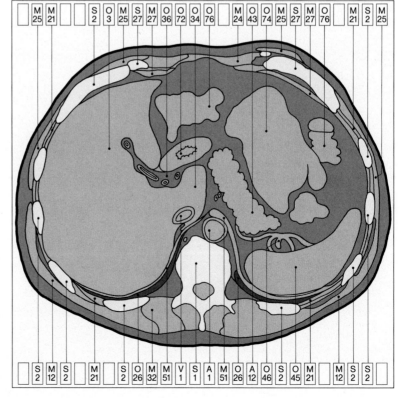

2-19/20

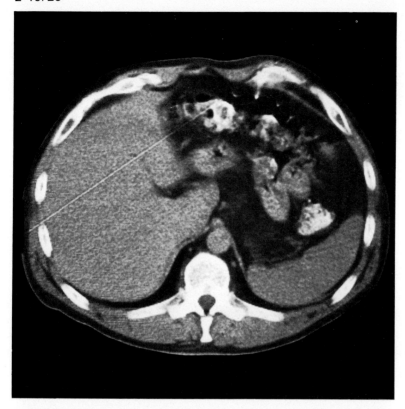

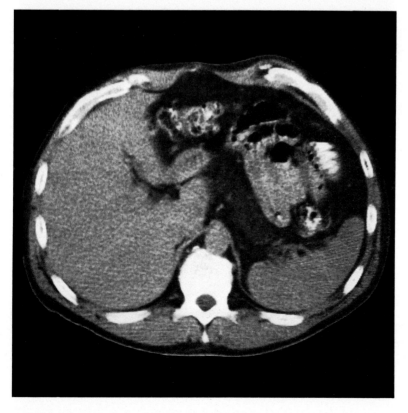

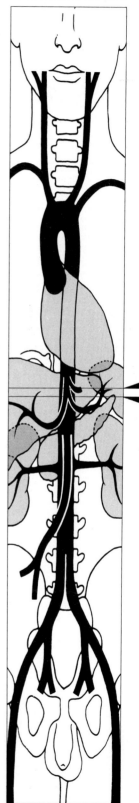

Anatomical outline

2-21/22

21/22

A 1	Aorta thoracica
A 11	A. hepatica
V 1	V. cava inferior
V 10	V. azygos
V 11	V. hemiazygos
V 12	V. lienalis
V 13	V. portae
O 3	Hepar
O 34	Lobus caudatus
O 36	Porta hepatis
O 37	Vesica fellea
O 41	Caput pancreatis**
O 43	Corpus pancreatis**
O 45	Lien
O 72	Gaster
O 74	Jejunum
O 76	Colon
O 77	Flexura colica
O 82	Glandula suprarenalis
M 12	M. latissimus dorsi
M 21	M. intercostalis (interior, intermedius, exterior)
M 22	M. serratus anterior
M 24	M. rectus abdominis
M 25	M. obliquus externus abdominis
M 27	M. transversus abdominis
M 32	M. erector trunci
M 51	Diaphragma
S 1	Vertebra
S 2	Costa (Corpus costae)
S 27	Arcus costalis

* = ramus
** = lipomatosis pancreatis

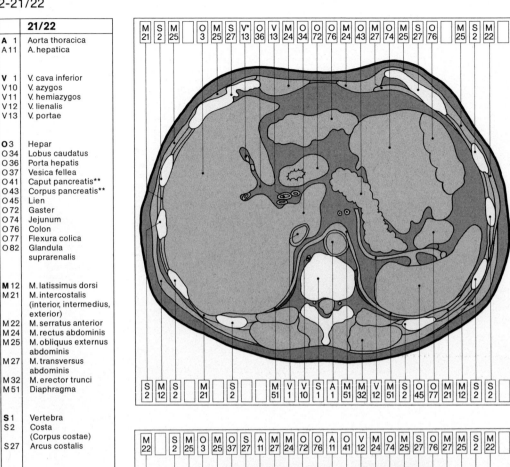

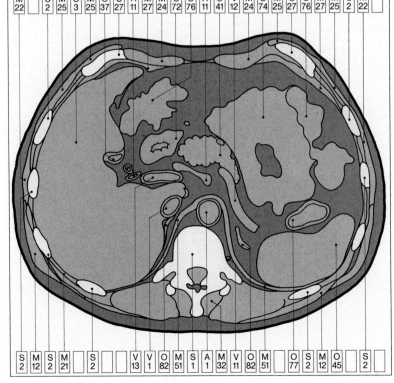

2-21/22

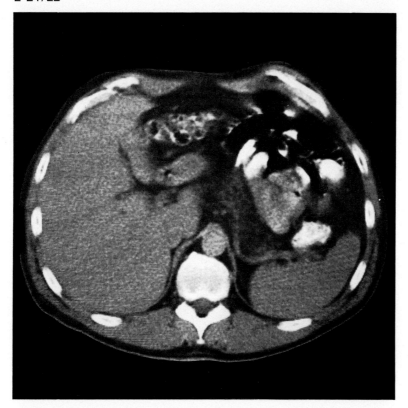

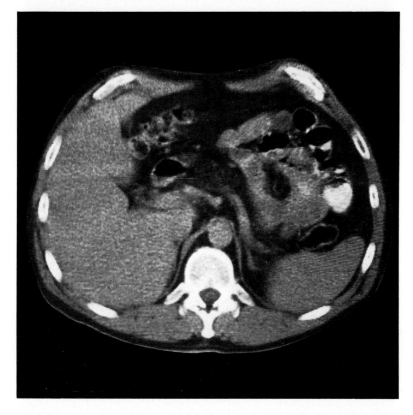

Anatomical outline

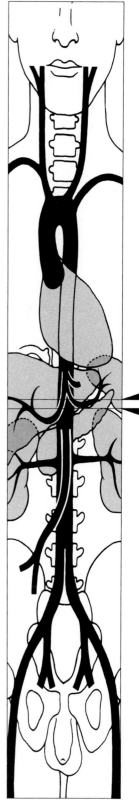

2-23/24

	23/24
A 1	Aorta abdominalis
A 14	A. mesenterica superior
V 1	V. cava inferior
V 11	V. hemiazygos
V 12	V. lienalis
V 13	V. portae
V 14	V. mesenterica superior
V 17	V. vertebralis
O 3	Hepar
O 37	Vesica fellea
O 41	Caput pancreatis**
O 45	Lien
O 5	Organa uropoetica (ren)
O 73	Duodenum
O 74	Jejunum
O 76	Colon
O 77	Flexura colica
O 82	Glandula suprarenalis
M 12	M. latissimus dorsi
M 21	M. intercostalis (interior, intermedius, exterior)
M 22	M. serratus anterior
M 24	M. rectus abdominis
M 25	M. obliquus externus abdominis
M 27	M. transversus abdominis
M 33	M. iliocostalis
M 34	M. longissimus dorsi
M 51	Diaphragma
S 1	Vertebra
S 2	Costa (Corpus costae)
S 27	Arcus costalis

* = ramus
** = lipomatosis pancreatis

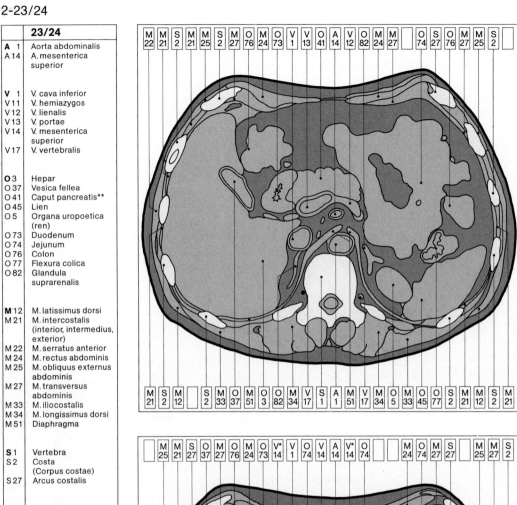

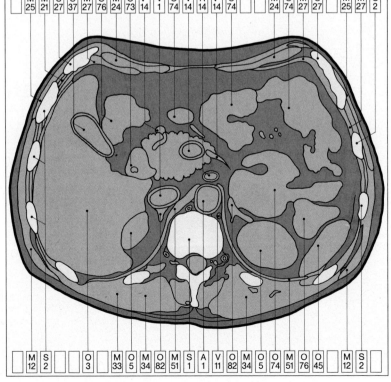

2-23/24

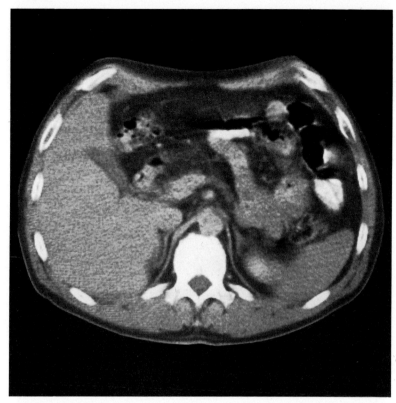

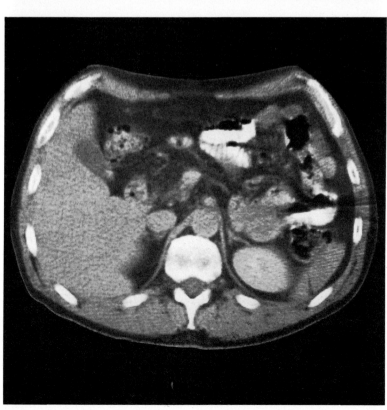

Anatomical outline

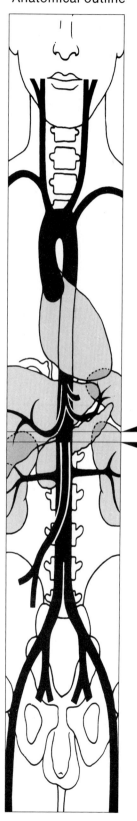

2-25/26

	25/26
A 1	Aorta abdominalis
A 14	A. mesenterica superior
V 1	V. cava inferior
V 10	V. azygos
V 14	V. mesenterica superior
O 3	Hepar
O 37	Vesica fellea
O 41	Caput pancreatis**
O 45	Lien
O 5	Organa uropoetica (ren)
O 54	Calices renales
O 55	Cortex, Medulla renalis
O 73	Duodenum
O 74	Jejunum
O 76	Colon
O 77	Flexura colica
O 82	Glandula suprarenalis
M 12	M. latissimus dorsi
M 21	M. intercostalis (interior, intermedius, exterior)
M 24	M. rectus abdominis
M 25	M. obliquus externus abdominis
M 27	M. transversus abdominis
M 29	M. psoas
M 33	M. iliocostalis
M 34	M. longissimus dorsi
M 51	Diaphragma
S 1	Vertebra
S 2	Costa (Corpus costae)
S 27	Arcus costalis
C 9	Linea alba

* = ramus
** = lipomatosis pancreatis

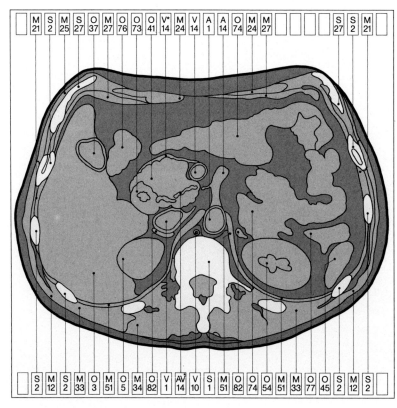

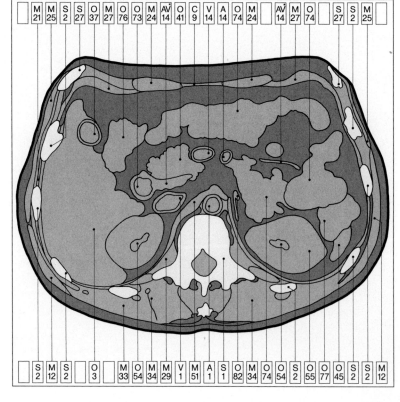

2-25/26

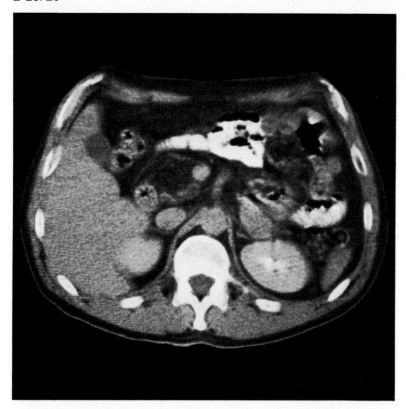

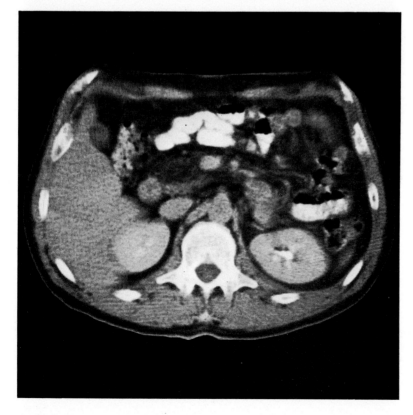

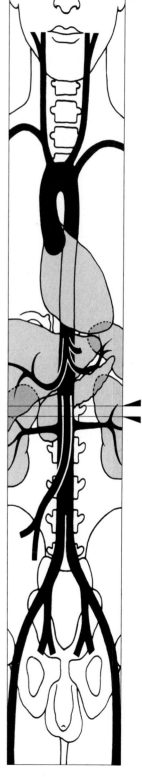

Anatomical outline

2-27/28

	27/28	
A 1	Aorta abdominalis	
A 14	A. mesenterica superior	
A 15	A. renalis	
V 1	V. cava inferior	
V 14	V. mesenterica superior	
V 15	V. renalis	
O 31	Lobus dexter	
O 41	Caput pancreatis**	
O 52	Sinus renalis	
O 53	Pelvis renalis	
O 54	Calices renales	
O 55	Cortex, Medulla renalis	
O 73	Duodenum	
O 74	Jejunum	
O 76	Colon	
O 77	Flexura colica	
M 12	M. latissimus dorsi	
M 21	M. intercostalis (interior, intermedius, exterior)	
M 24	M. rectus abdominis	
M 25	M. obliquus externus abdominis	
M 26	M. obliquus internus abdominis	
M 27	M. transversus abdominis	
M 28	M. quadratus lumborum	
M 29	M. psoas	
M 33	M. iliocostalis	
M 34	M. longissimus dorsi	
M 51	Diaphragma	
S 1	Vertebra	
S 2	Costa (Corpus costae)	
S 27	Arcus costalis	
C 9	Linea alba	

* = ramus
** = lipomatosis pancreatis

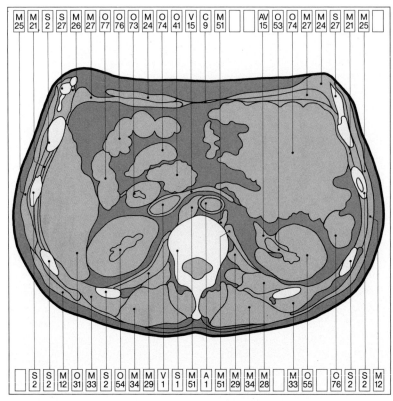

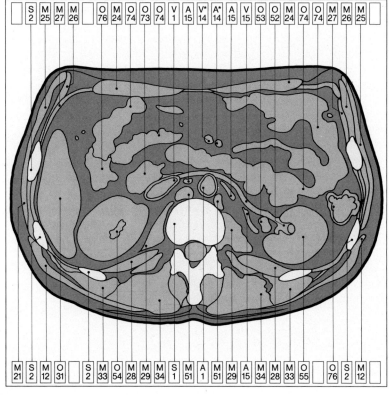

2-27/28

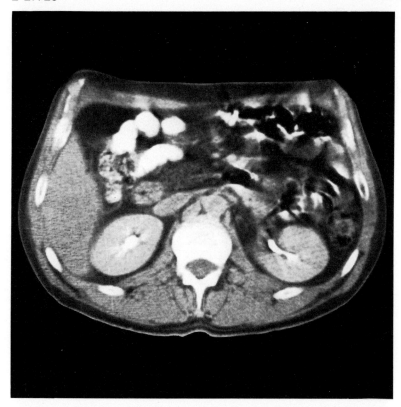

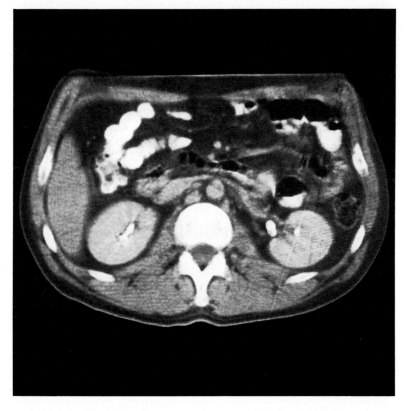

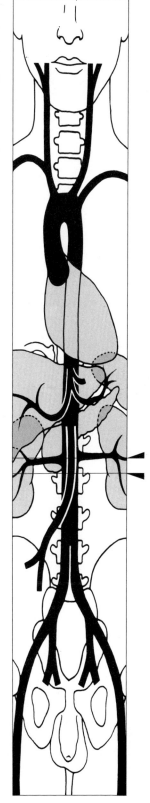

Anatomical outline

2-29/30

	29/30
A 1	Aorta abdominalis
A 14	A. mesenterica superior
A 15	A. renalis
A 16	A. lumbalis
V 1	V. cava inferior
V 14	V. mesenterica superior
V 15	V. renalis
V 17	V. vertebralis
O 3	Hepar
O 51	Hilus renalis
O 53	Pelvis renalis
O 54	Calices renales
O 55	Cortex, Medulla renalis
O 74	Jejunum
O 75	Ileum
O 76	Colon
M 12	M. latissimus dorsi
M 21	M. intercostalis (interior, intermedius, exterior)
M 24	M. rectus abdominis
M 25	M. obliquus externus abdominis
M 26	M. obliquus internus abdominis
M 27	M. transversus abdominis
M 28	M. quadratus lumborum
M 29	M. psoas
M 35	M. multifidus
M 51	Diaphragma
S 1	Vertebra
S 2	Costa (Corpus costae)
S 27	Arcus costalis

* = ramus

2-29/30

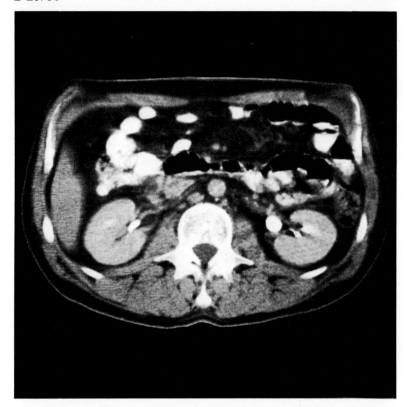

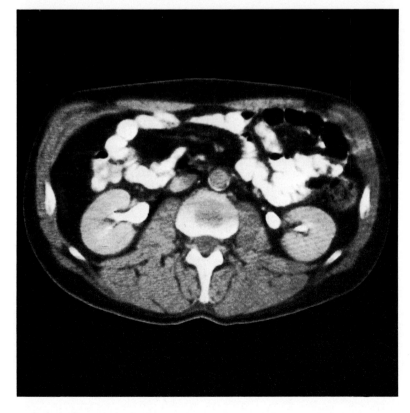

Anatomical outline

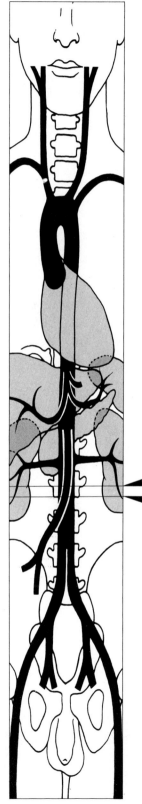

2-31/32

	31/32
A 1	Aorta abdominalis
A 16	A. lumbalis
V 1	V. cava inferior
V 16	V. lumbalis
O 54	Calices renales
O 56	Ureter
O 75	Ileum
O 76	Colon
M 12	M. latissimus dorsi
M 21	M. intercostalis (interior, intermedius, exterior)
M 24	M. rectus abdominis
M 25	M. obliquus externus abdominis
M 26	M. obliquus internus abdominis
M 27	M. transversus abdominis
M 28	M. quadratus lumborum
M 29	M. psoas
M 35	M. multifidus
S 1	Vertebra
S 11	Corpus vertebrae
S 17	Processus articularis inferior
S 2	Costa (Corpus costae)
C 9	Linea alba

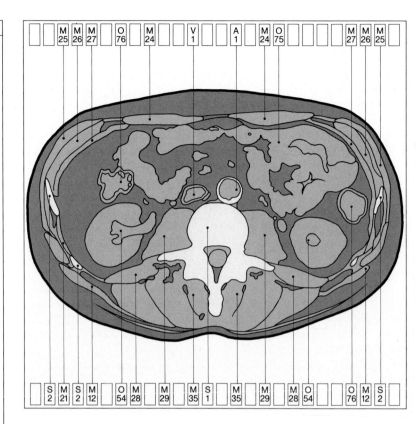

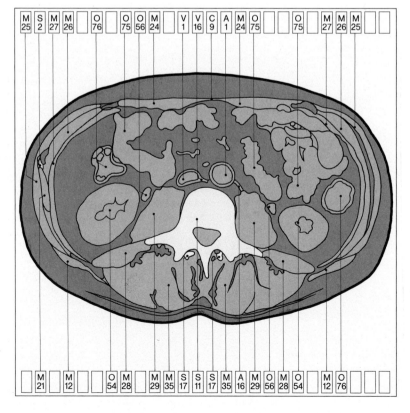

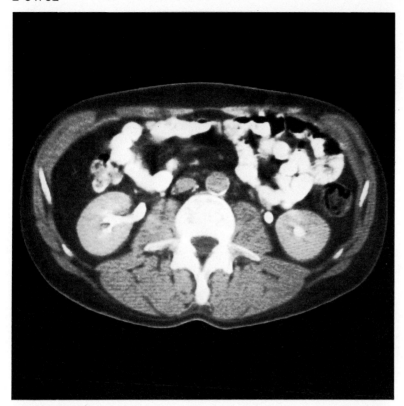
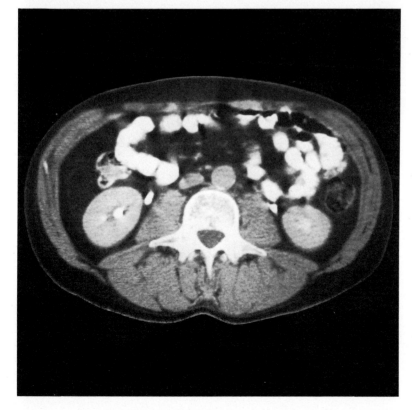
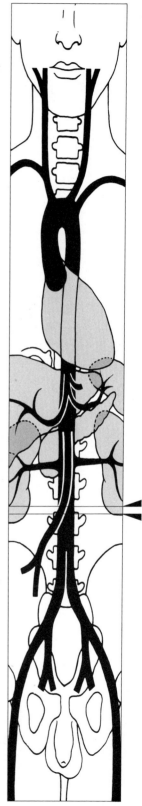

Anatomical outline

2-33/34

	33/34
A 1	Aorta abdominalis
A 14	A. mesenterica superior
A 17	A. mesenterica inferior
V 1	V. cava inferior
V 14	V. mesenterica superior
O 5	Organa uropoetica (ren)
O 56	Ureter
O 75	Ileum
O 76	Colon
M 24	M. rectus abdominis
M 25	M. obliquus externus abdominis
M 26	M. obliquus internus abdominis
M 27	M. transversus abdominis
M 28	M. quadratus lumborum
M 29	M. psoas
M 35	M. multifidus
S 1	Vertebra
	* = ramus

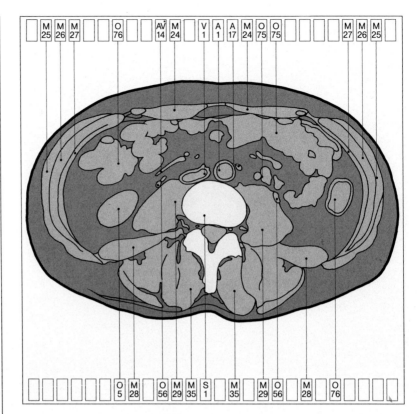

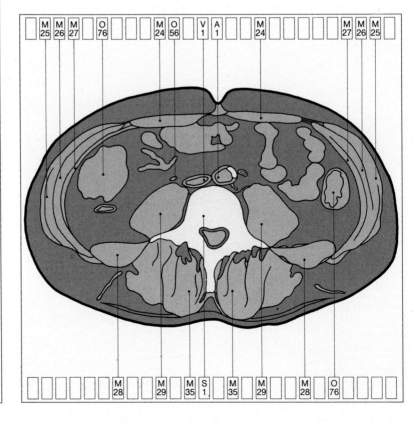

2-33/34

Anatomical outline

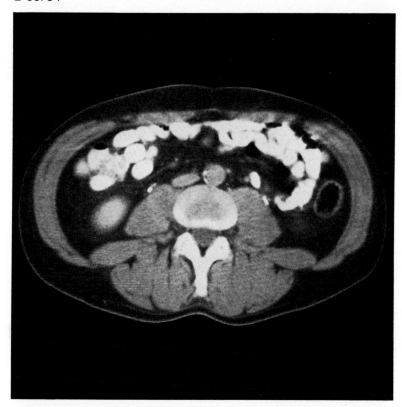

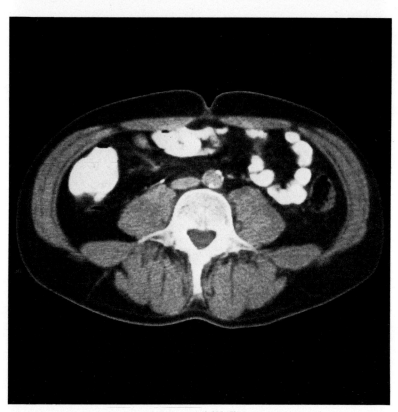

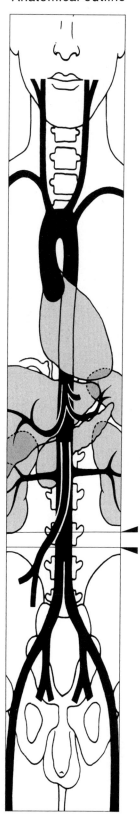

35/36

A 1	Aorta abdominalis
A 18	A. iliaca communis
V 1	V. cava inferior
O 56	Ureter
O 75	Ileum
O 76	Colon
M 24	M. rectus abdominis
M 25	M. obliquus externus abdominis
M 26	M. obliquus internus abdominis
M 27	M. transversus abdominis
M 28	M. quadratus lumborum
M 29	M. psoas
M 30	M. iliacus
M 35	M. multifidus
M 37	M. glutaeus medius
S 1	Vertebra
S 13	Articulatio intervertebralis
S 15	Processus transversus
S 41	Ala ossis ilium
C 9	Linea alba
C 10	Radix nervi spinalis

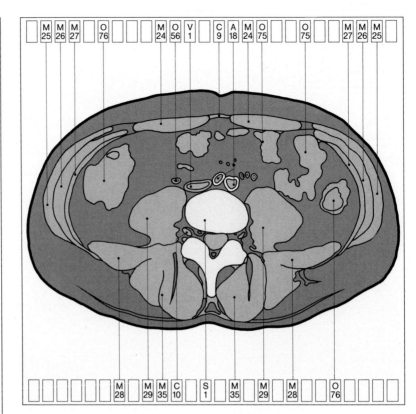

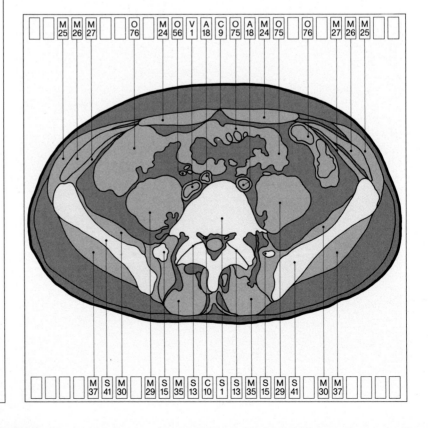

2-35/36
Anatomical outline

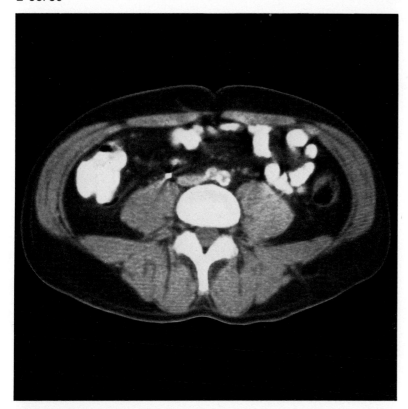
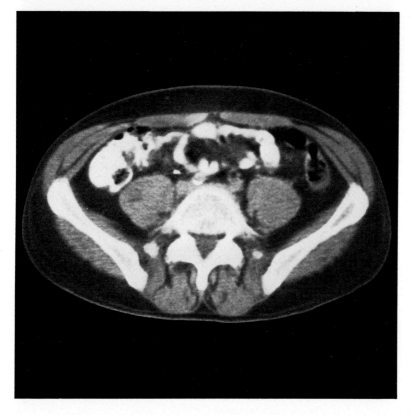
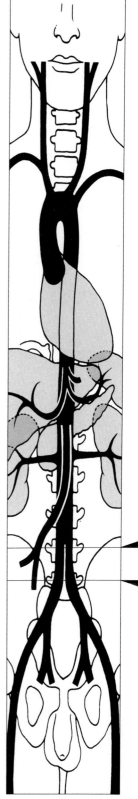

2-37/38

	37/38
A 18	A. iliaca communis
A 19	A. iliaca interna
A 20	A. iliaca externa
V 18	V. iliaca communis
V 19	V. iliaca interna
V 20	V. iliaca externa
O 56	Ureter
O 75	Ileum
O 76	Colon
M 24	M. rectus abdominis
M 25	M. obliquus externus abdominis
M 26	M. obliquus internus abdominis
M 27	M. transversus abdominis
M 29	M. psoas
M 30	M. iliacus
M 35	M. multifidus
M 36	M. glutaeus maximus
M 37	M. glutaeus medius
S 1	Vertebra
S 41	Ala ossis ilium
S 65	Articulatio sacroiliaca
C 4	Plexus lumbosacralis
C 9	Linea alba
C 10	Radix nervi spinalis

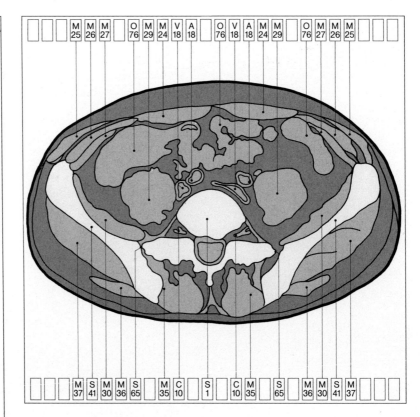

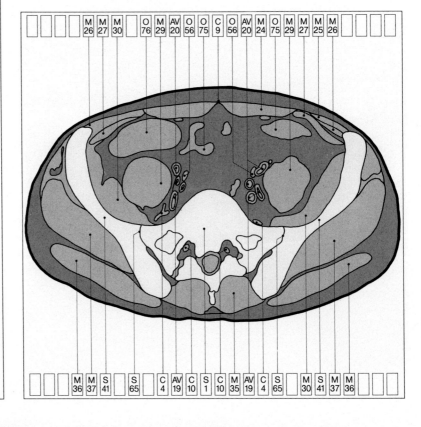

Anatomical outline

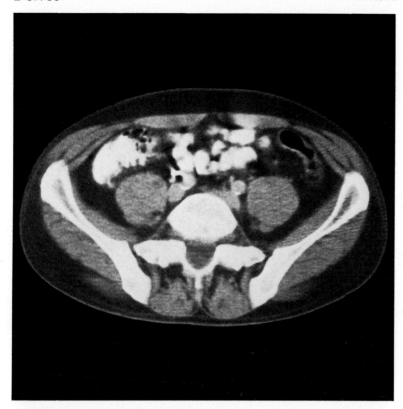

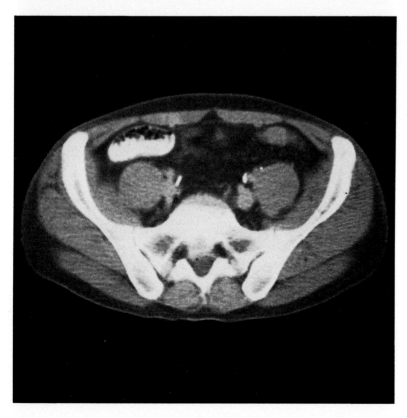

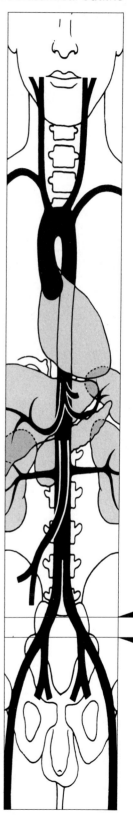

2-39/40

	39/40	
A 19	A. iliaca interna	
A 20	A. iliaca externa	
V 19	V. iliaca interna	
V 20	V. iliaca externa	
O 56	Ureter	
O 57	Vesica urinaria	
O 75	Ileum	
O 76	Colon	
O 78	Colon sigmoideum	
M 24	M. rectus abdominis	
M 26	M. obliquus internus abdominis	
M 27	M. transversus abdominis	
M 31	M. iliopsoas	
M 35	M. multifidus	
M 36	M. glutaeus maximus	
M 37	M. glutaeus medius	
M 38	M. glutaeus minimus	
S 41	Ala ossis ilium	
S 61	Foramina sacralia pelvina	
S 62	Crista sacralis	
S 65	Articulatio sacroiliaca	
C 4	Plexus lumbosacralis	
C 10	Radix nervi spinalis	

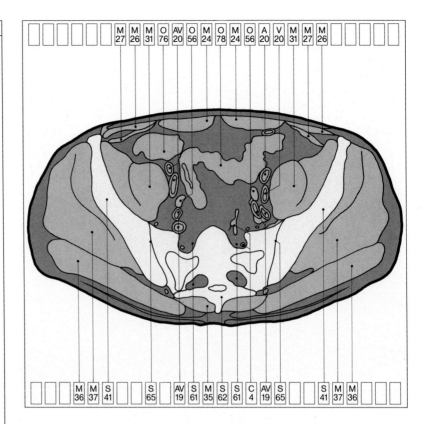

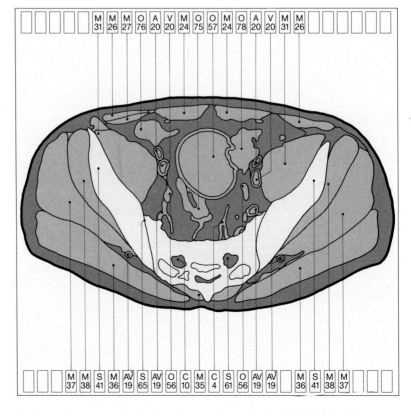

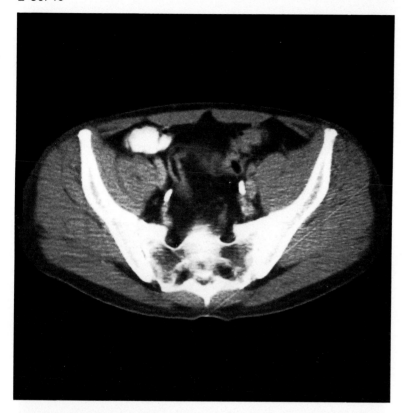
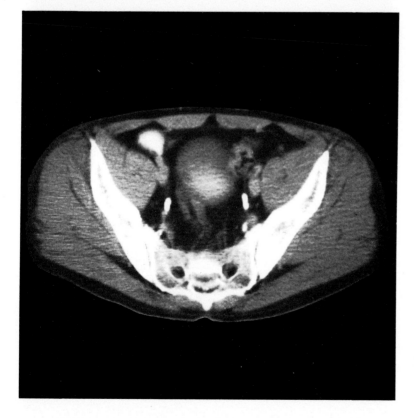
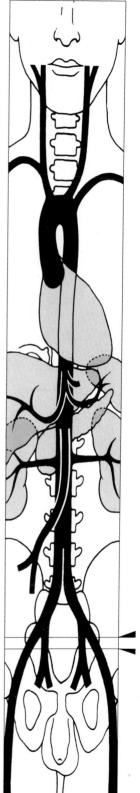

Anatomical outline

2-41/42

	41/42
A 19	A. iliaca interna
A 20	A. iliaca externa
V 19	V. iliaca interna
V 20	V. iliaca externa
O 56	Ureter
O 57	Vesica urinaria
O 6	Organa genitalia masculina
O 62	Vesicula seminalis
O 63	Funiculus spermaticus (Ductus deferens + vasa)
O 79	Rectum
M 24	M. rectus abdominis
M 26	M. obliquus internus abdominis
M 31	M. iliopsoas
M 36	M. glutaeus maximus
M 37	M. glutaeus medius
M 38	M. glutaeus minimus
M 39	M. piriformis
M 40	M. obturatorius internus
M 46	M. sartorius
M 47	M. rectus femoris
M 48	M. tensor fasciae latae
M 53	M. pyramidalis
S 4	Os coxae
S 42	Acetabulum
S 6	Os sacrum, Os coccygis
C 4	Plexus lumbosacralis
C 8	Nodus lymphaticus
C 9	Linea alba
* = ramus	

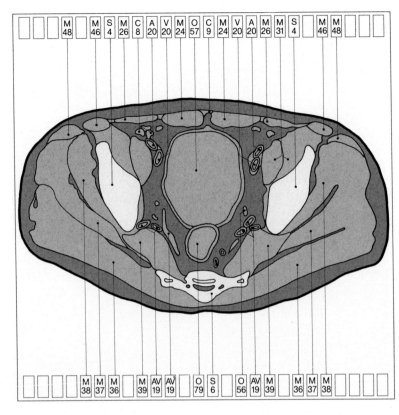

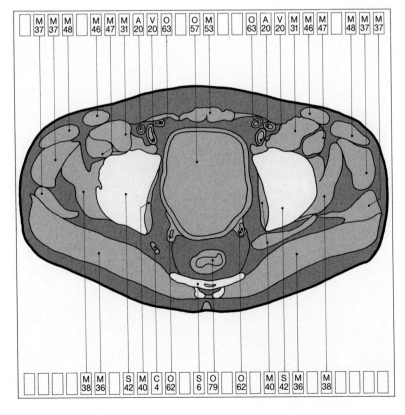

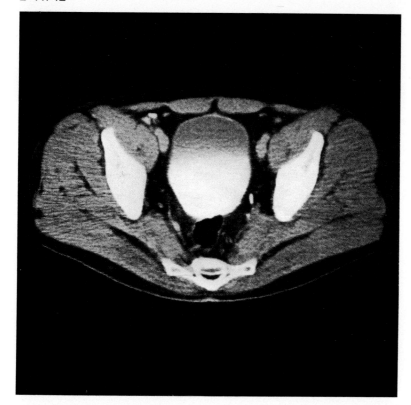
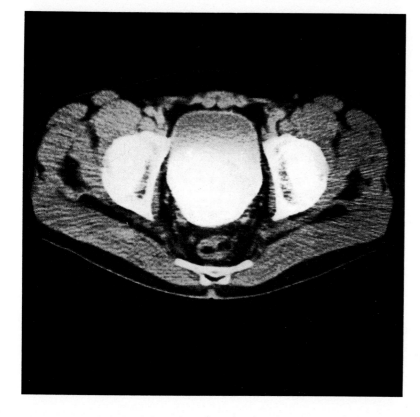
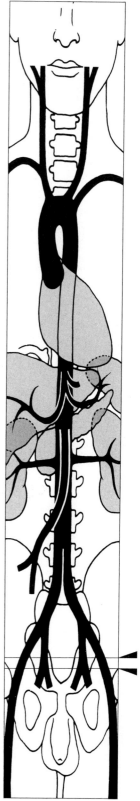

Anatomical outline

2-43/44

	43/44
A 20	A. iliaca externa
A 21	A. femoralis
A 22	A. pudenda
A 24	A. obturatoria
V 20	V. iliaca externa
V 21	V. femoralis
V 22	V. pudenda
V 24	V. obturatoria
O 57	Vesica urinaria
O 62	Vesicula seminalis
O 63	Funiculus spermaticus (Ductus deferens + vasa)
O 79	Rectum
M 31	M. iliopsoas
M 36	M. glutaeus maximus
M 37	M. glutaeus medius
M 40	M. obturatorius internus
M 41	M. gemellus (superior, inferior)
M 46	M. sartorius
M 47	M. rectus femoris
M 48	M. tensor fasciae latae
M 50	M. levator ani
M 53	M. pyramidalis
S 44	Corpus ossis ischii
S 46	Symphysis pubica
S 47	Ramus superior ossis pubis
S 51	Caput femoris
S 53	Trochanter major
S 54	Articulatio coxae
S 66	Os coccygis
C 1	N. ischiadicus
C 2	N. femoralis

2-43/44

Anatomical outline

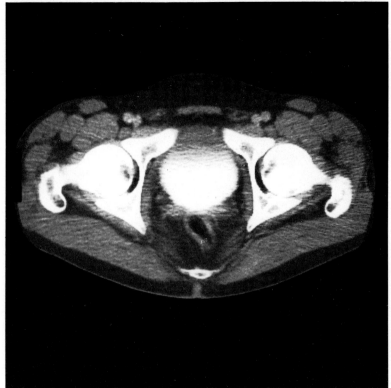
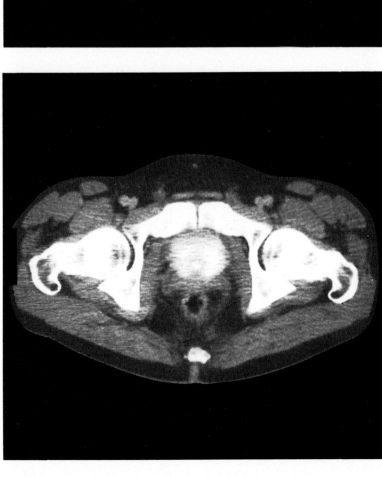
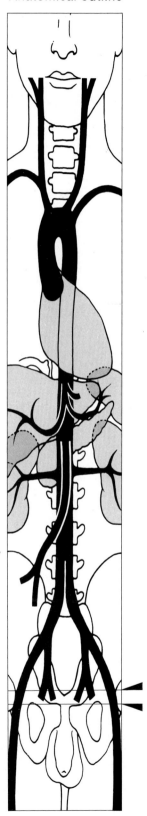

2-45/46

	45/46	
A 21	A. femoralis	
A 22	A. pudenda	
A 23	A. penis dorsalis	
V 21	V. femoralis	
V 22	V. pudenda	
O 58	Urethra	
O 61	Prostata	
O 63	Funiculus spermaticus (Ductus deferens + vasa)	
O 79	Rectum	
M 31	M. iliopsoas	
M 36	M. glutaeus maximus	
M 40	M. obturatorius internus	
M 41	M. gemellus (superior, inferior)	
M 42	M. obturatorius externus	
M 43	M. pectineus	
M 44	M. adductor longus	
M 45	M. gracilis	
M 46	M. sartorius	
M 47	M. rectus femoris	
M 48	M. tensor fasciae latae	
M 49	M. vastus lateralis	
M 50	M. levator ani	
M 54	M. quadratus femoris	
S 43	Tuber ossis ischii	
S 46	Symphysis pubica	
S 5	Femur	
S 52	Collum femoris	
S 53	Trochanter major	
S 66	Os coccygis	
C 1	N. ischiadicus	
C 5	Fossa ischiorectalis	

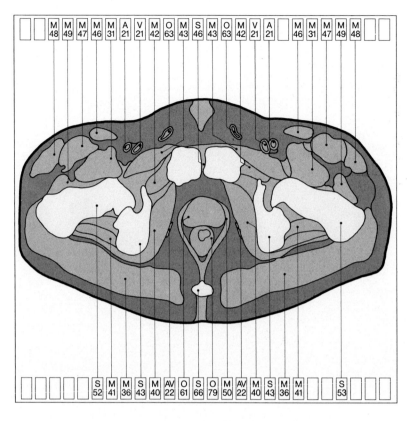

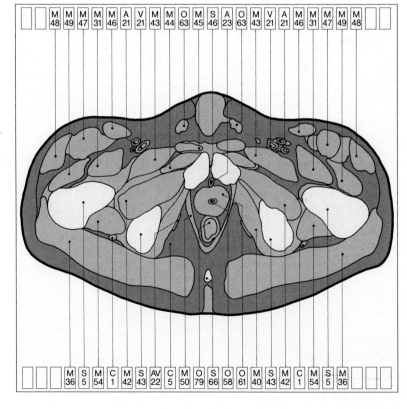

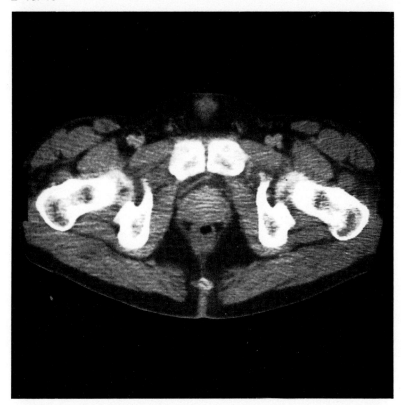
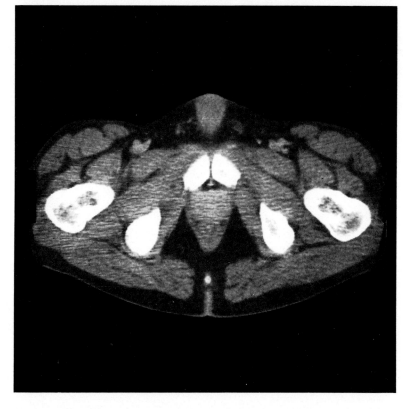
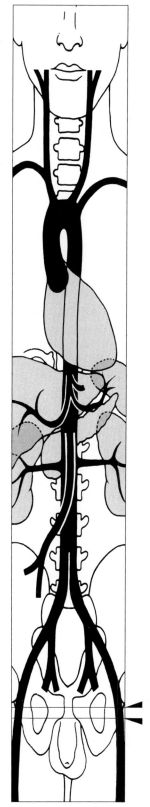

Anatomical outline

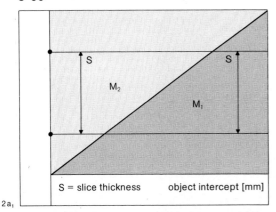

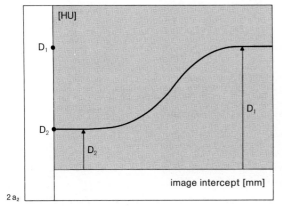

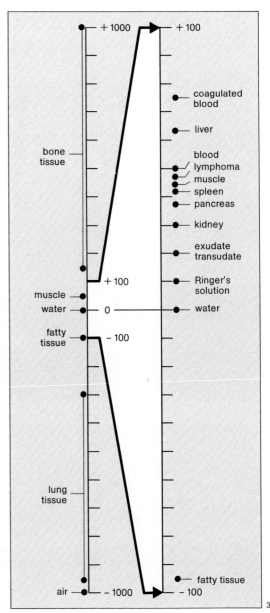

Fig. 3-2 a: Density value and partial volume effect. The boundary surface of two media (M_1, M_2) of radiodensity D_1 and D_2 running obliquely through the CT slice produces mixed values which lie between the density values D_1 and D_2. The density value reliably represents the measured homogeneous medium when the slice thickness (S) is completely filled.

Fig. 3-3 a: The Hounsfield scale.

Fig. 3-3 b: The radiodensity of different types of tissue and body fluids (reference values based on data from various authors [59, 94, 104, 105, 106, 681]).

Tissue	Standard value (HU)	Range (HU)	Fluids	Standard value (HU)
Bone (compact)	> 250		Blood (coagulated)	80 ± 10
Bone (spongy)	130 ± 100		Blood	
Thyroid	70 ± 10		(venous whole blood)	55 ± 5
Liver	65 ± 5	45 – 75	Plasma	27 ± 2
Muscle	45 ± 5	35 – 50	Exudate (>30 g protein/l)	>18 ± 2
Spleen	45 ± 5	35 – 55	Transudate	
Lymphoma	45 ± 10	40 – 60	(<30 g protein/l)	<18 ± 2
Pancreas	40 ± 10	25 – 55	Ringer's solution	12 ± 2
Kidney	30 ± 10	20 – 40		
Fatty tissue	−90 ± 10	−80 – (−110)		

Density measurement (3-00)

In addition to the morphological structures of the computed tomogram, the density values must be analysed and associated with the diagnosis. A knowledge of the reliability and pathomorphological substrate of the density value is a prerequisite for this.

Evaluation (3-10)
The evaluation units of the scanners permit measurement of the density over freely selectable areas of the computed tomogram (**regions of interest**[1]). The density value of the individual volume element is subject – depending on the photon flow during the data collection – to statistical variations which cause graininess (**image noise**[1]) in the computed tomogram. These statistical variations are expressed numerically as the **standard deviation**[1] around a mean value. The accuracy of the **mean value** can be improved by choosing regions of adequate size.

Falsification of density values (3-20)
A distinction must be made between the statistical inaccuracy inherent in the method of data collection and systematic errors. Systematic errors are caused mainly by movements of the patient during scanning, hardening of X-radiation and inaccuracies of image reconstruction. They are known collectively as **artifacts**[1]. Reliable density measurements can only be expected in artifact-free areas of the computed tomogram.

Since the density value represents a mean absorption value of the tissue contained in the volume element, the radiodensity of the tissue to be measured can only be stated with certainty when this tissue completely fills the entire slice thickness (Fig. 3-2a). Great care must therefore be taken that the tissue concerned fills the entire slice thickness when measuring densities at the boundaries of a structure. A **partial volume effect** (1-50) is always present in structures with a diameter smaller than the slice thickness, and this makes accurate density measurement impossible (**slice geometry**[1]).

Density scale (3-30) (Fig. 3–3a)
The density value is measured in **Hounsfield units** (HU) (1-40). The fixed points of the density scale are defined by air (= −1000 HU) and water (= 0 HU) and are therefore independent of the tube voltage used. The various kinds of tissue vary within certain limits in relation to the value of water, depending on the effective radiation energy employed, so that the tissue densities reported in the literature (in HU) must be regarded as standard values (Fig. 3-3b). In computerized tomography the density units are usually directly proportional to the linear attenuation coefficients.

Terminology (3-40)
In making a diagnosis, an important factor in addition to the actual numerical values is the **density of the tissue** (radiodensity) **relative** to the **surrounding tissue**. This has led to the establishment of the terms **isodensity** for identical tissue density in relation to the surrounding tissue, **hypodensity** for reduced tissue density and **hyperdensity** for increased tissue density. In the case of parenchymatous organs such as the brain, liver, kidney and pancreas it is frequently accepted by tacit agreement that the density value is measured relative to healthy tissue. Clear reference to this relation should, however, be made in the findings.

Pathomorphological substrate (3-50)
Body tissues in the living organism should not be regarded as static parameters, since they react in different ways to trauma, infection, tumours and metabolic changes. Some of these changes are visible in the computed tomogram.

Cystic contents, transudate, exudate (3-51)
Cysts – enclosed water-filled spaces – are found in a number of organs. The density value of the cystic contents is slightly above that of water, due both to a varying content of protein and to measuring inaccuracies and electrolytes (Fig. 3-3a). As can be seen in Fig. 3-5c, the content of protein causes a not inconsiderable increase of the density value. Density values of 20–30 HU can be achieved in the case of **exudates** which exhibit a protein content greater than 30 g per litre and which differ from **transudates** by virtue of this higher density.

Cysts are avascular spaces and do not enhance following **administration of contrast media** (4-50).

---

[1] see CT Terminology (97-00)

Blood – haematomas (3-52)

The **density value of blood,** which is determined primarily by the protein content of the blood corpuscles, is 55±5 HU in healthy persons with normal haematocrit and haemoglobin content. The haemoglobin content accounts for 40 HU (Fig. 3-5a), while 15 HU correspond to the density of plasma. The density values of plasma are distributed evenly between the protein and the electrolytes. As can be seen in Fig. 3-5a, the density value of blood is directly dependent on the haemoglobin content or the haematocrit. The iron content of the haemoglobin plays only a subordinate role (Fig. 3-5b). The calcium level of plasma has virtually no influence on the density value of blood (106).

When blood **coagulates,** haemoconcentration corresponding to an increased haematocrit value takes place as a result of the retraction of fibrin. In its fresh stage, a compact haematoma is therefore hyperdense in comparison to fresh venous blood. As Fig. 3-5d shows, this hyperdensity is demonstrable for up to 7 days after onset of the haemorrhage. The density value falls as a result of decomposition of the fibrin and blood corpuscles and the subsequent absorption of the protein bodies. In the case of larger haematomas which have formed a capsule from granulation tissue, the radiodensity can fall to within the range of water in accordance with the protein content (posttraumatic cyst). Clinical results show that the time relationship demonstrable in cerebral diagnosis is present to only a limited extent in the whole body sphere (Fig. 3-5d). The hyperdensity present in the fresh stage can be evaluated in the diagnosis. Hypodensity is equivocal and must be distinguished from other accumulations of fluid.

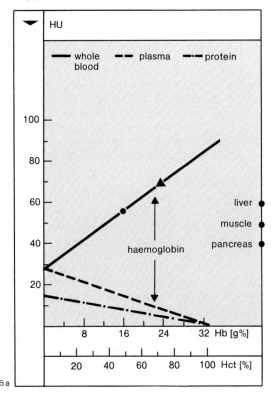

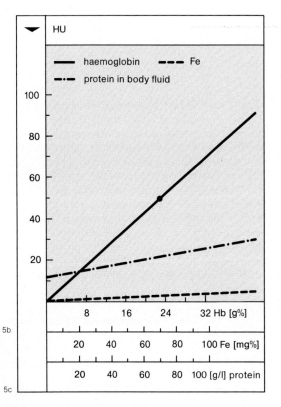

Fig. 3-5a: **The radiodensity of blood** and its fractions in relation to the haematocrit based on data from New (105), Norman (106) and Hübener (94). The increased density value of a fresh haematoma (▲) corresponds to an increased haemoconcentration, i.e. an increased haematocrit.

Fig. 3-5b: **The radiodensity of haemoglobin and serum iron** in relation to the concentration (g % and mg %, respectively).

Fig. 3-5c: **The radiodensity of body fluids.** It increases linearly in relation to the protein content.

Density measurement

Abscesses (3-53)

The reaction of the organism to an infection is **inflammation**, a process which is accompanied by local hyperaemia, exudation and leukocyte immigration and which is reversible as long as no tissue has perished. Tissue necroses, exudation and perished leukocytes are the pathological substrate of pus, the consistency of which can vary depending on its composition. The accumulation of pus becomes demarcated from the 3rd to the 5th day by invading granulation tissue, which eventually forms the membrane of the abscess. On successful antibiotic therapy, the sterile pus is absorbed and a (protein-rich) cyst develops. The granulation tissue forms a scar following incision or spontaneous discharge.

In keeping with these processes, the computed tomogramm reveals varying **density values** in the region of the abscess (95) (Fig. 3-5e). Slight hypodensity due to the concomitant oedema can sometimes be demonstrated by computerized tomography in the fresh stage of leukocytic immigration. The density falls distinctly following liquefaction, or pus-formation. The density values stabilize in this stage at about 30 HU. Depending on the therapy, one finds either discharge of the pus with the formation of a scar displaying density values in the connective-tissue range or the formation of a cyst rich in protein, the radiodensity of which gradually approaches the water range (see above).

Several additional diagnostic criteria can be obtained by the **administration of contrast medium** (4-50). Highly vascularized granulation tissue is recognizable by an opacified, hyperdense ring around the hypodense abscess. While enhancement can be very pronounced in fresh, inflammatory infiltration due to hyperaemia, it cannot be demonstrated in liquefied zones.

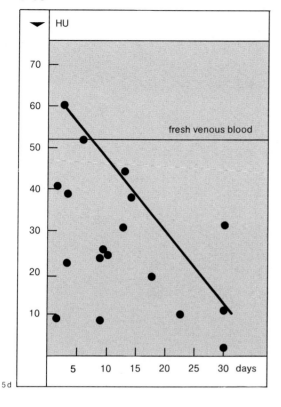

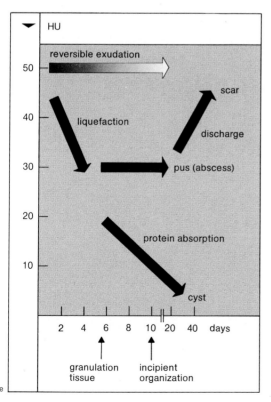

Fig. 3-5d: **The radiodensity of a haematoma** depends on the age of the accumulation of blood. The solid line represents Bergström's data (76). The measuring points entered below the curve represent personal measurements of haematomas, the age of which could be established, and those of Guertler (91).

Fig. 3-5e: **The radiodensity of an abscess** with reference to the various pathophysiological courses (after Hübener [95], modified).

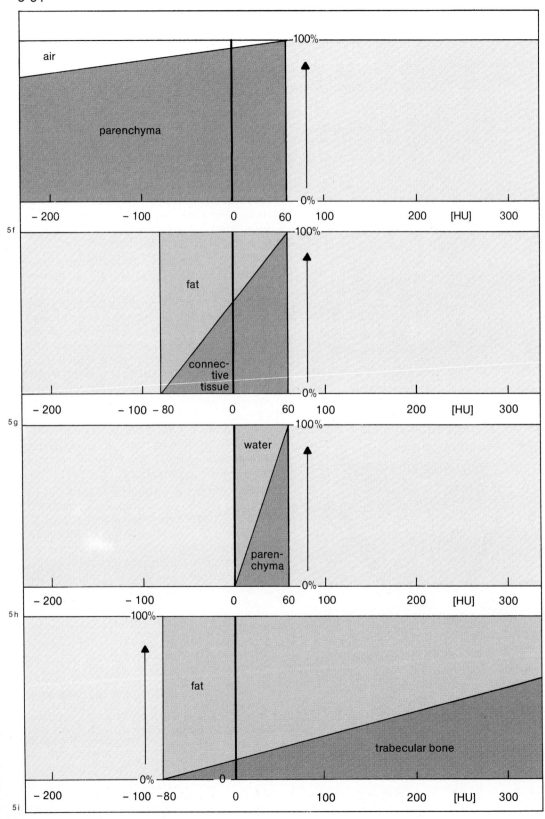

Solid tissue (3-54)

The density value of bone depends on its mineral content. In all other solid tissues (Fig. 3-5f–i), it is determined overwhelmingly by the content of protein, water and fat. Consequently, the protein-rich parenchyma of the liver, muscle and spleen displays higher density values than that of the kidney with its varying hydration. Fatty tissue displays a radiodensity of -80 to -100 HU and functions as filling material. For practical reasons, the term **soft tissue** is used when the radiodensity of fatty tissue is clearly exceeded (mostly muscle tissue).

The density value of **mixed tissues** is determined by the volume ratio of the different tissue components, and can be calculated in a simple (directly proportional) manner where two components are present. As Fig. 3-5g shows, a certain ratio of fatty to connective tissue can produce a density value of 0 HU. Homogeneous structures of water density can therefore also correspond to solid tissue. Analogously, the degree of fatty degeneration of the liver can be established directly from the density value (10% fatty degeneration $\triangleq$ 14 HU). A reduction of density of liver or muscle tissue can also be caused by accumulation of water (oedema). As an example, Fig. 3-5g,h shows that the build-up of fat or water can produce a value of 15 HU – a value which can also be present in accumulations of protein-rich fluid (Fig. 3-5c).

Pulmonary and osseous tissue are marked by wide ranges of density due to the varying addition of a high-contrast component (air, cortical bone) to the soft tissue.

Regressive change (3-55)

Calcifications in necrotic material or in denaturated proteins are a familiar radiological sign which is demonstrated more sensitively by computerized tomography than in the X-ray film. **Hyalinization** and **amyloidosis** are interstitial and intracellular depositions rich in protein which do not modify the density values of the organs concerned to any significant degree. On the other hand, liquefying **necrosis** leads to an unequivocal, varying reduction of density into the water range. It is found not only in inflammations (see above), but also and more importantly in rapidly expanding tumours, where it develops as a result of hypoxia or haemorrhagic perfusion and may display smooth demarcation ("cystic degeneration"). Gas is frequently demonstrated within aseptic necroses (e. g. following embolism of an organ artery) (571), and is in these cases not of bacterial origin. The incorporation of gas within cystic formations is usually regarded as pathognomonic for abscesses (formation of gas by anaerobes).

Fig. 3-**5f–i**: **The radiodensity of mixed tissues.** Assuming that a mixed tissue consists of two components, the percental composition can be concluded from the density value. For example, the content of air in the case of lung tissue (5f), the fat content in the case of fatty parenchyma (5g), the amount of water in the case of water accumulation (5h) and mineral-containing bone substance in the case of bone tissue (5i) can be determined if the density values of both components are definitely known.

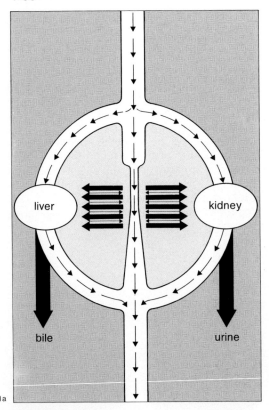

Fig. 4-1a, b: Distribution spaces of intravascularly administered contrast media.

1a: The contrast medium injected into the blood stream disperses into the extracellular space. The excretory processes via either the kidney or the liver commence at the same time.

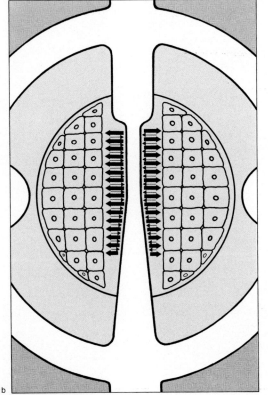

1b: The component of the contrast medium not bound to protein diffuses through the capillaries into the interstitial space (➡) and does not enter the cells. The blood level of contrast material falls as a result of the excretory processes. Redistribution of the contrast material into the blood stream (→) takes place once the level falls below the concentration of contrast medium in the interstitial space.

Contrast media (4-00)

Forms of opacification (4-10)
There are two different forms of administration for use in computerized tomography:

Intracavitary opacification

Intracavitary opacification is governed by simple laws. The intestinal tube, lumen of the urinary bladder and the cerebrospinal fluid space must be regarded fundamentally as enclosed spaces in which the contrast material mixes with the fluid present there. The degree of opacification is determined by the dose and the distribution volume.

Intravascular administration

Intravascular administration leads to complex, time-dependent distribution in various tissue spaces. The degree of opacification in the body organs is determined not only by the dose, but also by the pharmacokinetics (i. e. by the haemodynamics, the distribution between the tissue spaces and the route of excretion).

Intravenously administered contrast media undergo varying degrees of protein binding, a phenomenon which has a considerable influence on the excretory processes in the organism. For the greater part, the unbound portion diffuses from the vascular lumen through the capillary wall into the interstitial space (Fig. 4-1b). However, it is also withdrawn from the blood by glomerular filtration in the kidney. Tubular reabsorption of water results in an increased concentration of contrast material in the urinary tract, a phenomenon which forms the basis for the nephrographic effect. High protein binding of the contrast material prevents rapid glomerular filtration and mediates active uptake into the hepatocyte, which transports the contrast material to the bile ducts (cholegraphy). The plasma level of contrast medium falls as a result of these excretory processes, in response to which redistribution takes place from the interstitial into the intravascular space – up to complete elimination (Fig. 4-1b). Contrast media with varying protein binding have been developed to help achieve particular clinical objectives (cholegraphic and urographic agents). The good tolerance of renal contrast media is based on exclusive distribution in the extracellular space. Angiography exploits the pharmacokinetic phenomenon that intravascularly administered contrast medium does not enter the interstitial space immediately, but rather gradually. It therefore remains within the vessels in the phase required for angiography. In the case of computerized tomography, which can demonstrate individual organs directly, not only tried and tested, but also other, previously less heeded properties of contrast media contribute to the diagnosis:

● Opacification of a pathological lesion in the **brain** by loss of the blood-fluid barrier. This property applies only to cerebral diagnosis.

● **Parenchymal opacification**, which has previously been used only on a limited scale for total-body opacification. Following injection, uniform distribution of the contrast material in the extracellular space leads to an increase of density of the entire organ. In contrast, the term "parenchymal phase" commonly used in angiography means short-lasting opacification of the capillary bed.

● Concentration of the contrast medium in the **renal parenchyma** (nephrographic effect). The measurable renal function becomes a diagnostic criterion.

● Demonstration of the **intravascular space**. Various modes of administration opacify the lumen of larger vessels or, indirectly, highly vascular kinds of tissue or regions. The features distinguishing this from parenchymal opacification overlap.

● Concentration of the contrast material in the **bile** (biligraphic effect). The specific excretory capacity of the liver parenchyma can be used only within limitations (4-40).

These properties are exploited in various ways depending on the mode of administration and the examination technique. Adequate opacification of the structure to be demonstrated which lasts for the entire duration of the examination is desirable. Since contrast media can only be used in limited amounts, the time resp. flow rate for the administration is restricted. In turn, the mode of administration is determined by the degree of enhancement required.

Intracavitary contrast media (4-20)

Retrograde cystography (4-21)

The density of the bladder lumen can only be increased uniformly and specifically to a predetermined value of 150–200 HU by retrograde instillation of a defined solution of contrast material. If the bladder is filled until the patient reports a sensation of pressure, it can be demonstrated as an almost spherical shape, and compression effects by intestinal loops can be avoided (83-10). If catheterization is impossible, a small amount of a urographic agent can be injected intravenously instead (4-34).

Bowel opacification (4-22)

The shape and position of the greater part of the bowel can be recognized in the plain scan. Since, however, the contents of the bowel usually display soft-tissue density, interpretation of the plain scan is frequently difficult. The duodenum can simulate an enlarged head of the pancreas, while individual small bowel loops can resemble a mass in the tail region of the pancreas or lymph nodes. Pelvic organs in particular cannot be assessed in detail. Because of this, **oral opacification of the bowel** (Fig. 4-2b,c) soon became a routine method. Visualization of the upper gastrointestinal tract as far as the proximal ileum suffices for the epigastrium and, in particular, for the bed of the pancreas. The small and large bowel should be filled with contrast medium to achieve demarcation from the retroperitoneal space.

If artifacts are to be avoided, a limit must be set for the degree of enhancement of the intestinal lumen. Contrast of 150–200 HU is desirable if unequivocal identification of the bowel is to be achieved despite partial volume effects. The iodine content of the contrast medium administered should therefore lie between 5 and 15 mg iodine/ml, i.e. between 1.3 and 3.5 % v/v Gastrografin[1].

The measuring sensitivity of the scanners for iodine varies and depends primarily on differing effective radiation energy (tube voltage, filtration) (Fig. 4-2a). 2–4 % v/v Gastrografin has proved its value in practice. By comparison, diluted barium sulphate is less suitable because of uncontrollable high-contrast flocculation at the intestinal wall.

The degree of opacification actually achieved in the intestinal lumen is also influenced by the **absorption physiology**. Isotonicity (isoosmosis) occurs in the small bowel, since water diffuses passively through the intestinal wall proportionate to the osmotic pressure. Even a 4 % v/v Gastrografin solution is still highly hypotonic, which means that Gastrografin – which cannot be absorbed – becomes concentrated as a result of water absorption, resulting in greater opacification of the lumen. The absorption of water can be prevented by the addition of osmotic (non-absorbable) substances, as a result of which the opacification attainable with this solution does not alter. If, in addition, the amount of contrast medium swallowed is relatively large, dilution effects due to any fluids still present within the lumen can be ignored if the motility of the gastrointestinal tract is normal.

As an inert filling material, such an isotonic, non-absorbable contrast medium can lead to demonstration of the various sections of the bowel depending on the amount administered and the time. If **opacification of the entire bowel** is desired, the medium should be taken in portions and over an extended period up to the start of scanning. Filling of the rectum can

Type of scanner	Tube voltage (KV)	Measuring sensitivity for iodine (HU) per mg I/ml
EMI Mark I	100	34–32
	120	27–26
	140	21–22
EMI 5005	120	23
	140	19
(30 x 40 Ph)	140	17
Siretom 2000	125	19.5
	133	18.5
	141	17.5
Somatom 2	125	21.5
Delta 50	120	25–28.6
GE 8800	120	28.5

Fig. 4-2a: **Measuring sensitivity for iodine.** The individual scanners display a varying sensitivity depending on the tube voltage and filtration (effective radiation energy) used.

[1] In USA: Gastrovist® (Berlex Laboratories, Inc.)

Contrast media

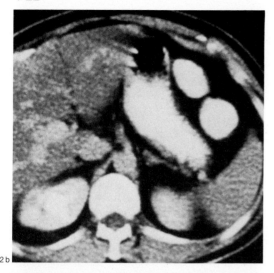

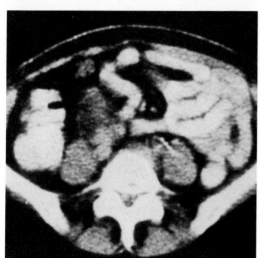

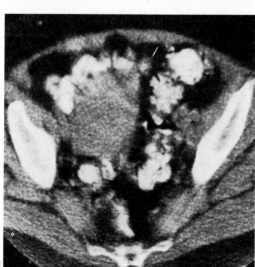

be expected after 60–80 minutes, since, as with osmotic laxatives, passage through the bowel is accelerated. The amount of contrast medium administered is eliminated in highly fluid form.

The disadvantages of the volume stress can be reduced by the administration of Gastrografin and granulate 24 hours before the examination. The colon then becomes identifiable by inhomogeneous opacification (Fig. 4-2d). The small bowel must also be opacified directly before the examination.

If unequivocal demarcation of the rectum or sigmoid cannot be achieved with the methods described above, a small **colonic enema** with 200–300 ml of a 2–4 % v/v solution of Gastrografin or Urografin 76 %[1] is to be recommended in diagnostically critical cases (136).

Oral administration should be preferred for practical reasons. Larger amounts of hypotonic solutions are, however, contraindicated in cardiac insufficiency, since the water absorbed into the circulatory system leads to additional stress on the heart. For as yet unexplained reasons, caution should be exercised in diarrhoea with the use of larger volumes of isotonic, strictly speaking inert contrast medium mixtures. The diarrhoea can otherwise be exacerbated with all the negative sequelae of an electrolyte shift or dehydration.

Fig. 4-**2b–d: Bowel opacification.**

2b: A diluted Gastrografin solution drunk evenly leads to uniform and artifact-free opacification of all sections of the bowel including the stomach and epigastrium.

2c: The entire bowel including the colon opacifies uniformly following oral administration of larger amounts of a diluted Gastrografin solution.

2d: Opacification of the large bowel after administration of Gastrografin and granulate 24 hours before the examination. The colon can be clearly identified by crumbly opacification (even without intestinal gas).

[1] In USA: Angiovist® 370 (Berlex Laboratories, Inc.)

Modes of administration (4-23)

● **Partial opacification of the bowel**

For opacification of the upper gastrointestinal tract:

Oral administration of 500 ml of a diluted Gastrografin solution (see below). The solution should be swallowed in portions up to the start of scanning.

● **Total opacification of the bowel**

Oral administration of approx. 1,000 up to 1,500 ml of a diluted Gastrografin solution (see below). The solution should be swallowed slowly and in portions over 60 minutes up to the start of scanning with the patient in the right lateral position.

● **Rectal demonstration of the colon**

Enema with 200–300 ml of a diluted solution of Gastrografin or Urografin 76 % (see below) directly before the examination.

●●●**Instructions for preparing the dilute Gastrografin solution:**

30 ml Gastrografin add 1,000 ml water. In addition, 35 g mannitol can be added to ensure isotonicity. The amount of mannitol to be added depends on the concentration of the Gastrografin solution (Fig. 4-2e). Urografin 76 % can be used instead of Gastrografin.

● **Oral opacification of the colon**

24 hours before the examination, the patient should drink 3 x 2 beakers of freshly prepared diluted Gastrografin swelling agent.

Preparation
Half a teaspoon of Gastrografin and 1 tablespoon of a swelling agent are added to a 250-ml beaker of water and stirred.

Peritoneography (4-24)

The method described by Dunnick (131) is used to assess the intraperitoneal distribution of fluid. In patients with peritoneal carcinosis a contrast medium is added to the dialysis fluid together with the chemotherapeutic agent. The diagnostic value of CT peritoneography is limited and uncertain (156).

Myelography (4-25)

The lumbar puncture is performed with the usual technique. Instillation of metrizamide with an iodine dose of 1.5–3 g (10 ml with 170 mg iodine/ml [fluid-isotonic], 20 ml with 85 mg iodine/ml or 13 ml with 260 mg iodine/ml [125, 657, 659, 661]). Opacification of the fluid spaces to be examined by appropriate repositioning of the patient.

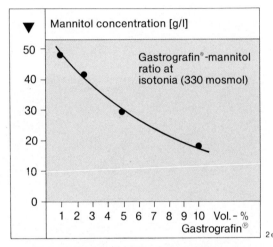

Fig. 4-**2e: Addition of mannitol** (g/l) in relation to the concentration of the Gastrografin solution (% v/v) to obtain an isotonic solution.

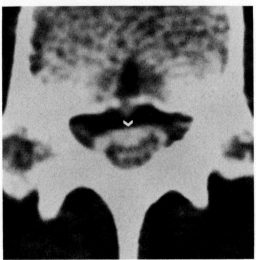

Fig. 4-**2f: Secondary CT myelography.** Demonstration of the subarachnoid space after instillation of metrizamide (>).

Renal contrast media (4-30)

Pharmacokinetics (4-31)

The time-related density above the abdominal aorta provides information about the opacification (enhancement) of the blood following a **bolus injection** of a renal contrast medium. Fig. 4-3a,b shows that the density decreases sharply in the first few minutes. Regardless of the rate of injection, intermixture of the contrast medium with the blood volume can be assumed 1 minute after the injection. The reduction of density decelerates distinctly after 2 minutes.

The radiodensity above the aorta is then determined by redistribution between the tissue spaces and the elimination via the kidneys. The initial increase and decrease of density are subject to haemodynamic factors. With brief injection times, the bolus is distributed centrally in a small volume of blood. Scanning must be commenced when the wave of contrast material reaches the veins of the target organs and is concluded after the wave has passed through the organ. This technique results in distinct opacification of the organ vessels (angio-CT). The following maxim applies for the degree of enhancement: **the shorter the injection time of a certain amount of contrast medium, the higher the – short-lasting – opacification of the organ**, which can be fully demonstrated only by exact timing of the start of scanning. Knowledge of the circulation time and of the time taken for the medium to pass through the arteriovenous system of the organ is of paramount importance for correct timing of the start of scanning (4-32).

This mainly intravascular phase is followed by parenchymatous opacification (Fig. 4-3c), which is brought about by diffusion of the contrast medium into the interstitial space. Enhancement of the blood and organ paren-

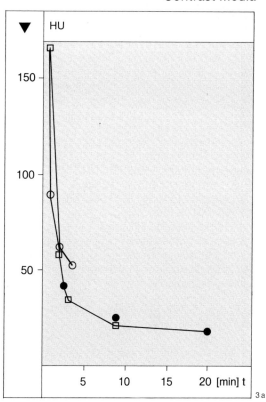

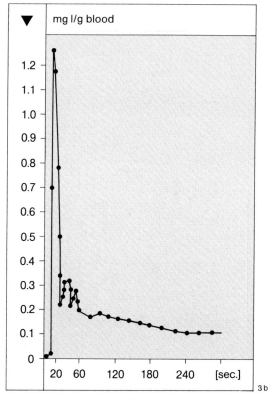

Fig. 4-3a: **Bolus injection.** Enhancement over the abdominal aorta. Results of various authors (□ Fuchs [132], ○ Marchal [475], ● Wegener [161a]).

Fig. 4-3b: **Bolus injection.** Iodine concentration in the external iliac artery following a rapid intravenous bolus injection of 5 ml Angiografin within 1 second. Maximum opacification is achieved after 16 seconds. Two further peaks indicate first and second recirculation.

chyma becomes equal as a result of the distribution processes of the contrast medium. **Infusion** of a renal contrast medium leads to a slow increase of intravascular enhancement, which is accompanied by synonymous but lesser opacification of the parenchyma (e. g. of the liver) (41). The contrast gradient vessel/parenchyma and the maximum enhancement which can be achieved are considerably lower after infusions than after bolus injections. Consequently, the administration technique determines the attainable intravascular and parenchymatous enhancement. Enhancement of at least 50 HU is required – and 60–80 HU is desirable – to achieve unequivocal identification of medium-calibre vessels. An increasing number of authors is aiming at achieving greater opacification for the demonstration of smaller focal parenchymal lesions (60).

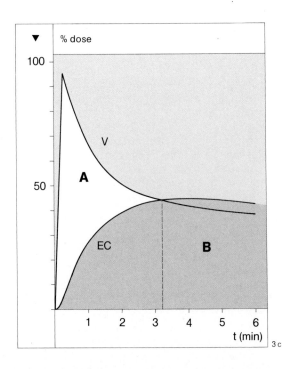

Fig. 4-3 c: **Bolus injection.** Relative distribution of the contrast medium (% dose) in the intravascular space (V) and the easily accessible extracellular space (EC). The concentrations in the two compartments equalize after 3 minutes. Predominantly intravascular (A) opacification can be distinguished from the parenchymatous (B). (Analog computer simulation based on transfer constants obtained experimentally in man using Rayvist 300.)

Fig. 4-3 d: **Infusion.** Enhancement following an even infusion of 250 ml Urovison within 10 minutes. It increases continuously over the kidney, blood and liver, and is most pronounced over the kidney due to accumulation of the contrast material.

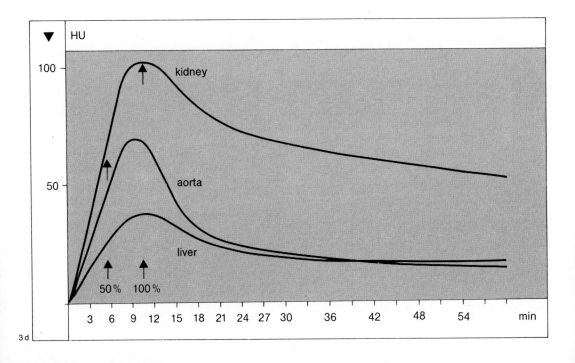

Guided bolus injection (4-32)

To achieve brief examination times with high opacification of the target organ, the volume of the organ is narrowed down, i. e. a limited number of body slices is chosen for guided opacification following a plain scan.

The method inaugurated by Hacker (137) is based on exact timing of the start of scanning following the intravenous bolus injection: scanning is commenced just after the wave of contrast material has passed through the target organ (arteriovenous passage, transit time). The injection time (length of the bolus) must be gauged in such a way that the target organ remains opacified during the scanning process (Fig. 4-3e, f).

This means:

> Time interval between start of injection
> and start of scanning =
> circulation time + arteriovenous transit time

whereby

> injection time =
> arteriovenous transit time + scanning
> (series) time

The scanning series time is the sum of the scanning and interscanning times of a scan series. The time interval between the start of the injection and the start of scanning is also known as the lead time.

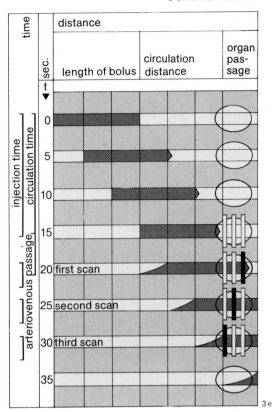

3e

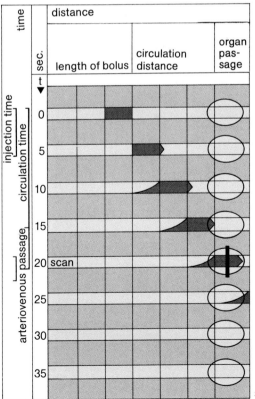

3f

Fig. 4-3 e, f: Time sequence for guided bolus injections.

3e: The injection time of 15 seconds permits a scan series of 3 slices at intervals of 5 seconds during maximum opacification of the organ.

3f: A shorter injection time of 5 seconds permits only one scan during maximum opacification of the organ. Note the asymmetrical spread of the bolus in the blood stream due to passage through the lung and heart, a phenomenon which permits further scans during non-maximum organ opacification.

Circulation time

The circulation time is defined as the time taken for an indicator injected into the blood to pass between two measuring points in the blood stream. In healthy adults at rest, the circulation time from the cubital vein to the central arteries (carotid artery, abdominal aorta) is 13–22 seconds. Optimal opacification can be expected at the time of maximum concentration (peak time Fig. 4-3g). Circulation times are dependent on the cardiac output. Because of a linear relationship between the so-called central blood volume and the stroke volume (141), Schad (157) reports that account can be taken of the influence of the cardiac output by measuring the circulation time in pulse beats (Fig. 4-3h). Determination of the decholin time is still recommended only in frank cardiac insufficiency.

Fig. 4–3g: **Circulation times** [seconds] in a healthy person.

Arm-ear time	
Appearance time	8–12
Peak time	13–22
Recirculation time	15–28
Lung-ear time	3– 5
Decholin time	10–16

Abb. 4–3h: **Circulation times** (t) [seconds] in pulse beats (n).

Arm – right ventricle	4
Arm – left ventricle	11
Arm – thoracic aorta	12
Arm – abdominal aorta	13
Arm – brain	13
Arm – iliac arteries	15
where $t = n \frac{60}{f}$ [seconds]	
f = heart rate [minutes^{-1}]	

Arteriovenous transit time

The arteriovenous transit time is defined as the interval between the time that the maximum contrast medium concentration enters the afferent artery of the organ and the time that it reappears in the efferent vein. The following values are based on circulatory measurements and experience in angiography:

Brain	6– 8 seconds
Kidney	8–12 seconds
Lung	4– 7 seconds
Liver (hepatic artery)	10–15 seconds
Liver (superior mesenteric artery)	15–30 seconds

A mean transit time of 7 seconds can therefore be assumed for the brain (137) and of 10 seconds for abdominal parenchymatous organs. The liver is a special case which is opacified sequentially by the hepatic artery and the branches of the portal vein (71-40).

Scan series time

The method described by Hacker referred initially to a single scan. Very brief scanning times ($\sim$ 2 seconds) permit a scan series during arteriovenous transit. Since, as stain dilution curves have shown, the length (injection time) of the intravenous bolus is extended by 10 seconds in persons with normal circulation because of transit through the lungs and heart, a scan series is frequently advisable to exploit the wave of contrast medium to the full. Moreover, a series of scans is of methodological advantage in that the uncertainty regarding the start of scanning due to varying circulatory times is restricted to the first slice, since the following scans are made during the time that the contrast medium bolus forms a plateau. The scan series time is made up of the scanning time, the number of scans and the minimum time between the scans (interscan time).

Alternatively, several short-lasting bolus injections can be given instead of a scan series, for each of which exact account must be taken of the circulation times (multiple bolus technique).

Contrast media

Sequential computerized tomography

A further development of angio-CT is the performance of a sequence of computed tomograms of the same body slice. As a result of the split mode of individual scanners, it is possible to achieve a rapid slice sequence of 1–2 seconds. The arrival and clearance of the contrast material provide quantitatively functional data about freely selectable regions of the organs (143). The rapid slice sequence permits differentiation of arterial and venous compartments. In sequential computerized tomography there is no need to wait for saturation of the organ with contrast material up to the veins, as suggested by Hacker.

Demonstration of the heart is a special case with regard to sequential computerized tomography. The same bolus injection is used to demonstrate the right ventricle in the first slice and the left ventricle in the next slice (157).

Guided bolus injection with scanning times of 15–20 seconds

Because of the longer scanning times of second generation scanners, bolus injections cannot be exploited to the full. The injection time depends on the scanning time (see above). The scan series time is prolonged by 10 seconds by the need for the patient to recover from holding his breath. In general, adequate opacification can be achieved for 2–3 slices. Opacification is generally poorer than with rapid scanners because of the extended bolus.

Administration technique

- Determination of the scanning region by plain scans.
- Injection of the contrast medium.

Dose: 1 ml Angiografin/kg bodyweight.
Injection time = scan series time (+ 10 seconds for parenchymatous organs).
Maximum rate of injection: 8 ml/second. The total dose is reduced in the case of very short injection times. 30 ml physiological saline solution should then follow at the same injection rate as vis a tergo. The total dose can be increased to 1.5 ml Angiografin/kg bodyweight in the case of longer scanning times

● Scanning Table

Start of scan for	Time after start of injection	
	Seconds	Pulse beats
Right heart	4	4
Left heart	11	11
Thoracic aorta	12	12
Abdominal aorta	13	13
Iliac arteries	15	15
Abdominal organs	20	13+10 sec.
Brain	22	13+ 7 sec.

Controlled bolus injection (4-33)

The object of this technique is to achieve distinct opacification of the intravascular and cardiac space over a period of approx. 3 to a maximum of 5 minutes (310). The controlled bolus injection is particularly suitable for examinations of the heart, in which fairly large sections must be scanned and during which patients with cardiopathies must be given time to relax between the scans. A condition for the use of the controlled bolus injection is immediate image reconstruction after every scan. The density values of the opacified lumen are read off on the monitor and the rate at which the contrast medium is injected is adjusted accordingly. The aim is to enhance the blood space by at least 100 HU. The scanning time should not be much longer than 5 seconds.

Administration technique cf. 62-20.

Reduced bolus injection (4-34)

A small amount of contrast medium is injected intravenously 10–15 minutes before the start of the examination to achieve opacification of the lumen of the urinary bladder. Substratification phenomena in the urinary bladder can be avoided if the patient moves round immediately before the examination or is rotated on the scanning couch.

Dose: 5–10 ml Urovison[1], Angiografin[2] or Rayvist 300[3].

---

[1] sodium diatrizoate and meglumine diatrizoate
[2] meglumine diatrizoate
[3] meglumine ioglicate

Infusions (4-35)

Normal-dose infusion

Since it leads to longer opacification of the organ to be examined, protracted administration of contrast material appears to be ideal for all investigations lasting longer than 3 minutes. As Fig. 4-3d demonstrates, intravascular enhancement increases only slowly under the usual free infusion of 25 ml/min (= 4g iodine/minute) and does not reach a value of 75 HU until after 10 minutes, which leaves 5 to a maximum of 10 minutes for the examination at this level of enhancement. Opacification of the liver and pancreas is distinctly lower. Adequate and long-lasting enhancement resulting from accumulation of the contrast material occurs only over the renal parenchyma, which makes the normal-dose infusion (42g iodine) appear suitable for computerized tomography of the kidney. The infusion rate should be increased if greater initial enhancement is desired (40).

High-dose infusion

If intravascular enhancement (of more than 60 HU) is to be maintained over a longer period of time, a maintenance dose must be administered during the examination itself. The total dose then increases in accordance with the length of the examination.

● Combined technique – bolus infusion

The rate of infusion determines the build-up of the enhancement. Since contrast medium enters the interstitial space even during this early phase and cannot therefore be used for the examination, a combined technique appears to be the most rational – particularly as it also offers the advantage of a speedy examination. The desired intravascular enhancement can be achieved by an intravenous injection of contrast medium within 1–2 minutes, followed by an infusion as a maintenance dose. The rate of infusion (maintenance dose) will depend on the desired level of contrast medium (Fig. 4-3 i, k).

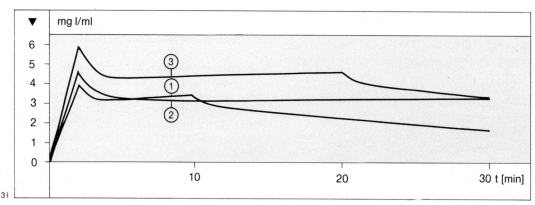

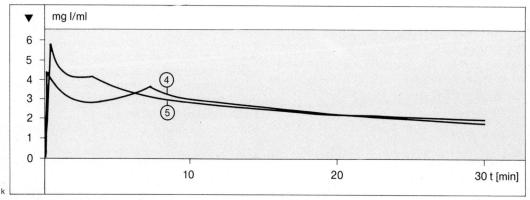

Forms of administration (4-36)

● **Normal-dose infusion**

Infusion of 250 ml Urovison for infusion or Rayvist 180[1] within 10 minutes. Start of scanning after about 7 minutes. Suitable for an examination time of 5–8 minutes.

For examination of the kidney: intravenous infusion of 125 ml Urovison for infusion or Rayvist 180 within 5 minutes. Even infusion of the remaining amount during the scanning process. Suitable for an examination time of up to 20 minutes.

● **High-dose infusion**

Infusion of 100 ml Urografin (= 37 g iodine) within 3–5 minutes. Maintenance dose of 6 ml Urovison/min (2 g iodine/minute).

Start of scanning after 3–5 mins.

Suitable for an examination time of up to 20 minutes.

● **Bolus infusion**

Injection of 80 ml Angiografin or Rayvist 350[2] within 1–2 minutes. Subsequently, infusion of 8 ml Angiografin or Rayvist per minute (2 g iodine/min).

Suitable for an examination time of up to 20 minutes.

Fig. 4-3 i, k: **Biphasic infusion and bolus infusion.** Mode of administration and intravascular iodine level (1 mg I/ml corresponds to 20–25 HU, cf. Fig. 4-2a). Desirable blood level during the examination: 3 and 4 mg I/ml (study by Schering AG West Germany, anologue computer simulation).

3 i: Biphasic infusion with rapid infusion for 2 minutes and even infusion of the remaining amount (with a total predetermined dose of 42 g I [e.g. Rayvist 300] and 75 g I [e.g. Urografin]).
① 75 % of the dose ($\triangleq$ 31 g I) within 2 minutes.
   25 % of the dose ($\triangleq$ 11 g I) within 8 minutes.
② 40 % of the dose ($\triangleq$ 30 g I) within 2 minutes.
   60 % of the dose ($\triangleq$ 45 g I) within 35 minutes.
③ 60 % of the dose ($\triangleq$ 45 g I) within 2 minutes.
   40 % of the dose ($\triangleq$ 30 g I) within 18 minutes.

3 k: Bolus infusion with a bolus injection within 12/24 seconds and even infusion of the remaining amount with a total predetermined dose of 42 g iodine.
④ 60 % of the dose ($\triangleq$ 25 g I) within 12 seconds.
   40 % of the dose ($\triangleq$ 17 g I) within 7 minutes.
⑤ 80 % of the dose ($\triangleq$ 33 g I) within 24 seconds.
   20 % of the dose ($\triangleq$ 9 g I) within 3 minutes.

---

[1] meglumine ioglicate
[2] meglumine ioglicate and sodium ioglicate

Biliary contrast media (4-40)

Biliary contrast media are taken up by the liver cells and transferred to the biliary tract by means of active transport mechanisms. The opacification above the liver tissue, which can be measured by computerized tomography, is therefore based on the one hand on intracellular accumulation and the content of contrast material in the bile ducts and, on the other, on the level of contrast material in the blood and interstitial space. Maximum enhancement is achieved by infusion or slow intravenous injection after 30–60 minutes (142, 132) but, at 10–15 HU, is still inadequate. Neither increasing the dose nor a combination with urographic agents can increase it any further. At the present time, therefore, biliary contrast media are employed only in special cases to demonstrate the efferent bile ducts.

Mode of administration

30 ml Biliscopin[3] by slow ($\geq$ 5 minutes) i.v. injection (iodine dose 5.4 g) or 100 ml by infusion (iodine dose 5.0 g).

Rapid bolus injections may not be used because of severe side effects.

Pathophysiological correlate (4-50)

As explained above, two different phases separated in time occur following injection of a urographic agent: predominantly intravascular and predominantly parenchymal opacification (Fig. 4-3c).

Angiographic criteria can be employed for **intravascular opacification**. The capillary bed is depicted in the angiographic parenchymal phase, which can be demonstrated with brief scanning times during the first passage of the contrast material. Areas of tissue displaying greater vascularity than the normal parenchyma of the organ are described as **hypervascular**. They can be present as:

1. Vascular neogenesis within neoplasms and
2. vascular dilation and invasion in inflammatory (granulation tissue) and absorptive processes (e. g. haematoma encapsulation).

During the phase of intravascular opacification, hypervascularized regions are depicted as **hyperdense** zones. Since certain kinds of tumour tend towards hypervascularization, the degree of vascularity can be (roughly) estimated via the increase of density and employed in the differential diagnosis.

---

[3] meglumine iotroxinate

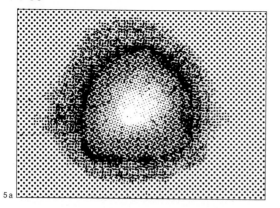

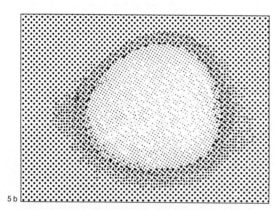

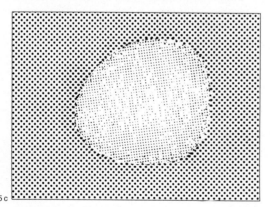

Areas of tissue displaying less vascularity than the surrounding organ parenchyma are described as **hypovascular**. They display less opacification than the surrounding parenchyma in the computed tomogram, i. e. they become **hypodense**.

Avascular areas do not participate in enhancement. They correspond with fluid-filled spaces (cysts, abscesses, haematomas etc.) and dead solid tissue (necrosis). Their demonstrability, which is determined by the plain contrast with the surrounding organ tissue, can be improved depending on the amount of contrast material.

Since regressive changes in the centre of a tumour lead to reduced perfusion, i. e. to hypodensity, tumour-induced hyperdensity can appear in a ring shape (Fig. 4-5a). Hyperdense zones due to granulation tissue can be recognized by the fact that they are situated primarily on (demarcating) boundary surfaces. The abscess membrane, the granulation tissue around a haematoma and absorptive surfaces in cavities of the body usually delimit avascular spaces, which do not participate in enhancement (Fig. 4-5b). The absence of (hyperdense) granulation tissue around cystic formations indicates an epithelialized cyst rather than an inflammatory haemorrhagic process (Fig. 4-5c). The dual (arterial and portal) vascularization of the liver is a special issue, since it creates special phases of opacification (71-40).

In the later phase of (predominantly) **parenchymal** opacification, which leads to assimilation of the intravascular and interstitial concentration of contrast medium, the degree of vascularity – although less pronounced – remains the yardstick for the enhancement (Fig. 4-5d, e). This basic pattern of opacification with its dependence on the degree of vascularity is superordinated in a complex manner by the varying diffusion capacity of the contrast medium in the interstitial spaces of normal and pathological tissue. In the case of parenchymal opacification, hyperdense areas are demonstrated only in exceptional cases.

Fig. 4-5 a–c: In predominantly **intravascular opacification,** hypervascularized regions appear hyperdense in the computed tomogram.

5 a: The peripheral parts of a hypervascular tumour frequently receive a greater supply of blood. The computed tomogram then reveals a ring shape, the enhancement in the centre of the tumour being determined by its vascularity.

5 b: Depending on the amount present, inflammatory granulation tissue, e.g. in an abscess, can likewise lead to ring-shaped hyperdense zones, the central regions of which do not participate in enhancement due to liquefaction. The hypodense zone displays sharp contours on development of an abscess membrane.

5 c: Missing hyperdense zones are the expression of a non-reactive process (e.g. in the vicinity of a benign cyst).

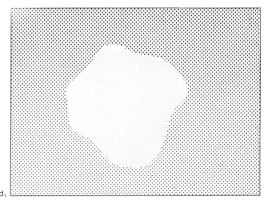
5d₁

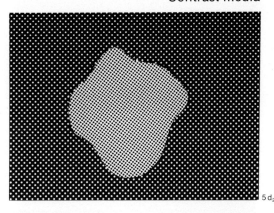
5d₂

5e₁

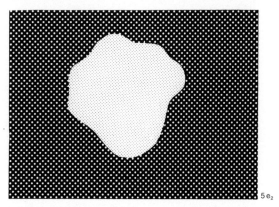
5e₂

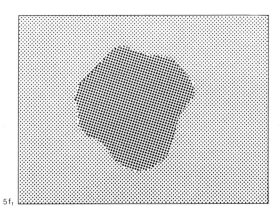
5f₁

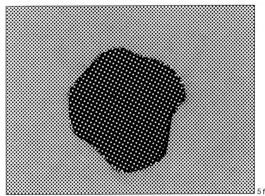
5f₂

Fig. 4-5 d–f: In **parenchymatous opacification,** the contrast medium has largely permeated the interstitial space in a uniform manner. In this phase, too, the enhancement of a lesion is determined predominantly by the degree of vascularity.

5 d: The density gradient increases if the vascularity of the lesion is less pronounced than that of the vicinity. A hypervascular lesion can disappear, i.e. become isodense, in the computed tomogram.

5 e: Hypovasuclar regions hardly participate in enhancement, which makes them stand out clearly from the opacified parenchyma.

5 f: In the brain, contrast medium does not diffuse into the interstitial space because of the blood-fluid barrier. If this barrier is broken down as a result of a pathological process, the contrast medium penetrates into the lesion, giving rise to a hyperdense zone. Note the varying pathophysiological basis for the development of hyperdense zones (Fig. 4-5a).

Indications for whole body computerized tomography (5-00)

	Detection	Evaluation (confirmation)	Differentiation	Localization, extent, infiltration	Guided biopsy	Preceding diagnostic procedures
Orbit						
Neoplasm	●	●	●	●		
Inflammation (incl. pseudotumours)	●	●	●	●		
Vascular malformation	●		●	●		
Trauma		●		●		R
Foreign bodies	●					R
ENT						
Neoplasm		○	○	●		R, To
Inflammation			○	●		R, To
Neck						
Neoplasm				●		
Foreign bodies				●		R
Retropharyngeal abscess		●		●		R
Mediastinum						
Neoplasm: primary	●	●	●	●	○	R, To
secondary	●			●	○	R, To
Hilar lymph nodes				●		To
Vessels:						
Anomalies	○	●				R
Aneurysm		●	●	●		R, US
Ectasia		●	●			To
Lipomatosis			●			R
Lung						
Neoplasm: primary	●			●		R, To
postpneumonectomy	●					R
secondary	●			●		R
Granuloma (tuberculoma)			●			R, To
Chest Wall						
Neoplasm				●	○	
Heart						
Vein graft occlusion	●					
Cardiac aneurysm		○				R, US
Cardiac vs. pericardiac processes			●			
Pericardial effusion	○		●	○		US
Liver						
Neoplasm: primary	●	●	●	●	○	US, RN
secondary	●	●	●	●	○	US, RN
Trauma	●	●		●		(US, RN)
Abscess	●	●	●	●	○	US, RN
Diffuse liver disease					○	US, RN
Fatty infiltration	●	●		●		(US, RN)
Haemochromatosis	●	●				
Glycogen storage disease	○					
Biliary Tree						
Obstructive vs. non-obstructive disease		●	●			US
Site of obstruction	●					US
Spleen						
Neoplasm	●	●	●			US, RN
Trauma	●	●		●		US
Abscess	●	●	●	●		US
Pancreas						
Neoplasm	●	●	●	●	○	(US)
Inflammation	●	●	●	●		US
Pseudocyst	●	●	●	●		US
Abscess	●	●	●	●		US

Indications for whole body computerized tomography

	Detection	Evaluation (confirmation)	Differentiation	Localization, extent, infiltration	Guided biopsy	Preceding diagnostic procedures
Kidneys (incl. perirenal space)						
Neoplasm: solid	●	●	●	●		UR, US
cystic	●	●	●	●		UR, US
Agenesia, aplasia	●	●				UR, (US)
Calculi	○	○				UR, US
Hydronephrosis	●	●		●		UR, US
Trauma		●		●		UR, US
Abscess	●	●	●	●		UR, US
Diffuse renal disease					○	US
Adrenal Gland						
Neoplasm	●	●	●	○		(US)
Hyperplasia	●	●	●			
Insufficiency	●					
Uterus, Ovaries						
Neoplasm		●	●	●	○	US
Inflammation		○	●	●		
Bladder, Prostate, Seminal Vesicles						
Neoplasm		○		●	○	
Retroperitoneum						
Neoplasm: primary	●	●	●	●	○	US
secondary	●	●		●		US

	Detection	Evaluation (confirmation)	Differentiation	Localization, extent, infiltration	Guided biopsy	Preceding diagnostic procedures
Vessels (aneurysm)	●	●	●	●		US
Trauma	●	●	●	●		US
Abscess	●	●	●	●	○	US
Peritoneum						
Fluid collections	●		●	●		US
Abscess	●	●		●		US
Neoplasm	○			○	○	US
Spine						
Spinal stenosis	●	●		●		R
Dysraphic abnormalities		●		●		R
Paraspinal neoplasm				●		R
Trauma (fragments)	○			●		R
Paraspinal inflammation				●		R
Herniation of nucleus pulposus	○			○		R
Muscle, Skeletal System						
Bone neoplasm: primary		○		●	○	R, To
secondary	●			●		R, RN, To
Joint abnormalities		○				R
Soft tissue neoplasm	○	●	●	●	○	

Indications (●) for whole body computerized tomography under consideration of the proposals of the Society for Computed Body Tomography (AJR 133 [1979] 115–119).
○ = rare indication

R = Standard radiographs
US = Ultrasound
UR = Urography
RN = Radionuclids
To = Conventional tomography

Cranium, neck (50-00)

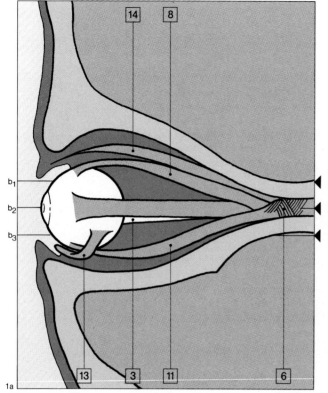
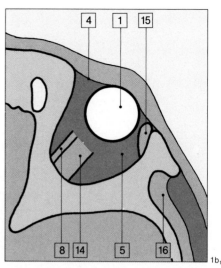
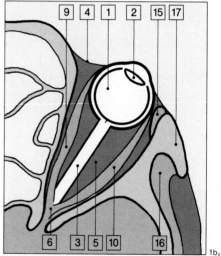
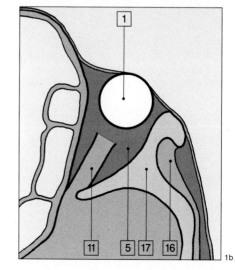

Fig. 51-**1a,b: Anatomy of the orbit.** In horizontal sections (b).

Key
1 Ocular bulb
2 Lens
3 Optic nerve
4 Orbital septum
5 Adipose body of the orbit
6 Common tendinous arch
7 Intermuscular membrane
8 M. rectus superior
9 M. rectus medialis
10 M. rectus lateralis
11 M. rectus inferior
12 M. obliquus superior
13 M. obliquus inferior
14 M. levator palpebrae
15 Lacrimal gland
16 Temporal muscle
17 Wing of the sphenoid

Orbit (51-00)

Anatomy and imaging (51-10)

The orbit, which is about 35 mm high, 40 mm wide and 40 mm deep in the adult, is formed by various bones of the base of the skull. The pyramidal cavity converges on the optic canal. The **musculi recti** originate at a common tendinous ring surrounding the optic nerve in the optic foramen, run forwards in a straight line and insert in front of the maximum circumference of the eyeball in the sclera. The **musculus obliquus superior** lies above the musculus rectus medialis, passes above the osseous trochlea and connects with the sclera at the posterosuperior surface of the eyeball. The **musculus obliquus inferior** originates at the medial wall of the orbit, crosses below the ocular insertion surface of the musculus rectus inferior and radiates laterodorsally into the sclera. The musculi recti are connected in the anterior orbit by an **intermuscular membrane,** the cranial parts of which are more pronounced (Fig. 51-1f). This membrane is usually no longer present in the tip of the orbit, in which the muscles converge. It divides the orbital fatty tissue, which displays varying consistency, into a central and a peripheral section. The orbit is closed ventrally by the **orbital septum.** The orbital septum also covers the **lacrimal gland,** which lies directly against the osseous orbit in the upper, outer angle. The intraorbital diameter of the **optic nerve** measures 3–4 mm. With indifferent gaze position, the optic nerve meanders slightly in a craniocaudal direction. It deviates from its central position depending on the gaze shift, the deviation being particularly pronounced directly retrobulbar.

● **CT**

Demonstration of the orbital structures in the computed tomogram depends on the technique employed. The customary method is to try to lay the CT slices parallel to the **neuroocular plane** (NOP), which is formed by the lens, the papilla and the optic canal with the eye in an indifferent gaze position. It runs almost parallel to **Reid's** base-line or the **infraorbitomeatal line** (OML) (Fig. 51-1c). This projection permits clear and reproducible demonstration of the optic nerve, the musculi recti and the maximum circumference of the eyeball. However, the craniocaudal tortuosity of the optic nerve can simulate alterations of the calibre due to partial volume effects. With

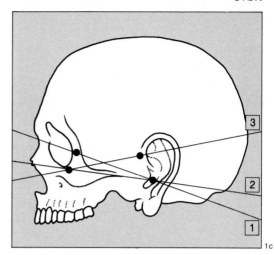

Fig. 51-1c: Horizontal planes and their fixed external points.
1. Orbitomeatal line: lateral canthus – middle of the external auditory meatus.
2. Infraorbitomeatal line (Reid's line, Frankfurt-Virchow line) –10° to the orbitomeatal line: lower orbital margin – upper limit of the external auditory meatus.
3. –20° to the orbitomeatal line (after Unsöld [213]): lower margin of the orbit – upper insertion of the auricle.

Fig. 51-1d: Course of the optic nerve. The nerve meanders when the gaze is neutral, but straightens out when the gaze is lifted by 40°. The stretched nerve is then intercepted by a slice projection of –10° to the Reid's line without any apparent fluctuations of calibre.

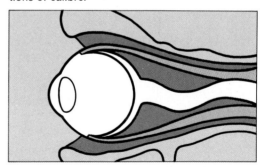

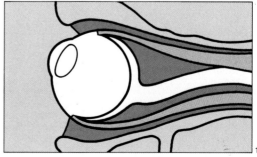

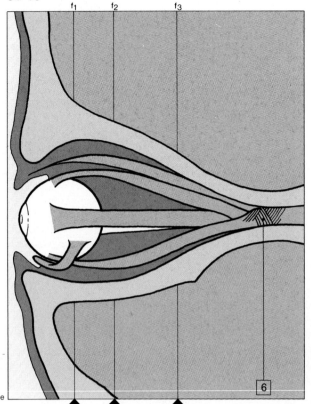
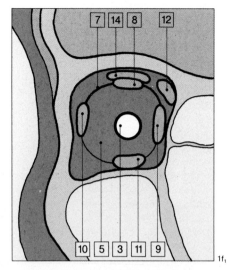
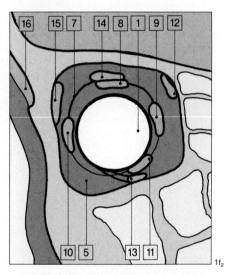
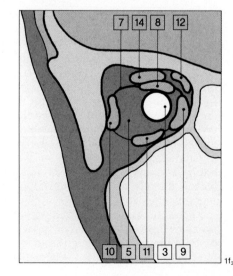

Fig. 51-1e–g: **Anatomy of the orbit** in coronal slices.

Key
1 Ocular bulb
2 Lens
3 Optic nerve
4 Orbital septum
5 Adipose body of the orbit
6 Common tendinous arch
7 Intermuscular membrane
8 M. rectus superior
9 M. rectus medialis
10 M. rectus lateralis
11 M. rectus inferior
12 M. obliquus superior
13 M. obliquus inferior
14 M. levator palpebrae
15 Lacrimal gland
16 Temporal muscle
17 Wing of the sphenoid

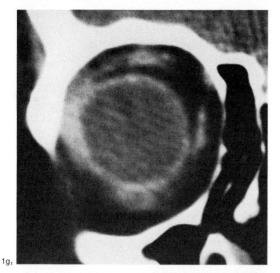

1g₁

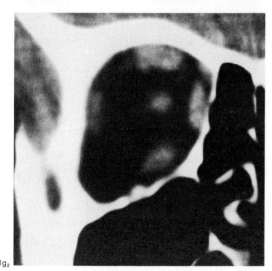

1g₂

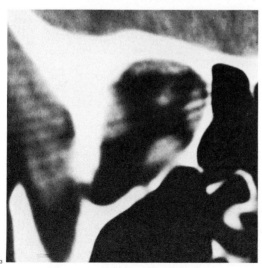

1g₃

slice thicknesses of 5–8 mm in the horizontal projection, the musculi recti superior and inferior are clearly demarcated only retroocularly. The **musculus levator palpebrae** cannot be separated from the musculus rectus superior. On the other hand, if a specific search is made it is frequently possible to demonstrate a superior **ophthalmic vein** of normal width, which runs between the optic nerve and the musculus rectus superior. A **lacrimal gland** of normal size cannot always be unequivocally identified because of overshadowing by soft tissues of the upper eyelid and the osseous curvature of the orbital angle, while the sclera, lens and vitreous body of the eyeball always stand out clearly. The individual structures can be differentiated better and more sharply if thin slices of 2–5 mm are used, since partial volume effects in horizontal fissures are avoided. The technique demands exact alignment of the sectional planes (e. g. with the neuroocular plane) in order to avoid apparent fluctuations of calibre of the optic nerve due to partial volume effects. Because of this, it has been suggested that the examination should be carried out in upgaze or downgaze position, since this leads to stretching of the nerve. Depending on the line of fixation, the sectional plane must then be angled by 10° in relation to Reid's base line (Fig. 51-1d).

Coronal slices: a vertical projection into the infraorbitomeatal line is desirable. This is usually only possible with a tiltable gantry, since retroflection of the head is subject to physiological (age-related) limitations. In practice, therefore, it is frequently only possible to achieve projections at an angle of 50–70° to the infraorbitomeatal line. If the technique is perfect, the optic nerve and the retroocular muscles run almost vertically through the CT slice. The musculi obliquus inferior and superior are usually clearly identifiable. Since these retrobulbar structures completely fill the slice thickness, the density measurement is more reliable than in horizontal computed tomograms and is also reproducible. **Multiplanar reconstruction** is another way of obtaining frontal computed tomograms (cf. **secondary slices** [97-00]). Any sectional planes at all can be composed (interpolated) in a single series of adjacent scans if very thin slice thicknesses and small picture elements (small volume elements) are chosen.

Histology	%	of these primary (%)	of these secondary (%)
Vascularised tumours	12		
Haemangiomas		8.1	
Haemangiopericytomas		1.7	
Reticuloendothelial tumours	10		
Malignant lymphomas		3.6	4.7
Carcinomas	28	3.2	24.9
Pseudotumours (inflammatory)	8		
Meningeomas	7	3.0	3.8
Cystic tumours	5		
Dermoid cysts			
Epidermoids		2.8	
Mucoceles			1.5
Malignant melanoma	5	0.4	4.0
Neural tumours	5		
Neurofibromatosis		2.1	
Neurolemmoma		1.3	
Neurofibroma		0.8	
Mixed tumours	5		
malignant		1.5	1.0
benign		1.9	
Neuroglial tumours	4		
Optic nerve glioma		3	
Retinoblastoma			1.3
Mesenchymal tumours			
Fibroma, Fibrosarcoma etc.	3		
Fibrous dysplasia	1		
Osteoma, Osteosarcoma etc.	2		2
Rhabdomyosarcoma	2	1	1
Lipoma, Liposarcoma	1		

Fig. 51-3a: **Tumours of the orbit.** Distribution of 465 orbital tumours from a study by Henderson (20).

Examination technique (51-20)

● **Preparation of the patient** is unnecessary.

● **Scanning**
With slice thicknesses of 5 – (max.) 8 mm and an adjacent slice sequence.

Horizontal slices
a) Parallel to the infraorbitomeatal line.
b) At an angle of –10° to the infraorbitomeatal line with the patient's gaze fixed upwards (40°) for demonstrating the optic nerve.

Coronal slices
Hyperreflection of the head with the patient in the abdominal or dorsal position. Appropriate tilting of the gantry so that the projection is about vertical (at least 60°) to the infraorbitomeatal line.

First slice: 1 cm dorsally of the root of the nose.

● **Intravenous contrast medium administration** (facultative)
As an infusion (4-36) or as the guided bolus technique (4-32).

Tumours of the orbit (51-30)

A study by Henderson (Fig. 51-3a) of 465 orbital masses which included primary and secondary tumours as well as pseudotumours produced the following findings: the largest group, accounting for 25% of cases, comprises of metastatic carcinomas or carcinomas invading the orbit directly. Primary neoplasias display a broad histological spectrum. Only haemangiomas, which account for 8% of cases, occur as a homogenous subgroup. According to recent statistical studies, pseudotumours appear to occur more frequently than was assumed in the era before computerized tomography. The incidence of orbital tumours reported by Henderson is 0.43‰ of the registered patients of the Mayo clinic.

For reasons of expediency, orbital masses are subdivided into tumours situated predominantly within **(intraconal)** and outside **(extraconal)** the cone of the extraocular muscles.

Intraconal tumours (51-40)

Intraconal tumours are defined as masses situated within the cone of the extraocular muscles.

Haemangiomas (51-41)

Haemangiomas are the most frequent benign orbital tumours. In childhood they consist of primitive endothelial cords (hypertrophic haemangiomas) without a blood-filled cavity system, which develops increasingly in adults. Haemangiomas, which are usually cavernous, are subject to regressive changes (sclerosis, thrombosis, fibrosis) which lead to obliteration of the blood spaces. Damage to the optic nerve can result from displacement by growth.

● **CT**
The computed tomogram reveals a well delineated mass which displaces the optic nerve and which can usually be demarcated from the latter by thin coronal sections. Enhancement following contrast medium administration, although depending on the state of development of the blood spaces (see above), is usually distinctly demonstrable (218).

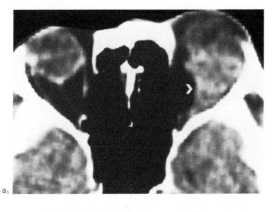
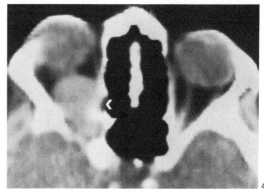
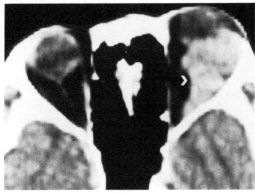

Fig. 51-4 a, b: Haemangiomas.

4 a: Multilobate mass right which does not fill the tip of the orbit and displays distinct enhancement of 37 HU after administration of contrast medium (a_2).

Fig. 51-4 c–e: Tumours of the optic nerve.

4 c: Glioma of the optic nerve. Spindle-shaped enlargement retrobulbar in the region of the optic nerve with dilation of the tip of the orbit including the optic canal.

4 d: Meningeoma of the optic nerve sheath with calcifications in the region of the optic sheath (>). No enlargement of the optic nerve is visible in this slice.

4 b: Sharply delineated, smooth-bordered mass right retrobulbar-intraconal, slightly hyperdense in comparison to the cerebral tissue.

4 e: Recurrence of a glioma of the optic nerve. The left orbit is virtually filled with tumour tissue which has completely eroded the orbital fatty tissue.

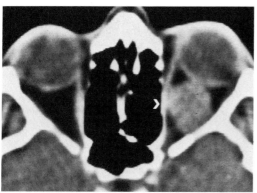
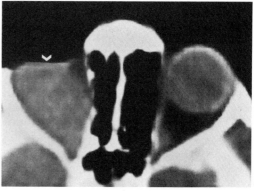

Tumours of the optic nerve (51-42)

Gliomas of the optic nerve occur – sometimes bilaterally – in more than 75% of cases in the first 10 years of life (187) and are associated with Recklinghausen's disease in 10–50% of cases. The incidence of the meningeoma of the optic nerve is about the same. The histology is similar to that of the intracranial meningeoma, which calcifies typically (psammoma bodies) and which differs from the glioma in its clinical course. Exophthalmos is rare in meningeoma and glioma (194).

● CT

The computed tomogram usually reveals generalized expansion or sharply contoured spindle-shaped enlargement of the optic nerve, which cannot usually be demarcated within the mass. However, its structure can sometimes be recognized in cases of Recklinghausen's disease when thin slices are used. While contrast medium enhancement of gliomas is very moderate (187), it is pronounced in meningeomas. Since the intracranial extent of both tumours can be considerable, a positive finding in the orbit necessitates detailed investigation of the optic canal, the chiasm and geniculate bodies.

Neurinomas (51-43)

Neurinomas, which result from diffuse proliferation of the Schwann's cells, likewise frequently occur in association with Recklinghausen's disease.

● CT

In the computed tomogram, neurinomas lead to a lobulated mass around the optic nerve with relatively sharp demarcation from the surrounding fatty tissue. Marked enhancement following contrast medium administration has been described (197).

Malignant lymphomas (51-44)

Malignant lymphomas, which account for 7–15% of neoplasias (57), are encountered relatively frequently in the orbit. Since lymphatic tissue is restricted to the subconjunctival area and around the lacrimal glands, lymphocytic forms are found in front of the orbital septum and reticulocytic forms, which display good vascularity in the angiogram, in the retrobulbar space (57).

● CT

Malignant lymphomas give a structurally homogenous appearance in the computed tomogram. They are usually asymmetrically situated, circumscribed soft tissue masses which surround or displace the optic nerve and which can mask the extraocular muscles (198, 209). Isolated leukaemic infiltration of the optic nerves leading to diffuse, smoothly bordered expansion of one or both optic nerves has been reported (212).

Other malignant intraconal tumours (51-45)

Primary malignant tumours, e.g. carcinomas, sarcomas, spindle-cell and round-cell sarcomas in adulthood and rhabdomyosarcomas and neuroblastomas in childhood, are rare.

Secondary malignant tumours are usually haematogenous metastases from tumours of the breast, kidney, prostate, uterus, thyroid, pancreas and lung.

● CT

Computerized tomography reveals solitary or multiple masses which initially leave the optic nerve and eyeball intact, thus permitting demarcation of the structures. Unless bone destruction is present, they cannot be distinguished at this stage from benign masses. Diffuse opacification of the retrobulbar fatty tissue – without protrusion of the bulb – has been reported in metastatic mammary carcinoma (209). Enophthalmos can develop in basal cell carcinoma (194). Multiplicity of the round foci is an indication of metastases. In sarcomas of childhood with aggressive growth (rhabdomyosarcoma) and in neuroblastomas, frequently the only use of computerized tomography is to determine the extent of tumour growth for palliative therapy.

Retinoblastoma, melanoma (51-46)

Progressive retinoblastomas and melanomas of the ocular bulb can invade the retrobulbar space. The extent of the tumours can be accurately determined by computerized tomography. Retinoblastomas display marked enhancement following administration of contrast medium (187), while melanomas are hyperdense even in the plain scan (218).

Extraconal tumours (51-50)

Extraconal tumours are defined as masses arising from the structures surrounding the orbit and from the lacrimal gland.

Meningeomas (51-51)

Meningeomas are the commonest type of extraconal tumour and originate mainly from the large sphenoid bone and less frequently from the tubercle of sella turcica or the olfactory

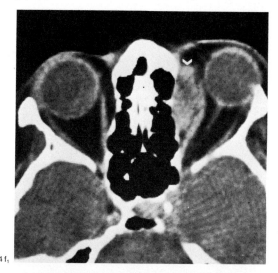

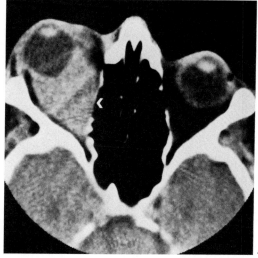

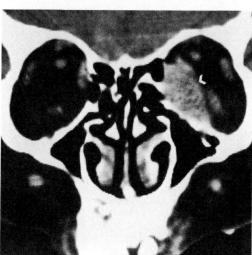

Fig. 51-**4 f–i: Malignant lymphomas.**

4 f: The medial lesion can be demarcated from the medial extraocular muscles and the almost exclusively extraconal location determined both in the horizontal (f_1) and frontal (f_2) slice.

4 g: Similarly homogeneous structure of a lateral malignant lymphoma (polymorphic immunocytoma) situated within and outside the muscle cone and masking (probably infiltrating) the musculus rectus lateralis.

4 h: A mainly intraconal malignant lymphoma with enlargement of the muscle cone extending into the tip of the orbit. Again homogeneous tissue density.

4 i: Plasmocytoma with infiltration of the retrobulbar fatty tissue and destruction of the osseous orbit (>).

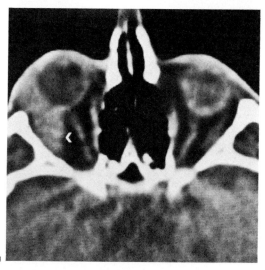

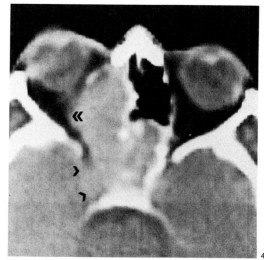

sulcus. Histologically they are surrounded by a fibrous capsule, frequently display calcification and occasionally undergo cystic degeneration.

● **CT**

The appearance in the computed tomogram is marked by signs of displacement (musculus rectus lateralis bulbi in the case of a sphenoid meningeoma) and by thickening and sclerosis of the bone concerned. The typical detailed structure of the bone in the tabula externa and interna is also obliterated. The intracranial, temporal and orbital extents of the tumour can be determined simultaneously. Following contrast medium administration, meningeomas display marked enhancement which provides excellent demarcation of the tumour from surrounding soft tissue, including the brain.

Tumours of the lacrimal gland (51-52)

The histology of lacrimal gland tumours is pleomorphic. More than half of them are benign mixed tumours (pleomorphic adenomas), while the carcinomas are just as varied (cystadenoid carcinoma, pleomorphic carcinoma, mucoepidermic carcinoma etc.). Even the benign mixed tumours can infiltrate the bones of the fovea lacrimalis (218).

● **CT**

A mass in the upper external quadrant is regarded as a typical but non-specific CT sign of a lacrimal gland tumour. Since benign neoplasms also tend to erode bone, it is not always possible to distinguish them from malignant ones. As the tumour grows it also invades intraconal structures. Not infrequently, the lacrimal gland is also the site of origin of a malignant lymphoma or pseudotumour (51-44, 51-64). Dacryoadenitis must be considered if the lacrimal gland enlargement is bilateral (51-63).

Periorbital malignant tumours (51-53)

On progression, both bone metastases from the base of the skull and paranasal malignant tumours, which originate most commonly from the maxilloethmoidal angle, invade the orbit.

● **CT**

Computerized tomography can demonstrate periorbital neoplasias, their expansion into the orbit and signs of displacement of intraorbital structures. In particular, it can aid the planning of therapy by revealing the distance remaining between the tumour and the optic nerve or whether the latter has already been invaded.

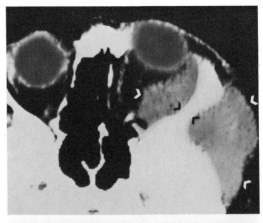

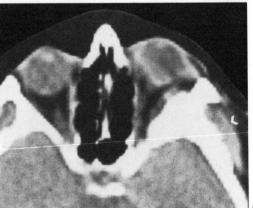

Fig. 51-**5a–c: Meningeomas.**

5a: Meningeoma of the right wing of the sphenoid, which is distinctly thickened (><). The dense tumour tissue extends into both the right orbit and the temporal fossa (>).

5b: Meningeoma of the sphenoid with slight constriction of the orbit right and enlargement of the major wing of the sphenoid. The soft-tissue component is less pronounced than in 5a.

5c: Recurrence of a sphenoid meningeoma. In addition to the thickened wing of the sphenoid, demonstration of tumour tissue right in the temporal fossa and retrobulbar.

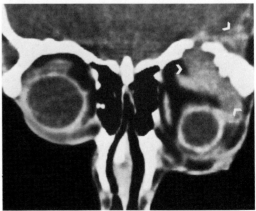

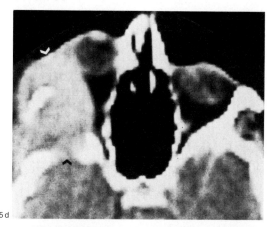

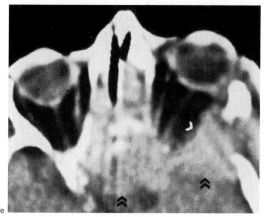

Fig. 51-**5d, e: Periorbital malignant tumours.**

5d: Metastasis from a liver cell carcinoma. Destruction of the major wing of the sphenoid. The tumour mass is sharply demarcated and displaces the bulb.

5e: Metastastic cancer of the breast with destruction of the entire osseous orbital infundibulum. The density of the tumour tissue (≫) differs from that of the brain.

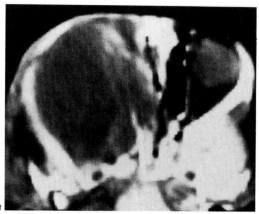

Dermoid cysts (51-54)

Dermoid cysts, which usually contain sebaceous material, are frequently sited in the fovea lacrimalis or at the roof of the orbit. They are congenital and do not become clinically manifest until later in life when they enlarge and begin to displace other structures. Involvement of the adjacent bone is usual.

● **CT**

Computerized tomography demonstrates a smoothly bordered, round mass in the upper external quadrant of the orbit or at the roof of the orbit. The density values vary depending on the composition of the tissue. Although soft tissue density can be measured in mainly solid tissue (197), the sebaceous or lipoid content usually reduces the density values well down into the negative range (204, 209). The diagnosis can be made fairly safely on the basis of the localization and density value, although herniation of retrobulbar fatty tissue (usually classified as a lipoma [209]), must be considered in the differential diagnosis.

Fibromas (51-55)

Like dermoid cysts, fibromas are also congenital, and are located in the region of the bony orbital structures, usually at the roof of the orbit.

● **CT**

Fibromas stand out in the computed tomogram from other orbital structures as sharply demarcated masses and are frequently best demonstrated by the coronal slice technique. They usually display distinct enhancement following contrast medium administration.

Neurofibromas (51-56)

The plexiform neurofibroma frequently occurs together with dysplasia of the large sphenoid bone. It appears as either a circumscribed or diffuse mass of soft tissue density which can be situated inside and outside the muscle cone.

Fig. 51-**5f: Recklinghausen's disease.** Extensive mass with deformation of the left visceral cranium. The orbit can no longer be demonstrated on the right. The mass displays cystic components.

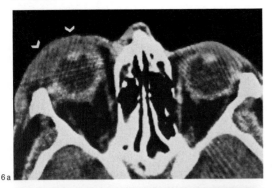

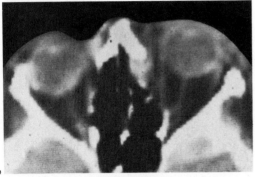

Fig. 51-**6a, b: Exudative lesions.**

6a: Phlegmonous inflammation of the left eye, but mainly in front of the orbital septum.

6b: Autopsy-confirmed orbital phlegmon right with moderate exophthalmus. In neither case (a, b) is the density value of the retrobulbar fatty tissue increased to any significant extent.

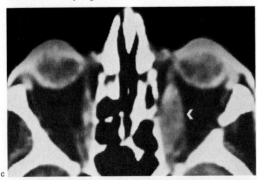

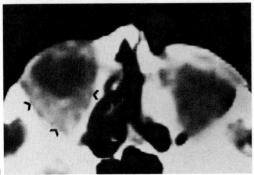

Inflammations (51-60)

Acute inflammations of the retrobulbar space (51-61)

In the majority of cases, acute inflammations invade the orbit from the paranasal sinus and lead to phlegmonous invasion of the retrobulbar fatty tissue.

Paranasal inflammation (particularly ethmoiditis) first of all invades the orbital tissue adjacent to the sinus. Expanding **phlegmon** later leads to an increase of density of the entire fatty body with consecutive masking of the retrobulbar structures. In rare cases, acute – usually infectious – **dacryocystitis** spreads from the nasal canthus to the retrobulbar space (197).

Granulomatous changes (51-62)

Granulomatous inflammation can occur outside the muscle cone, involve the extraocular muscles themselves or invade the retrobulbar fatty tissue. The main etiological possibilities are sarcoidosis, histiocytosis and Wegener's granulomatosis (51-64).

● **CT**

Computerized tomography reveals thickening of individual muscles (usually in sarcoidosis) and partial or total obliteration of the fatty tissue with exophthalmos (197).

Dacryoadenitis (51-63)

Bilateral dacryoadenitis is found mainly in the Sjögren and Mikulicz syndromes. Unilateral acute inflammations of the lacrimal gland are usually caused by infection (viral, bacterial) (cf. Pseudotumours 51-64).

● **CT**

Computerized tomography reveals a distinctly enlarged lacrimal gland which stands out sharply from the orbital structures. Bilateralism suggests the Sjögren or Mikulicz syndrome, both of which display only slight enhancement following administration of contrast medium (196). Exophthalmos depends on the extent of the increase of volume of the lacrimal gland tissue. Differential diagnosis is usually aided by the clinical picture.

(Idiopathic) pseudotumours (51-64)

Pseudotumours represent an important group of primary orbital masses (Fig. 51-3a). They

Fig. 51-**6c: (Non-exocrine) ocular myositis** (>) which regressed within 6 weeks under cortisone therapy.

may be the expression of a systemic disease (Wegener's granulomatosis, xanthogranuloma, collagenosis and sarcoidosis) or the result of an intraorbital foreign body. The term pseudotumours is used in its narrower sense in numerous cases in which the cause cannot be clarified (idiopathic pseudotumours [68]). Histological and topographical aspects permit differentiation between lymphoid, plasma cell-containing and sclerosing forms on the one hand and disturbances involving primarily the muscles, lacrimal glands and vessels on the other. Pseudotumours accompanied by acute signs of inflammation of the eyelid, conjunctiva or lacrimal gland are marked by a relatively acute clinical onset in patients aged 30–80 years. The complaints disappear again after 2–3 months, and it is this acute aspect which distinguishes the pseudotumour from the more insidious course of a neoplastic mass. The majority of authors are agreed that unilateral occurrence is the rule (68, 197, 193). In general, idiopathic pseudotumours can only be diagnosed by an exclusion process.

● CT

Computerized tomography can discriminate between myositic and non-myositic forms. The former stand out in the computed tomogram as enlargement of individual sections of muscle, although diffuse involvement of all muscles is also possible. The boundaries of the relatively dense, partly lobular masses are usually well demarcated. Pseudotumours without muscle involvement appear as diffuse, circumscribed densities or as opacities encircling the bulb. They can extend as far as the lacrimal gland or even involve the gland exclusively. Enhancement within pseudotumours is generally moderate and does not usually reveal any new diseased areas of tissue. Better differentiation of individual pseudotumours can be expected in the future from the coronal slice technique or from specific multiplanar reconstruction in the direction of the individual extraocular muscles.

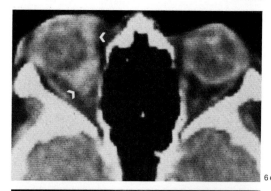
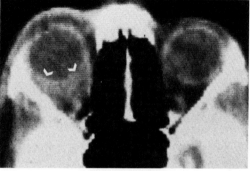

Fig. 51-6 d–f: Pseudotumours (d, e of the lympho-plasmocellular type). The retrobulbar space is almost completely (d), partially (e) or only in the peribulbar region (f) filled by a soft-tissue zone.

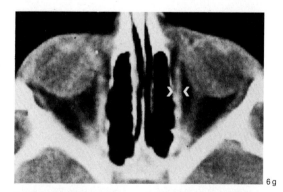
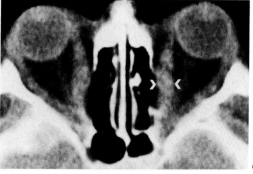

Fig. 51-6 g, h: Endocrine ophthalmopathy.

6 g: Moderate, relative swelling of the musculus rectus medialis in comparison to the musculus rectus lateralis which is demonstrable on several slices.

6 h: Considerable swelling and meandering of the musculi recti, enlargement of the medial muscle being greater than that of the respective lateral muscle.

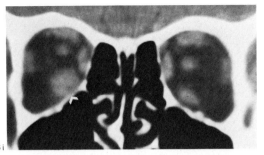

Fig. 51-6i: **Endocrine ophthalmopathy.** Isolated swelling of the musculus rectus inferior left. This finding is made most reliably in a frontal projection (>).

Fig. 51-6j–l: **Mucocele, pyocele.**
6j: Mucocele of the right ethmoid bone, the walls of which have lost bone density and are thickened. Ventrolateral displacement of the bulb.
6k: Pyocele right (similar appearance to 6j).
6l: Status after surgery for a pyocele with orbital phlegmon left. Distinct sclerosis of the walls of the ethmoid bone right and compacted soft-tissue zone retrobulbar (≫).

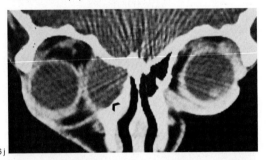

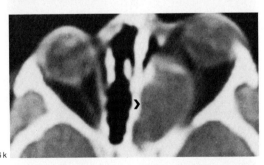

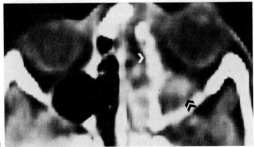

Endocrine ophthalmopathy (51-65)

The thyrotoxic form leads to inflammatory infiltration of orbital soft tissue with increased deposition of mucopolysaccharides. Fatty degeneration and oedema of the muscles are an expression of incipient myopathy. The thyrotropic form (malignant exophthalmos) leads to marked formation of oedema and culminates in fibrosis of the inflammatory retrobulbar tissue with increasing protrusion of the ocular bulb.

● **CT**

The principle sign in the computed tomogram is diffuse or spindle-shaped thickening of the extraocular muscles. Involvement is bilateral in the majority of cases and symmetrical in about 75%. The musculi rectus medialis and inferior are affected much more frequently than the musculi rectus lateralis and superior, and there have not yet been any observations of isolated swelling of the musculus rectus lateralis (193). In about half the cases of clinically unilateral ophthalmopathy computerized tomography also reveals a change on the opposite side. Enzmann observed negative CT findings in 10% of cases of clinically unequivocal ophthalmopathy (193). The value of contrast medium administration in endocrine ophthalmopathy is disputed.

Retrobulbar neuritis (51-66)

No definite correlation with the clinical findings has been found in the majority of cases which have so far been reported. Isolated cases of moderately discrete thickening or tortuosity of the optic nerve have been described (195).

Mucocele, pyocele (51-67)

Obstruction of a paranasal sinus by an osteoma, scars or swelling leads to congestion of secretion and, finally, to dilation of the closed cavity. The frontal sinuses and ethmoid cells are affected most frequently, the maxillary sinuses less frequently. The surrounding bones are expanded and protrude into the orbit. A pyocele develops if the congested secretion becomes infected.

● **CT**

Computerized tomography reveals a mass within a paranasal sinus with density values between those of water and soft tissue (25-40 HU). Malignant tumours of the paranasal sinuses invade the orbit in a similar way, but they consist of solid tissue. The bony contour of the mucocele or pyocele is frequently only paper-thin and cannot always be recognized even if the CT unit has good spatial resolution, thus the picture can be that of a destructive growth. The density values of a pyocele are the same as or higher than those of a mucocele (52-41).

Vascular processes (51-70)
Arteriovenous malformations (51-71)
● CT

In contrast to haemangiomas, arteriovenous malformations display poorly defined limits and vascular convolutions produce an inhomogenous pattern of densities. Amorphous calcifications have been described in some of the cases (218). Enhancement is usually distinct following contrast medium administration. Despite exophthalmos and specific investigation, the vascular malformation can escape CT detection, making angiography necessary (218).

Thrombophlebitis or **varicosis** leads to discrete masses of soft tissue density in the region of the optic nerve. Phleboliths are a not infrequent finding (206).

Trauma (51-72)
● CT

A fresh retrobulbar haematoma following blunt trauma can appear as a circumscribed hyperdense zone in the retrobulbar space. In fractures of the bone, the concomitant haematoma protrudes – frequently concentrically – into the orbit with typical signs of displacement. Fractures can be reliably recognized only if fragments are displaced. The dilated superior ophthalmic vein, which opacifies clearly following contrast medium administration, can frequently be demonstrated in a carotid cavernous sinus fistula if thin slice thicknesses are employed.

Foreign bodies (51-73)
● CT

A number of foreign bodies can be localized by computerized tomography in the intraocular and extraocular spaces if a rapid slice technique is used to avoid artifacts due to eye movements. Demonstration depends on the particle size (partial volume effect) and the radiodensity of the foreign body material. Wood and glass particles as well as metal splinters can be detected (199).

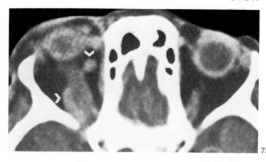
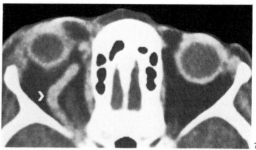

Fig. 51-7a: **Carotid sinus-cavern fistula.** Demonstration of a considerably dilated ophthalmic vein taking a curved course to the bulb between the musculus rectus superior/musculus levator palpebrae and the optic nerve.

Fig. 51-7b: **Trauma.** Fracture of the lateral wall of the orbit (≫) with saturation of the retroorbital fatty tissue with fluid (opacification of the retrobulbar fat and exophthalmus).

Fig. 51-7c: **Foreign body.** Foreign body with the density of metal (gunshot wound) in the tip of the orbit.

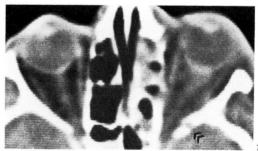
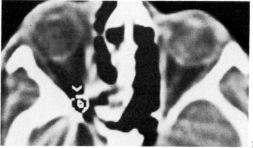

Visceral cranium (52-00)

Anatomy and imaging (52-10)

The **bony structures** of the visceral cranium are depicted in the frontal computed tomogram in a similar way as in the conventional antero-posterior tomogram. A **horizontal** projection produces better visualization of axially aligned boundary surfaces, in particular the anterior and posterior walls of the paranasal sinuses including the pterygoid process. Assessment in the horizontal plane of horizontal or semi-axial structures such as the roof and floor of the orbit, the alveolar recess of the maxillary sinus, the ethmoidal plane, the clivus and others is unsatisfactory even if thin slice thicknesses (of 4 mm) are chosen. Workers are still undecided about the diagnostic value of a frontal reconstruction from thin horizontal slices. If at all, only part of the upper section (towards the inferior orbital fissure) of the **pterygopalatine fossa** – a space which contains vessels and nerves (pterygopalatine ganglion) – can be demonstrated by computerized tomography (231).

Computerized tomography can demonstrate soft tissues far better than conventional tomography, and permits differentiation of the muscles of the visceral cranium. Depending on the direction in which they run, these muscles can be easily assessed to varying degrees in horizontal or frontal planes.

The **retromaxillary space** is divided up by muscles and fasciae. The strong pharyngeal fascia (pharyngobasilar fascia) inserts at the base of the skull and the medial lamina of the pterygoid process and runs caudalward in the shape of a tube to its junction with the buccopharyngeal fascia. In the epipharynx it extends laterally up to the styloid process and covers at some distance the prevertebral fascia, which invests the musculi longi capitis and colli. The lateral pterygoid muscle originates from the lateral lamina and runs slightly cranialward to the intervertebral disc of the tempero-mandibular joint, while the medial pterygoid muscle originates medial to it at the lateral lamina and runs caudalward to the inner surface of the angle of mandible. The temporal muscle inserts into the coronoid process of mandible.

The **infratemporal fossa** is bounded by the mandible, the lateral lamina of the pterygoid process and the styloid process. It is incompletely closed ventrally by the masseter muscle. The lateral boundary to the **parapharyngeal space** is not well defined. The parapharyngeal space extends laterally from the lateral wall of the pharynx up to the pterygoid muscles and the ramus of mandible and dorsally up to the styloid. It is divided into a prestyloid and poststyloid compartment by the pharyngeal fascia (Fig. 52-1a). The poststyloid compartment contains the internal jugular vein with lymph nodes, the internal carotid artery and the bundle of nerves consisting of the glossopharyngeal nerve, hypoglossal nerve, sympathetic nerve and vagus nerve. The prestyloid compartment contains branches of the maxillary artery and the maxillary ramus of the trigeminal nerve. The **retropharyngeal space** – which also contains lymph nodes – lies between the (basi)pharyngeal and the prevertebral fascia.

The shape and configuration of the epipharynx must be considered in the assessment of the parapharyngeal space. The auditory (eustachian) tube, which can only be demonstrated when it contains air, ends in front of the prominent torus tubarius, which consists of cartilaginous tissue. The pharyngeal recess (Rosenmüller's cavity) lies at a varying depth behind the torus. Medial to the medial pterygoid muscle, the tensor and levator muscle of the velum palatini runs caudalward within the pharyngeal fascia. The submucous muscle layer of the constrictor muscle of the larynx continuously increases in thickness in the direction of the hypopharynx. Slight asymmetry of the epipharynx can be regarded as a normal variant as long as the deeper parapharyngeal structures appear symmetrical and are not masked.

The **parotid gland,** which encircles the ascending ramus of mandible dorsally, appears as a hypodense, smoothly bordered zone and is bounded ventrally by the posterior surface of the masseter muscle. The sternocleidomastoid muscle lies against it dorso-caudally.

The **floor of the mouth** and the soft palate are best assessed in the frontal plane because they are predominantly horizontally aligned muscle surfaces. The individual muscle layers of the floor of the mouth, e. g. the digastric muscle, the mylohyoid muscle, the geniohyoid muscle and the genioglossus muscle, can usually be delineated from each other. The

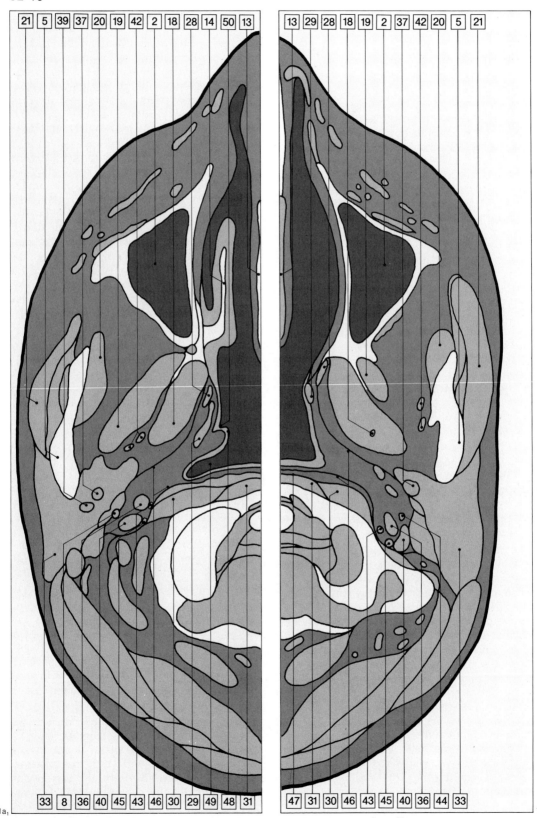

Visceral cranium

Fig. 52-1a,b: Topography of the visceral cranium.

1a: Horizontal sections at the level of the parapharyngeal space. Sectional plane of a_2 about 2 cm caudal of a_1.

1b: Horizontal computed tomograms. The sectional planes of b_1 and b_2 approximate those of a_1 and a_2; b_4 is at the level of the soft palate.

Key
Osseous structures
1 Maxilla
2 Sinus maxillaris
3 Palatum durum
4 Os zygomaticum
5 Mandibula
6 Capitulum mandibulae
7 Processus coronoideus
8 Processur styloideus
9 Processus mastoideus
10 Clivus
11 Sinus sphenoideus
12 Cellulae ethmoidales
13 Septum nasi
14 Concha nasalis
15 Lamina medialis proc. pterygoidei
16 Lamina lateralis proc. pterygoidei
17 Hamulus proc. pterygoidei

Muscular structures
18 M. pterygoideus medialis
19 M. pterygoideus lateralis
20 M. temporalis
21 M. masseter
22 M. buccinator
23 M. constrictor pharyngis sup.
24 M. digastricus
25 M. mylohyoideus
26 M. geniohyoideus
27 M. genioglossus
28 M. tensor veli palatini
29 M. levator veli palatini
30 M. longus capitis
31 M. longus colli
32 Palatum molle

Glands
33 Glandula parotis
34 Glandula submandibularis
35 Glandula sublingualis

Vessels, nerves, fasciae
36 A. carotis interna
37 A. carotis externa
38 A. lingualis
39 V. retromandibularis
40 V. jugularis interna
41 V. facialis
42 N. mandibularis
43 N. vagus
44 N. hypoglossus
45 N. accessorius
46 Fascia pharyngea
47 Fascia praevertebralis

and
48 Torus tubarius
49 Recessus pharyngeus lateralis
50 Tuba Eustachii (orificium)
51 Orbita
52 Spatium parapharyngeum
53 Spatium retropharyngeum
54 Fossa infratemporalis

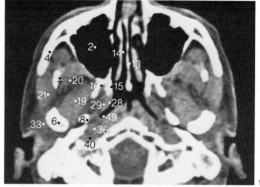
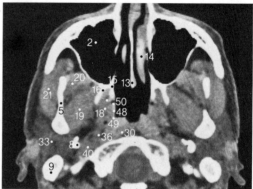
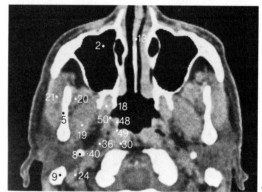
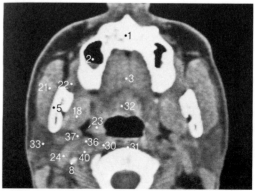

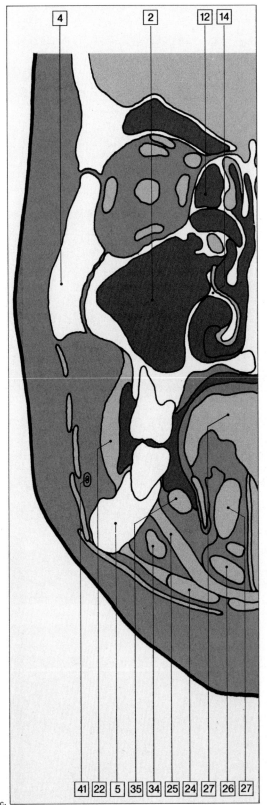
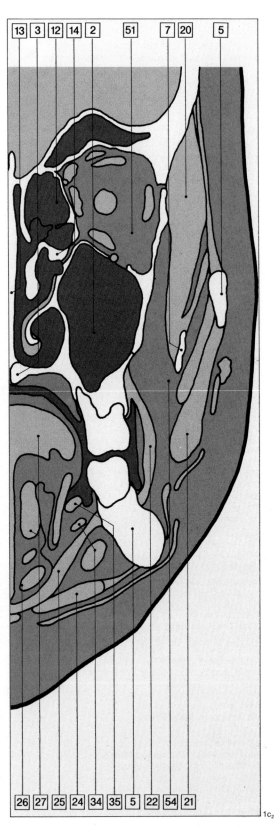

Fig. 52-1 c, d: **Topography of the visceral cranium.**

1c: Frontal section through the anterior visceral cranium. The sectional plane of c_1 is 1.5 cm in front of that of c_2.

1d: Coronal computed tomograms. Sectional plane continuous from dorsal (d_1) to ventral (d_4).

Key
Osseous structures
1 Maxilla
2 Sinus maxillaris
2 Palatum durum
4 Os zygomaticum
5 Mandibula
6 Capitulum mandibulae
7 Processus coronoideus
8 Processus styloideus
9 Processus mastoideus
10 Clivus
11 Sinus sphenoideus
12 Cellulae ethmoidales
13 Septum nasi
14 Concha nasalis
15 Lamina medialis proc. pterygoidei
16 Lamina lateralis proc. pterygoidei
17 Hamulus proc. pterygoidei

Muscular structures
18 M. pterygoideus medialis
19 M. pterygoideus lateralis
20 M. temporalis
21 M. masseter
22 M. buccinator
23 M. constrictor pharyngis sup.
24 M. digastricus
25 M. mylohyoideus
26 M. geniohyoideus
27 M. genioglossus
28 M. tensor veli palatini
29 M. levator veli palatini
30 M. longus capitis
31 M. longus colli
32 Palatum molle

Glands
33 Glandula parotis
34 Glandula submandibularis
35 Glandula sublingualis

Vessels, nerves, fasciae
36 A. carotis interna
37 A. carotis externa
38 A. lingualis
39 V. retromandibularis
40 V. jugularis interna
41 V. facialis
42 N. mandibularis
43 N. vagus
44 N. hypoglossus
45 N. accessorius
46 Fascia pharyngea
47 Fascia praevertebralis

and
48 Torus tubarius
49 Recessus pharyngeus lateralis
50 Tuba Eustachii (orificium)
51 Orbita
52 Spatium parapharyngeum
53 Spatium retropharyngeum
54 Fossa infratemporalis

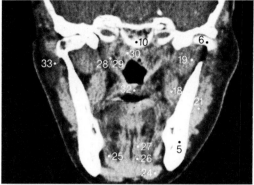
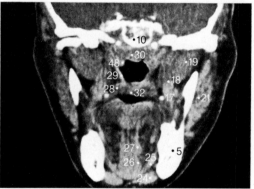
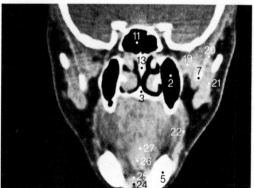
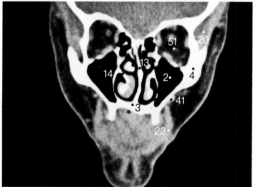

submandibular gland, which lies for the greater part beneath the mylohyoid muscle close to the lower jaw, can be identified as a hypodense zone – particularly after administration of contrast medium. The bed of the palatine tonsil is marked by the palatoglossus muscle and the pharyngopalatine muscle.

The **vessels** are only partly identifiable even when adequate amounts of fat are interposed, although administration of contrast medium (infusion) always leads to demonstration of the internal carotid artery and the internal jugular vein. Not infrequently, the opacified internal carotid artery can be seen together with the retromandibular vein within the carotid gland behind the ramus of mandible, and its branches are recognizable on careful analysis. For example, the administration of contrast medium leads to demonstration of sections of the facial artery lateral to the maxillary sinus, of the maxillary artery in the infratemporal fossa and of the lingual artery lateral to the genioglossus muscle.

The **nerves** themselves are not usually recognizable, but their location can be assumed from the course of the vessels.

Examination technique (52-20)

● Preparation of the patient is unnecessary. A fasting state is advisable because contrast medium administration is probable.

● **Scanning** with slice thicknesses of 5–8 mm and an adjacent slice sequence.

Scanning area: dependent on the clinical problem (including the regional groups of lymph nodes).

Horizontal slices parallel to the infraorbitomeatal line.

Frontal (coronal) slices about vertical to the infraorbitomeatal line.

Hyperreflection of the head and tilting of the gantry (51-20).

The patient must be positioned so that he can breath comfortably.

The swallowing reflex must be suppressed as much as possible (artifacts).

● **Intravenous contrast medium administration**

As a bolus injection (4-32) for differentiation of the lesion.
As an infusion (4-36) in extensive processes, for delimitation of the lesion, to clarify the vascular relationship, in the search for enlarged lymph nodes etc.

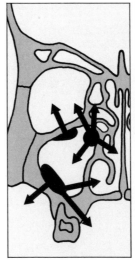
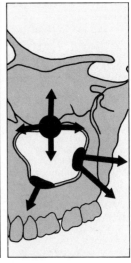

Fig. 52-3 a: **Pathways of infiltration of malignant tumours of the maxillary sinuses.**

Fig. 52-3 b: **Retothelial sarcoma** of the left maxillary sinus with destruction of virtually the entire wall. Infiltration of the soft tissues of the face (>) and of the retromaxillary space (≫). Obstruction of the left main meatus of the nose.

Fig. 52-3 c: **Cylindroma** of the left maxillary sinus under irradiation. Destruction of the medial and dorsal walls of the sinus. Recalcification of the swollen lateral sinus wall (><). The retromaxillary space does not appear to be infiltrated.

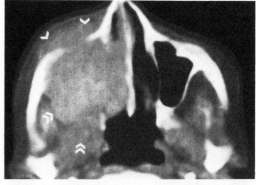
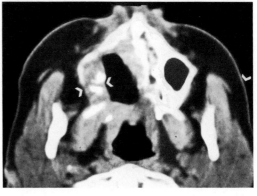

Tumours of the paranasal sinuses
(52-30)

Cystic forms (52-31)

Serous (non-secretory) cysts and dentogenic (primordial, follicular and radicular) cysts are localized primarily in the maxillary sinus. They occur much more frequently than cholesteatomas (epidermoids). Congenital meningoceles and encephaloceles are occasionally found in the frontal and ethmoid sinus. The rare dermoid cysts have no site of predilection. Common to all these cystic masses is more or less marked expansive growth, which is encountered in particular in dentigerous follicular cysts.

- **CT**

In dermoid cysts and cholesteatomas (epidermoids), computerized tomography often reveals reduced density values, which are an indication of an increased fat content. The other cystic masses display density values which lie between those of water and soft tissue. Concentric dilatation of the sinus concerned, which can even lead to erosion of the walls of the bone, is found in expansive growths.

The finding at the level of the alveolar process is important for odontogenic cysts, but this can be assessed better in the conventional radiological projections and by pluridimensional tomography. In neurogenic cysts, which represent herniation of meninges through a defect of the visceral cranium, the site of origin can be determined in the computed tomogram when the osseous defect is displayed tangentially (sphenoid sinus and ethmoid cells in a horizontal plane).

Benign solid tumours (52-32)

The ratio of benign to malignant tumours is 1:3. The non-calcifying or non-ossifying forms include papillomas, adenomas, myomas, lipomas, fibromas, juvenile angiofibromas, neurofibromas, giant-cell tumours and plasmocytomas. Circumscribed calcifications are found in haemangiomas (phleboliths) and in osteochondromas. Like certain odontogenic tumours, ossifying fibromas, osteomas and meningeomas are marked by dense, calcium-containing structures.

- **CT**

Smaller masses can be demarcated in the computed tomogram using the usual horizontal slice technique when they lie against the walls of the bone which are aligned in the axial

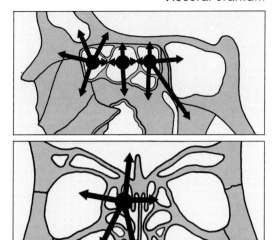

Fig. 52-3 d: **Pathways of infiltration of malignant tumours of the ethmoid bone.**

Fig. 52-3 e: **Carcinoma** of the right ethmoid bone with infiltration of the orbit, the right main meatus of the nose and the sphenoid sinus ($e_2 \gg$).

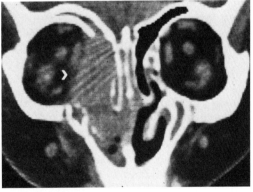

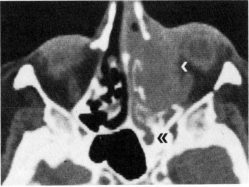

plane. They can escape detection on horizontal boundary surfaces, making additional coronal slices necessary (52-10). Computerized tomography is superior to conventional tomography in the demonstration of dorsal expansion of the lesion into the retromaxillary space, the orbit and the sella turcica, and can provide additional valuable information prior to major therapeutic intervention. Of the masses of soft-tissue density, only the very rare lipoma can be demarcated by virtue of its **radiodensity**. The high **vascularity** of juvenile angiofibromas, haemangiomas and meningeomas, which manifests itself as increased enhancement following contrast medium administration, can be employed in the differential diagnosis. There are a number of tumours or tumour-like changes, e. g. fibrous dysplasia, Paget's disease, osteomas and odontogenic tumours, in which computerized tomography usually yields no additional information.

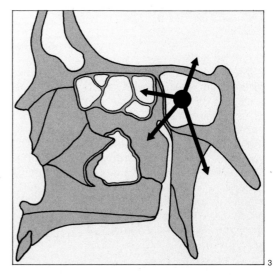

Fig. 52-3 f: **Pathways of infiltration of malignant tumours of the sphenoid.**

Malignant tumours (52-33)

Malignant tumours of the paranasal sinuses are rare (0.2% of cancer morbidity) and display a broad histological spectrum. **Carcinoma** (usually squamous cell carcinoma) accounts for 80% of cases, while malignant lymphomas account for 10%. Other types of carcinoma (adenocarcinoma and cylindroma), soft-tissue and bone **sarcomas**, malignant melanomas and plasmocytomas are numerically of secondary importance. In addition to these primary malignant lesions, tumours of the orbit, nasopharynx and sella turcica can spread to the paranasal sinuses. **Haematogenous dissemination** of tumours of the breast, lung, kidneys and prostate has been described. Overall, 60–80% of malignant tumours originate in the maxillary sinus. Regional lymph flow takes place retropharyngeally, partly subarachnoidally and cervically via the choanal lymph tract. Malignant lesions of the paranasal sinus metastasize relatively late via these lymphatic pathways.

The **pathway of infiltration** also depends on the localization of the tumour. Initially, the tumour invades the bone locally. Later on, with increasing size, it also involves adjacent walls. Tumours of the endosinus originating from the mucosa display expansive growth with gradual erosion of the walls. This finding is frequently made in the region of the sphenoid and frontal sinuses.

Fig. 52-3 g: **Epipharyngeal carcinoma.** Obstruction of the epipharynx by an extensive soft-tissue mass. Erosion of the clivus from a ventral direction (g_1 ≫). The soft-tissue mass fills the sphenoid sinus almost completely (g_2).

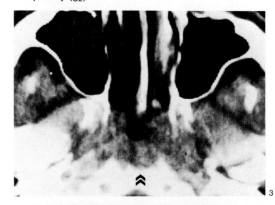

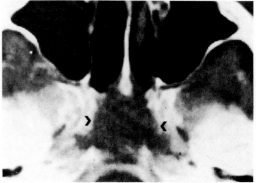

● CT

The tumour is recognizable in the computed tomogram as a soft-tissue zone. Destruction of the axially aligned osseous lamellae can usually be clearly demonstrated (52-10). Above and beyond the bone destruction, a great part of which can be demonstrated by pluridimensional tomography, the tumour tissue can also be depicted in anatomical spaces, the structure of which is not formed by air and which are assessable, e. g. in tumour expansion into the retromaxillary space, infiltration of the orbit and penetration of the tumour through the dorsal wall of the frontal and sphenoid sinuses. Coronal projections also permit assessment of the roof and floor of the orbit, the roof of the ethmoid bone and the hard palate (52-10) and, hence, of their destruction and tumour expansion beyond these structures.

Malignant tumours of the maxillary sinus invade the orbit in 25 % of cases (234) and, less frequently, the retromaxillary space, where the infiltration leads to masking of the contours of the medial and lateral pterygoid muscles. Tumour infiltration of the dorsal contour of the lateral pterygoid muscle means that branches of the ramus of mandible (N. V) have already been invaded. Further expansion leads to encasement of the internal carotid artery and the internal jugular vein, including cerebral nerves IX–XII. These vascular structures can be visualized by means of contrast medium.

Rarely, the **ethmoid cells** are the site of origin of a local malignant tumour which, depending on its position (anterior, medial and posterior cells), can invade the orbit, maxillary, frontal and sphenoid sinuses and the anterior cranial fossa. The ethmoid cells are not infrequently subject to secondary infiltration by adjacent lesions.

The **sphenoid sinus**, too, is usually invaded secondarily. Primary sphenoid tumours infiltrate the posterior orbit, nasopharynx, ethmoid cells and the sella turcica. In malignant lesions of the **frontal sinuses**, the dorsal walls and, hence, expansion of the tumour into the anterior cranial fossa can be assessed particularly well. Infiltration of the orbit and ethmoid cells is best depicted by coronal projections.

It must be borne in mind as regards the **differential diagnosis** that, in Wegener's granulomatosis – in which the inflammation usually causes opacity in the paranasal sinuses – bone destruction can occur relatively early and spread to the hard palate. **Sclerosis** of a paranasal wall can correspond to an osteoblastic reaction to tumour invasion and must be viewed critically in the absence of inflammatory changes in the sinus concerned.

Inflammations of the paranasal sinuses (52-40)

Inflammations of the paranasal sinuses with mucosal swelling or exudation are readily accessible to conventional radiological diagnosis and, in contrast to the following conditions, are not an indication for CT.

Mucoceles, pyoceles (52-41)

Mucoceles affect the frontal sinuses and ethmoid cells at a ratio of about 2 : 1. They seldom occur in the region of the sphenoid and maxillary sinuses, the incidence being up to 10 % of cases (251, 252). They develop as a result of an accumulation of mucus which cannot drain away due to obstruction of the paranasal ostium. The pressure of the secretion in the mucus-filled sinus leads to concentric usurption of the osseous walls and enlargement of the sinus. The osseous lamella eventually becomes paper-thin or even erodes. Infection of the secretion leads to a pyocele.

Occlusion of the ostium is caused most frequently by inflammation (infectious, allergic) or by intralumenal masses (polyps, osteomas) (252). Scars following trauma or surgery are a less frequent cause of the obstruction of flow. Exophthalmos is the guiding clinical symptom (51-67).

● CT

Computerized tomography reveals opacity of a paranasal sinus, the walls of which are concentrically expanded. Delicate osseous boundaries, e. g. the membrana papyracea, give way to the intracavitary pressure at an early stage, creating a small-arched protrusion. A thick-walled, sclerotic boundary to the deformed sinus can be demonstrated in chronic lesions, while a thin osseous lamella or the absence of an osseous boundary is found in rapidly expanding processes. The direction of the expansion is the same as that of malignant lesions (52-33), which means that a coronal projection may be necessary for exact visualization of the protrusion of the orbital floor and roof, floor of the sella, cribriform lamella, ethmoid roof etc. Particular attention must be paid to the boundary of the dorsal wall of the frontal sinus – the lateral border of the sphenoid (superior orbital fissure syndrome) – in the horizontal projection.

The **density values** of the lesions are frequently isodense with cerebral tissue (25-40 HU [232]) and usually higher than those of water. Mucoceles display neither peripheral nor central enhancement following contrast medium administration. Expansion of the lesions into the cranial fossa in the direction of the dura calls for the administration of contrast medium to achieve better demarcation from meningeal and cerebral structures (232). Pyoceles display higher central density values (45-85 HU [232]) than mucoceles and occasionally exhibit rim enhancement following contrast medium administration as a sign of extensive granulation tissue.

Mucocele vs tumour (52-42)
The diagnostic demarcation of a mucocele from sinusitis, serous cysts and antrochoanal polyps is simple if air is demonstrable within the sinus. In the absence of this sign, differentiation may be impossible if destruction of the osseous walls is also absent. Malignant lesions infiltrate the surrounding structures, whereas the expansive growth of mucoceles and pyoceles leads to displacement, leaving adjacent tissue planes, e. g. intraorbital fatty tissue, intact (232).

In contrast to mucoceles and pyoceles, some solid lesions display distinct enhancement in keeping with their degree of vascularity. Differentiation from mucoceles may be impossible in hypovascular benign and malignant tumours with primarily expansive growth (52-32, 52-33).

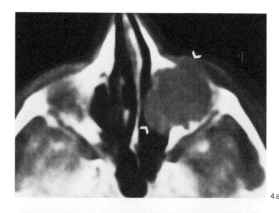

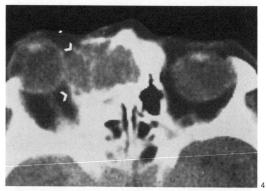

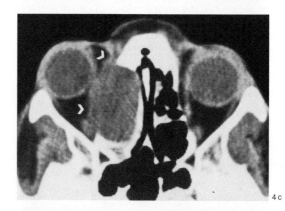

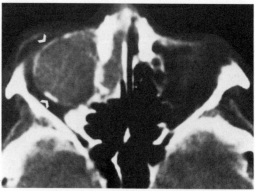

Fig. 52-4 a–d: **Mucoceles.** Concentric growth is also demonstrable where the osseous contours have been eroded or cannot be recognized (a, c). Expansion into adjacent spaces, the orbit in particular, can be exactly evaluated. Flattening of the osseous contours is demonstrated in some cases (b, d). The lesions do not enhance after administration of contrast medium. The density values range from 4–36 HU.

Tumours of the nasopharynx (52-50)

Benign tumours (52-51)

The benign tumours are the same as those described in 52-32. Of particular interest are chordomas and juvenile angiofibromas.
Chordomas, which originate from the sphenoid bone, the occipital bone and the cervical vertebrae as vestigeal tumours, lead early on to destruction of the adjacent bone up to the dorsum sellae. This can create the appearance of a carcinoma, although chordomas are primarily benign and rarely degenerate.
Juvenile angiofibromas, which usually occur and are detected in the second decade of life, originate at the roof of the pharynx and are marked by high vascularity and expansive growth with displacement of the adjacent osseous structures.

● CT

The computed tomogram reveals a tumour of soft-tissue density which does not usually permit diagnosis of the nature of the tumours mentioned under 52-32. Benign tumours (chordomas, angiofibromas) should be considered if bone destruction is demonstrated in this region. In juvenile patients, distinct enhancement following contrast medium administration is an indication of an angiofibroma. Not infrequently, delicate calcifications are demonstrated in chordomas. A cyst of the pharyngeal bursa should be considered in cystic masses of the roof of the pharynx.

Malignant tumours of the epipharynx (52-52)

Malignant lesions of the epipharynx are rare, though somewhat more frequent than those of the paranasal sinuses. Carcinomas are involved in about 50% of cases, malignant lymphomas (including reticuloendothelial sarcomas) in 45%. The histological spectrum is the same as that of the malignant neoplasms described under 52-33.

Malignant epipharyngeal tumours can spread contiguously in various directions and into various spaces:

1. Into the (lateral) parapharyngeal space (Fig. 52-1a) (prestyloid compartment) with the mandibular ramus of the trigeminal nerve and/or into the poststyloid compartment with the internal carotid artery, the internal jugular vein, the 9th–12th cerebral nerves and the lymph nodes.

2. Cranialward in the direction of the base of the skull causing invasion of the medial cranial

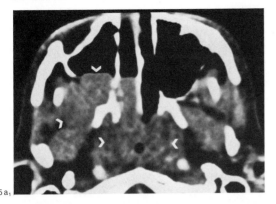

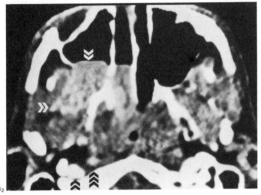

Fig. 52-**5a: Epipharyngeal tumour** (juvenile angiofibroma). Tumour of soft-tissue density with destruction of the dorsal wall of the maxillary sinus left, occupation of the entire epipharynx including the choanae. Infiltration of the left parapharyngeal space/infratemporal fossa. After contrast medium administration, signs of marked vascularization in some areas of the tumour (a_2 ≫). (Internal jugular vein ≫, internal carotid artery ≫.)

Fig. 52-**5b: Glomangioma.** Demonstration of an extensive soft-tissue mass left with infiltration of the parapharyngeal space and dorsal wall of the left maxillary sinus (≫). Obstruction of the choanae and left main meatus of the nose (>). A hypervascular tumour was found at angiography.

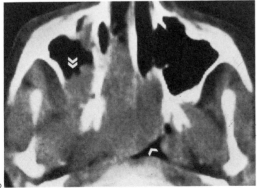

fossa (directly or through the foramina of the base of the skull).

3. In a dorsal direction into the retropharyngeal space, which is formed by the (bucco-)pharyngeal fascia and the prevertebral membrane of the deep cervical fascia and which contains lymph nodes (particularly the lateral retropharyngeal lymph nodes).

Lymphatic dissemination takes place early on into the cervical lymph nodes, usually via the upper internal jugular groups. Malignant epipharyngeal lesions metastasize at an early stage and, frequently, via the haematogenous pathway.

● CT

These small masses are usually asymmetrical and are normally detected by endoscopy. In extensive processes — which can even cause displacement of the nasopharynx, computerized tomography can complement the findings of the lateral X-ray film by demonstrating the soft-tissue zone itself and the displaced pharyngeal structures. The position and shape of the torus tubarius frequently reveal whether the eustachian tube or its direct vicinity has been invaded (Fig. 52-5c). Similarly, expansion and masking of the retropharyngeal structures indicate tumour invasion. The expansion of the tumorous soft-tissue zone into the parapharyngeal space and its compartments can be described in detail, particularly if thin slices are used. Intravenous injection of contrast medium should be given to opacify the large vessels and to improve the demarcation of the mass.

The extent of bone destruction can be depicted in detail. An intracranial soft-tissue component can be recognized in addition to the destruction of the base of the skull (the cribriform lamina, clivus, tips of the pyramids and the carotid canal, the foramen lacerum and others). Isolated sclerosis of the base of the skull in the region of the nasopharynx is also indicative of a malignant process, particularly if soft-tissue components or enlarged cervical lymph nodes are demonstrated. Cf. 52-10 and 52-33 for the value of the use of coronal slices.

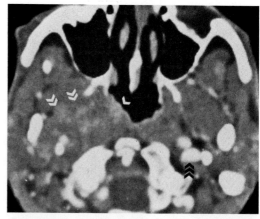

Fig. 52-5c: **Epipharyngeal tumour** (esthesioneuroblastoma). Demonstration of a mass in the left parapharyngeal space (>) with masking of the retromaxillary muscles (≫). After a bolus injection, patchy enhancement of the tumour, no opacification of the ipsilateral internal jugular vein and internal carotid vein as a sign of vascular occlusion. No demonstration of bone destruction. Internal jugular vein, internal carotid artery right (≫).

Fig. 52-6a: **Carcinoma of the floor of the mouth.** The tumour appears in the plain scan as a hypodense zone with displacement of the genioglossal muscle to the right (≫). It enhances distinctly following administration of contrast medium.

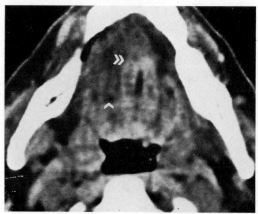

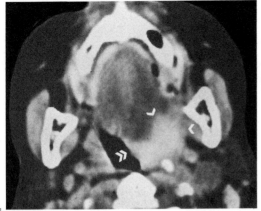

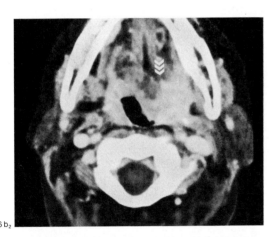

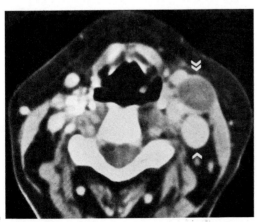

Fig. 52-6b: **Tonsillar carcinoma.** Demonstraton of a distinct soft-tissue mass in the bed of the tonsil deforming the mesopharynx and displacing it to the left (b_1 ≫). The well-supplied tumour demarcates from the muscles of the floor of the mouth following administration of contrast medium (b_2≫). Nodular structures cannot always be distinguished from vessels because of marked fluctuations in the calibre of the internal jugular vein, so that contrast medium is required (b_3: internal jugular vein >, lymph node metastasis ≫).

Tumours of the oro- and mesopharynx (52-60)

After carcinoma of the larynx, tonsillar carcinoma is the most common tumour of the upper respiratory tract. In about 80% of cases malignant tonsillar tumours are carcinomas of varying differentiation. Next in order of frequency are malignant lymphomas. As with tumours of the epipharynx, regional lymph node metastases are frequently found at the initial examination. The tomour invades adjacent tissue at an early stage, eroding first of all the retrolingual region and glossopalatine arch before spreading both cranially and caudally.

Carcinoma of the tongue is the most common malignant growth of the **oropharynx** (buccal cavity, tongue, upper and lower jaws), followed by tumours of the alveolar processes, the floor of the mouth, the hard and soft palate and the cheek. The neoplasms, which are initially superficial, spread via the paralingual space into the parapharyngeal space and craniodorsally in the direction of the base of the skull. The regional submandibular and cervical groups of lymph nodes are found homolaterally in the early stage and contralaterally in the advanced stage.

● **CT**

The usual role of computerized tomography is to determine the extent of the tumour and its relationship to the large vessels.

The tumour is recognized as a soft-tissue zone, the density value of which in the plain scan differs only slightly from that of muscle tissue. Masking of normal anatomical structures is a sign of tumour infiltration. A guided bolus injection or an infusion usually leads to better demarcation of the tumour. Administration of contrast medium is also required to opacify the large vessels, since this leads to more reliable identification of paravascular lymphomas (particularly those of the internal jugular group). Since, following surgery or irradiation, the demonstration of tumour recurrence is frequently rendered difficult by secondary inflammation, basal findings should be planned for later follow-up examinations.

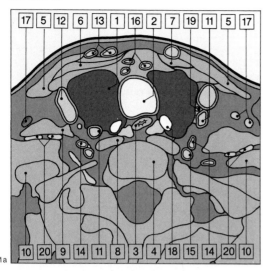

Fig. 53-1a, b: **Normal thyroid.**
1a: Topography of the thyroid.
1b: Computed tomogram of a normal thyroid.
Key
1 Thyroid
2 Trachea
3 Oesophagus
4 Cervical vertebra
5 M. sternocleido-
  mastoideus
6 M. sternothyreoideus
7 M. sternohyoideus
8 M. longus colli
9 M. scalenus anterior
10 M. scalenus medius
  et posterior
11 A. carotis communis
12 V. jugularis interna
13 V. jugularis anterior
14 A. vertebralis
15 V. vertebralis
16 Vv. thyreoideae imae
17 Lymphonodi
  cervicales profundi
18 Glandula para-
  thyreoidea inferior
19 N. vagus
20 Plexus cervicalis

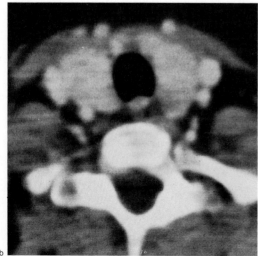

Thyroid (53-00)

Anatomy and imaging (53-10)

The **thyroid**, which encircles the trachea and thyroid cartilage ventrally in a convex-concave manner, is usually identified in the computed tomogram as a smooth and homogeneous soft-tissue structure. There is frequently no sufficient difference between the density of the internal jugular vein, the calibre of which varies, and that of the thyroid tissue, whereas the common carotid artery, which lies medio-dorsally next to the internal jugular vein, is clearly demarcated. The iodine content of a normal thyroid – 0.65 mg/g tissue – increases the tissue density of the thyroid tissue to 70 ± 10 HU, a value which exceeds the radiodensity of muscle tissue. The good vascularity results in marked enhancement of the thyroid tissue following administration of contrast medium (295).

Examination technique (53-20)

● **Scanning** with an adjacent slice sequence at a slice interval of 5–8 mm.

Scanning area dependent on the size of the thyroid.

● **Intravenous contrast medium administration** for demonstration of circumscribed lesions or for differentiation:
as infusion (4-36)
as the guided bolus technique (4-32)

Diffuse diseases of the thyroid (53-30)

Hyperplasia (iodine deficit, hyperthyroidism) and inflammations (Riedel, Hashimoto) lead to general enlargement of the gland.

● **CT**

Computerized tomography can be used to determine the extent of the enlargement as well as signs of displacement (trachea). Following administration of contrast medium, hyperthyroid strumata, which are isodense with the surrounding muscle tissue, display only slight enhancement in comparison to the normal thyroid. Inhomogeneous enhancement has been described in inflammations.

Focal disease of the thyroid (53-40)

Nodular changes are found in the iodine-deficiency struma (struma nodosa) and in isolated adenomas of varying histology. Carcinomas constitute the largest group of malignant le-

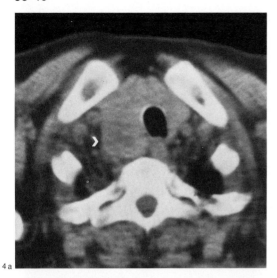

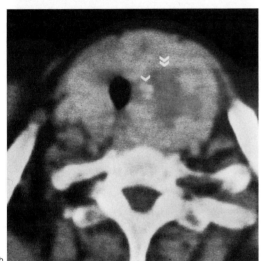

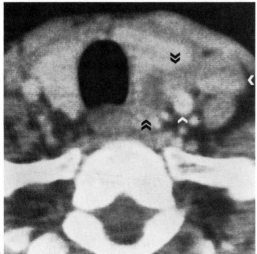

sions. They metastasize early via the lymphogenous route into the regional lymph nodes.

● **CT**

The density of **cysts** in the computed tomogram varies because of the varying content of protein and iodine and can even be higher than that of the surrounding muscle tissue. They display no enhancement and are well demarcated. **Adenomas** are frequently isodense with the surrounding muscle tissue and stand out smoothly from the thyroid tissue. An increase of density is usually recognizable after administration of contrast medium, although it is less than that of normal thyroid tissue. Enhancement is frequently missing in **malignant lesions.** Irregular demarcation from the thyroid tissue and isodensity with the surrounding muscles of the neck are regarded as further indications of a malignant lesion, although this assumption is as yet based on only a few cases (248).

Diagnosis of the thyroid, which is easily accessible to palpation and puncture, is largely covered by nuclear-medical methods. Computerized tomography can provide some additional information if there is no uptake. The experience so far gained in this sphere is limited (248, 247).

Fig. 53-**4 a, b: Focal diseases of the thyroid.** Demonstration of a strumous node originating from the right lobe of the thyroid (a >). Adenoma of the thyroid gland with enlarged left thyroid lobe with regressive changes (calcifications b >, liquefaction b ≫). Displacement of the trachea to the opposite side.

Fig. 53-**5 a: Adenoma of the parathyroid.** Demonstration of a hypodense mass behind the left thyroid lobe (≫). Common carotid artery (>), internal jugular vein (>).

Thorax (60-00)

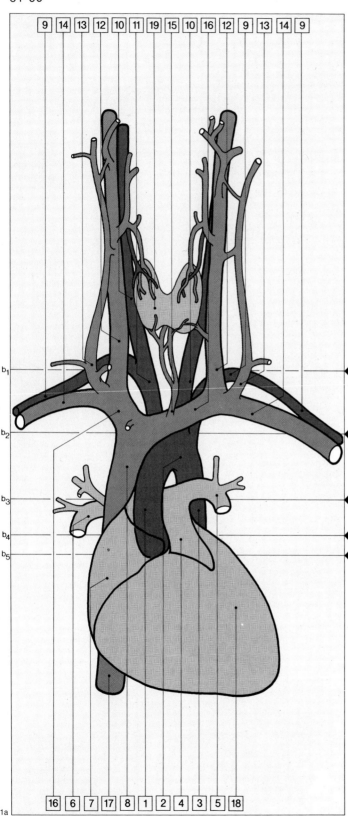

Fig. 61-1a,b: **Mediastinal vessels.**
1a: Situs
1b: Transverse sections (cf. 1a for levels)

Key
1 Aorta ascendens
2 Arcus aortae
3 Aorta descendens
4 Conus pulmonalis
5 A. pulmonalis sinistra
6 A. pulmonalis dextra
7 Auricula dextra
8 V. cava superior
9 A. subclavia
10 A. carotis communis
11 Truncus brachio-cephalicus
12 V. jugularis interna
13 V. jugularis externa
14 V. subclavia
15 V. thyreoidea ima
16 V. brachiocephalica
17 V. cava inferior
18 Heart
19 Thyroid
20 V. azygos

Mediastinum (61-00)

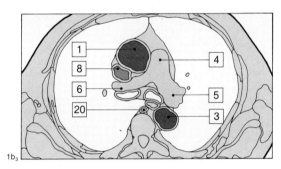

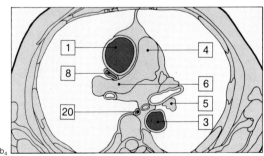

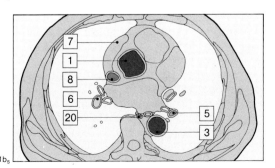

Anatomy and imaging (61-10)

The mediastinal spaces (61-11)
Individual authors (17, 39, 46, 7) propose different ways of dividing the mediastinum spatially according to anatomical, pathogenetic and diagnostic aspects. Since computerized tomography can depict the morphology of the mediastinum in detail, the value of a rigid division into spaces cannot yet be properly estimated. For reasons of tumour topography (61-40 to 61-60), a division into anterior, middle and posterior mediastinum (Fig. 61-4a) was chosen which is based on the proposal of Fraser-Paré and which modifies the division of Twinning and Zuppinger.

The mediastinal vessels (61-12)
The large vessels create a distinctive structure in the mediastinum and are best demonstrated in the computed tomogram when they run axially. As can be seen in Fig. 61-1a,b, this prerequisite is met in different ways for the individual sections of the vessels. Analysis of the image should always commence with the **aorta**, which is always unequivocally identifiable. Its brachiocephalic branches are intersected axially and can therefore likewise be clearly recognized. The veins are situated ventrally relative to these arterial structures. The left **brachiocephalic vein** (anonyma) is demonstrated obliquely in front of and above the aortic arch (Fig. 61-1b). Its junction to the **superior vena cava** is usually recognizable in the computed tomogram. The superior vena cava, which runs axially, can easily be followed laterodorsally to the ascending aorta up to its point of entry into the right atrium. In contrast, unequivocal identification of the **subclavian vein** and the **internal and external jugular vein** is rarely possible in the region where they branch. Overall, the veins appear to have a wide calibre, particularly the subclavian vein and the internal jugular vein. Even when it is looked for specifically, it is possible to demarcate the external jugular vein in only a few cases and frequently only after the administration of contrast medium.

The effluent pathways of the right ventricle and **pulmonary trunk** are usually readily identifiable because they are embedded in sub-

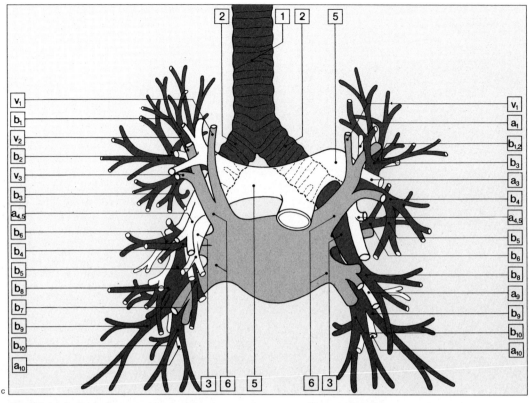

Fig. 61-1c,d: Bronchovascular structures of the pulmonary hilum.

1c: Situs seen ventrally

1d: Transverse sections (from cranial [d_1] to caudal [d_5])

Key
1 Trachea
2 Main bronchus
3 Lobar bronchus
4 Segmental bronchus
   b_1–b_{10} segmental bronchus 1–10
5 Pulmonary artery
   a_1–a_{10} segmental arteries 1–10
6 Pulmonary vein
   v_1–v_{10} segmental veins 1–10

Nomenclature of the segmental bronchi (SB).

b_1 = apical SB (UL)
b_2 = posterior SB (UL)
b_3 = anterior SB (UL)
b_4 = lateral SB (ML)
b_5 = medial SB (ML)
b_4 = superior SB (L)
b_5 = inferior SB (L)
b_6 = superior SB (LL)
b_7 = medial basal SB (LL)
b_8 = anterior basal SB (LL)
b_9 = lateral basal SB (LL)
b_{10} = posterior basal SB (LL)

(UL = upper lobe, ML = middle lobe, L = lingula, LL = lower lobe)

epicardial fatty tissue. The right **pulmonary artery** swings around the ascending aorta and then runs caudalward dorsal to the superior vena cava and ventrolateral to the bronchus intermedius after giving off the branch of the upper lobe. The left pulmonary artery, only a short stretch of which is situated within the pericardium, crosses **over** the left main bronchus and then, together with the branch of the lower lobe, runs in a caudal direction **behind** the bronchus close to the descending aorta (Fig. 61-1c).

If a suitable window setting is chosen, the pulmonary veins of the lower lobes can be followed separately up to the left atrium. The veins of the upper lobes run **in front** of the arteries and bronchi to the heart.

Depending on the amount of fatty tissue in the posterior mediastinum the **azygos vein**, which ascends on the right paravertebrally and retrocardially, can be demonstrated from a diameter of 3–5 mm. At the level of the 4th and 5th thoracic vertebrae it runs lateral to the oesophagus and medial to the right upper lobe bronchus and the right upper lobe artery to the right tracheobronchial angle. In the transverse section this is depicted as a lateroconvex arch. Above the azygos arch, the pleura invaginates to varying depths medially behind the trachea and forms the supra-azygos recess. Beneath

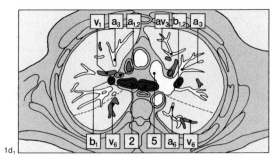
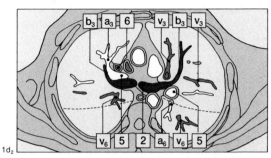
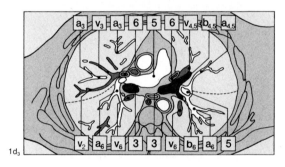
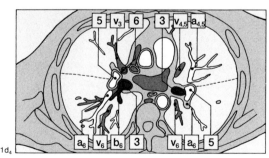
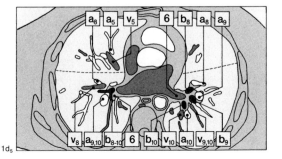

the arch, at the level of the hilum and heart, is a similar pulmonary protrusion, the azygooesophageal recess, which reaches the median line to varying degrees or can extend behind the oesophagus to the opposite side.

Trachea, oesophagus (61-13)
The **trachea** lies directly against the right mediastinal pleura both laterally and dorsally. The soft-tissue mantle between the lumen of the trachea and the lung usually measures 4 mm (19). Any increase of fatty tissue and constitutional variants, which can lead to widening of the trachea, are easily recognizable in the computed tomogram, although it must be ensured that the azygos arch is not included in the measurement. Because it contains air, the **oesophagus** is frequently easy to identify. Oral administration of diluted Gastrografin (4-23) may be necessary if the fatty mantle surrounding it is inadequate. In the upper mediastinum, the oesophagus is marked by its close proximity to the dorsal wall of the trachea. At the level of the tracheal bifurcation it lies approximately in the median line and then runs slightly to the left, crossing in front of the descending aorta retrocardially in a ventral direction.

The phrenic **nerves**, the vagus nerve and the **thoracic duct** cannot be recognized directly in the computed tomogram. Their position can only be assumed relative to the adjacent organs.

Fasciae (61-14)
As in the retroperitoneal space, the fascial boundaries in the mediastinum determine the pathways of expansion in haemorrhagic-exudative processes. According to Marchand (19), the oesophagus and trachea are surrounded by a common, thin integument of loose connective tissue which is invested by the **perivisceral fascia**. This **perivisceral space** is a continuation of a cervical compartment formed by the pretracheal and buccopharyngeal fascia and containing the larynx, trachea and pharynx. It continues as a fissure along the bronchi and into the periphery of the lung and communicates with the subepicardial fatty tissue of the heart. The periaortic adventitia is connected to the perivisceral fascia by connective tissue.

The **prevertebral fascia**, which runs from the base of the skull to the sacrum, surrounds the paravertebral connective tissue. It is the first barrier to vertebral and paravertebral inflammatory processes and explains the tendency for them to spread craniocaudally.

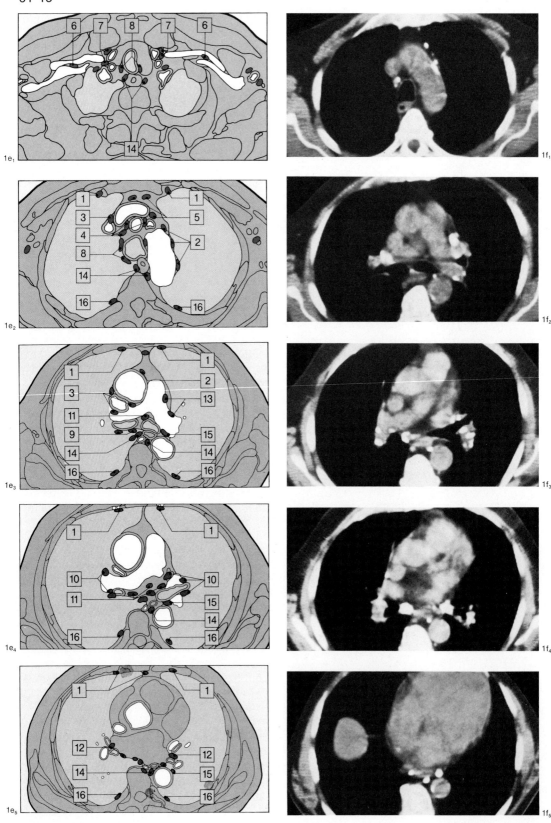

Lymph nodes (61-15)

Two separate groups of lymph nodes are found in the anterior mediastinum, the **sternal** (anterior parietal or mammary internal) group, which lies bilaterally behind the costal cartilage, and the **prevascular** (anterior mediastinal) group, which lies somewhat retrosternally (pericardially) but usually around the large vessels superior vena cava, anonymous vein and ascending aorta (including the left common carotid artery). In the posterior mediastinum, the **intercostal** group lies against the heads of the ribs and communicates with the **posterior mediastinal** group, which runs along the lower oesophagus and the descending aorta. In the mid-mediastinum, the parietal lymph nodes, which are situated at the lower circumference of the pericardium and alongside the pulmonary ligaments, are numerically far inferior to the visceral lymph nodes. Depending on their position, the latter are known as the **tracheobronchial, bifurcation (carinal) and bronchopulmonary groups**. Only a few **paratracheal** lymph nodes are found in front of the trachea, most of them being situated on the right side. They drain the bifurcation and, in addition, the bronchopulmonary groups.

In analogy to the anatomical situation in the retroperitoneal space (86-15), lymph nodes can be demonstrated from a diameter of 0.5–1 cm if favourable scanning conditions, i. e. the interposition of adequate fatty tissue, are present. This means that normal-sized – usually 0.3–0.6 cm – mediastinal lymph nodes cannot be depicted in the computed tomogram. The trachea, ascending and descending aorta, the superior vena cava, the oesophagus and the azygos vein offer readily identifiable axial boundary surfaces (Fig. 61-1a). Consequently, slight enlargement of lymph nodes is easily demonstrable if they are situated as follows: paratracheally (particularly at the right dorsolateral circumference), paracavially, preaortically (ascending aorta, aortic arch), perioesophageally, paraaortically (descending aorta), paravertebrally and retrosternally. The boundary surfaces of the main bronchi, pulmonary cone and the central pulmonary and brachiocephalic veins offer poor or unfavourable scanning conditions. Between these structures are horizontal or oblique fissures which can be clearly depicted by computerized tomography only if great amounts of fat are interposed. This applies in particular to the boundary surfaces pulmonary vein/bronchus, bronchus/pulmonary artery, tracheal bifurcation/left atrium and pulmonary trunk/aortic arch. The (intramediastinal) aortopulmonary window can consequently be assessed by computerized tomography only when it is situated at a reasonable distance ($\geq$ 1.5–2 cm) from the pulmonary trunk. The acute-angled azygooesophageal recess becomes deformed by enlargement of bifurcation (subcarinal) lymph nodes.

The poor scanning conditions for the blood vessels emerging at the hilum mean that the recognition of bronchopulmonary lymph node enlargement is frequently more difficult in the computed tomogram than in standard X-ray films, in which the spatial course of the ramifying vessels is easier to follow. For example, an increase in calibre of the pulmonary artery can be due to the rigid slice geometry of the computed tomogram or be caused by a moderately enlarged lymph node. A guided **bolus injection**, which clearly opacifies the vascular lumen, is frequently required for differentiation.

Fig. 61-1e, f: **Mediastinal lymph nodes.**
1e: Topography in the transverse section (cf. Fig. 61-1b)
1f: Calcified lymph nodes in the computed tomogram

Key

Anterior mediastinum
1 **Sternal** (mammary) **lymph nodes**
2–7 **Prevascular lymph nodes**
 2 Periaortic lymph nodes
 3 Pericaval lymph nodes
 4 Lnn. trunci brachiocephalici
 5 Lnn. v. anonymae
 6 Lnn. v. subclaviae
 7 Lnn. v. jugularis internae

Middle mediastinum
 8 Paratracheal lymph nodes
 9 Tracheobronchial lymph nodes
 10 Bronchopulmonary lymph nodes
 11 Bifurcation (carinal) lymph nodes
 12 Lnn. v. pulmonalis
 13 Lnn. ducti Botalli

Posterior mediastinum
 14 Paraoesophageal lymph nodes
 15 Paraortic lymph nodes
 16 Intercostal lymph nodes

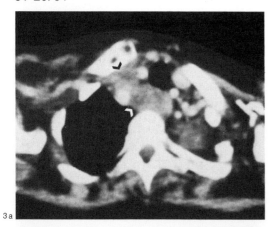

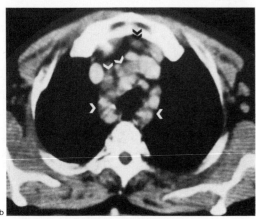

Fig. 61-3 a–d: **Malignant lymphomas.**
3a: Demonstration of structureless soft tissue masses retrotracheal and retroclavicular right (>). Displacement of the cervical soft tissues to the left.
3b: Demonstration of paratracheal lymph node enlargement, diameter of 2–3 cm bilaterally (>). Retrosternal lymphomas (≫) and lymphomas of the prevascular lymph node group.
3c: Extensive, structureless soft-tissue masses in front of the aortic arch and right retrocaval-paratracheal with displacement of the veins in a ventral direction. Contrast medium administration leads to unequivocal identification of mediastinal vessels.

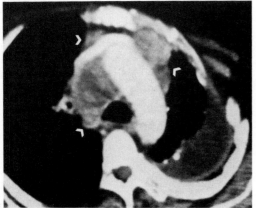

Examination technique (61-20)

● Preparation of the patient is unnecessary. A fasting state is advisable in case contrast medium administration is necessary.

● **Scanning** with slice thicknesses of 8–10 mm.
In localized processes adjacent slice sequence. In extensive processes (including systemic diseases) slice interval 20 mm.

● **Scanning area:** Dependent on the problem and clinical finding.

● **Intravenous contrast medium administration.** As an infusion (4-36) in non-circumscribed processes (pre-contrast scan unnecessary in the search for enlarged lymph nodes).

Guided bolus injection (4-32) in localized processes for further differentiation (pre-contrast scan essential).

Lymph node enlargements (61-30)

Malignant lymphomas (61-31)

Hodgkin's disease represents the largest group of malignant lymphomas, accounting for 53% of cases confirmed by biopsy. The age distribution of the morbidity is bimodal with an initial peak in the 3rd and a second in the 6th–8th decade of life. An intracanalicular form of dissemination from one lymph node to the next is typical. Extranodal invasion of the adjacent tissue is demonstrable in up to 15% of the reported cases, and haematogenous dissemination in the later course of the disease in 5–10%.

Non-Hodgkin's lymphomas represent a histologically heterogeneous group which is classified in different ways. Lukes considers malignant lymphomas and leukaemias to be different forms of the same disease (38). With the exception of lymphatic lymphoblastomas, non-Hodgkin's lymphomas occur most frequently in the 6th and 7th decades of life. The disease spreads in the same way as Hodgkin's disease. In contradistinction to the latter, however, there is a different pattern of involvement and a higher proportion of extranodal involvement and of the occurrence of a dissemination stage at the start of the disease.

Non-Hodgkin's lymphomas exhibit thoracic manifestation – usually as part of a generalized disease, but in more than 50% of cases in the late stage. Rosenberg reports primary disease of mediastinal lymph nodes in 3% of cases, and secondary disease of the lungs without thoracic lymph node involvement in 4.8 % (14). Not infrequently, the mediastinum escapes involvement during dissemination of the disease (mediastinal skip). Mediastinal and hilar lymphomas are found in about 25 % of patients with leukaemic forms – mainly the lymphocytic form. Overall, there are no fundamental differences between Hodgkin's disease and non-Hodgkin's lymphomas which would be of any material assistance in the differential diagnosis of the pattern of mediastinal involvement. Because of the contagious form of dissemination of the disease, however, the preferred primary involvement of the cervical lymph nodes in Hodgkin's disease leads to more frequent involvement of the anterosuperior mediastinum including the paratracheal chain of lymph nodes right, the anatomical number of which is greater than elsewhere. Primary manifestation of Hodgkin's disease in the mediastinum is rare (accounting for 5–7% of reported cases), and pulmonary involvement without thoracic lymphadenopathy is the exception. Pulmonary involvement – usually in the sense of direct hilofugal dissemination – in the course of the disease can be demonstrated in less than 30 % of cases.

● **CT**

Enlarged lymph nodes appear in the computed tomogram as nodular or structureless zones of soft-tissue density. The paratracheal, paravertebral, retrocrural (level of the diaphragm), pericaval, preaortic and retrosternal lymph node chains can be demonstrated particularly sensitively (61-15). In the upper thoracic aperture, ectatic vessels, particularly veins, and the thyroid lobe must be differentiated by exact comparison of the slices – possibly following administration of contrast medium. Calcification of lymph nodes is rare and occurs only in chronic forms, usually as a consequence of irradiation. Displacement of the trachea, bronchi and vessels is not infrequent in extensive lesions.

The **radiodensity** of lymphomas is within or slightly below the range of that of soft tissue. Cystic or necrotic areas must be regarded as a particular pathological constellation (61-42). Enhancement following the rapid injection of contrast medium is very limited because of the poor vascularity of the lymphomas.

Differential diagnosis
Primary mediastinal neoplasias should be

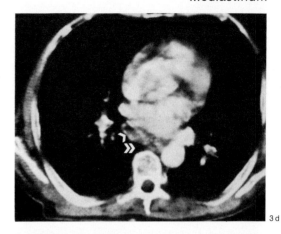

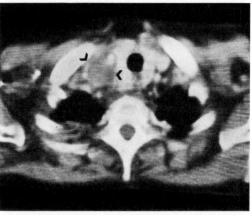

Fig. 61-3 d: **Malignant lymphomas** (cont.).
3 d: Demonstration of soft-tissue masses behind the left atrium with deformation of the azygo-oesophageal recess (≫).

Fig. 61-3 e, f: **Lymph node metastases** (from a bronchial carcinoma).
3 e: Soft-tissue mass right next to the thyroid, which enhances markedly following administration of contrast medium, enlargement of the internal jugular group of lymph nodes (><).
3 f: Soft-tissue mass right paratracheal with ventral displacement of the brachiocephalic vessels.

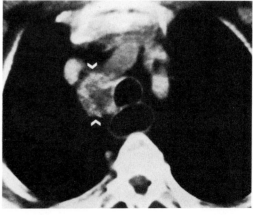

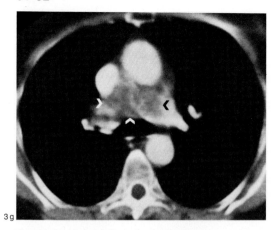

Fig. 61-3g–i: **Lymph node metastases.**

3g: Soft-tissue structures above the pulmonary outflow tract which demarcate clearly only after contrast medium administration (>). Metastases from an oropharyngeal carcinoma.

3h, i: Regional metastases from a bronchial carcinoma. Subcarinal group of lymph nodes with deformation of the azygooesophageal recess. They proceed in a caudal direction as a smoothly bordered zone. The hypodensity is a sign of necrobiotic processes (squamous cell carcinoma).

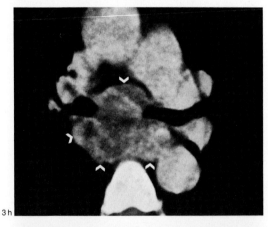

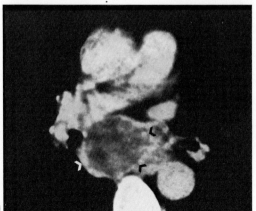

considered in solitary masses of soft-tissue density (Fig. 61-4a).

Lymph node metastases (61-32)
The form of lymphatic dissemination of a malignant lesion is determined by the position of and the drainage of lymph from the organ concerned. Enlarged lymph nodes are caused by metastases from an intrathoracic or extrathoracic tumour in only 20% of cases (14). The most common cause is bronchial carcinoma which, in the late stage, produces lymph node metastases in more than 80% of cases, followed by malignant lesions of the gastrointestinal tract (oesophagus, stomach, pancreas), mammary glands, kidneys, testes, prostate, thyroid and larynx. Lymph node involvement in bronchial carcinoma is asymmetrical – due to crossed lymphatic channels, the right bronchotracheal chain of lymph nodes is affected even when the tumour is localized on the left (Rouvière). In the case of lymphatic dissemination, extrathoracic tumours frequently spread by continuation to the mediastinal groups, and metastases of the retroperitoneal and cervical lymph nodes are then demonstrable. Carcinomatous lymphangitis of the lungs is found in carcinoma of the breasts, stomach, pancreas, thyroid and larynx, and is usually accompanied by hilar lymphadenopathy. In comparison to carcinomas, sarcomas rarely metastasize to the mediastinum via the lymphatic route.

● **CT**
Like malignant lymphomas, metastatic lymph node enlargements appear in the computed tomogram as soft-tissue structures. However, dissemination is not as great as with malignant lymphomas and early symptoms are caused even on slight enlargement of the lymph nodes due to invasion of the nerves and vessels (recurrent paresis). In keeping with the drainage zones, attention must be paid to the sternal groups of lymph nodes in mammary carcinoma, to the posterior (mediastinal) groups in tumours of the gastrointestinal tract, kidneys, testes and prostate and to the lymph node groups of the upper mediastinum in carcinoma of the larynx and thyroid. The intravenous administration of contrast medium may be necessary in the individual case for better differentiation from vessels. Unless the oesophagus is filled with air, the oral administration of diluted Gastrografin or insertion of a polyethylene tube is recommended for better demarcation.

Primary tumours of the anterior mediastinum (61-40)

Mesenchymal tumours (61-41)
Mesenchymal tumours are encountered in all three spaces of the mediastinum, but are found most frequently in the anterior compartment.

Lipomas and **lipomatosis**, the overall incidence of which is low, are generally more pronounced on one side of the mediastinum. They can leave the mediastinal cavity caudalward and cranialward, thereby assuming an hourglass shape. On the other hand, omental fatty tissue can herniate into the lower posterior mediastinum (267). Because of their soft consistency, lipomas do not lead to signs of displacement of the adjacent organs and are frequently a chance clinical finding. Lipomatosis can also be caused iatrogenically by corticoid therapy.

Lipo-(fibro-) sarcomas, which are extremely rare, are usually localized in the posterior mediastinum, where they can cause considerable displacement of the adjacent organs (265).

Fibromas do not give rise to clinical complaints until they have achieved a considerable size. Concomitant pleural effusion is occasionally demonstrated in **fibrosarcomas**, which tend to lie in the posterior mediastinum, and in fibromas.

Haemangiomas (cavernous haemangioma, haemangioendothelioma, haemangiosarcoma) are rare neoplasms and are localized in the anterior mediastinum in two thirds of cases. They are of variable shape, surrounded by a connective-tissue capsule and can occur in multiples. Phleboliths are frequently found within the tumours.

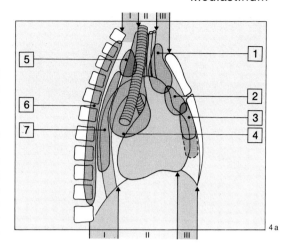

I = posterior mediastinum
II = middle mediastinum
III = anterior mediastinum

Fig. 61-4 a–c: Primary tumours of the mediastinum.

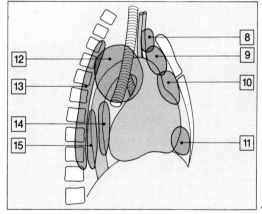

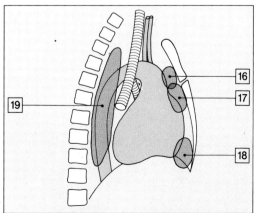

Key
4a: Solid lesions.
1. Retrosternal goitre
2. Thymoma, thyroid adenoma, haemangioma (lymphogranuloma)
3. Teratoma, disgerminoma (fibroma)
4. Primary malignant lymphomas
5. Retrotracheal goitre
6. Neurogenic tumours
7. Oesophageal tumours, fibrosarcomas

4b: Cystic lesions.
8. Thyroid cysts
9. Thymus cysts
10. Cystic teratomas
11. Mesothelioma (lymphangioma)
12. Bronchogenic cyst
13. Meningoceles
14. Neuroenteral cysts
15. Lymphangiomas

4c: Lipoid lesions
16. Thymus lipoma
17. Dermoid cysts
18. Lipoma
19. Liposarcoma

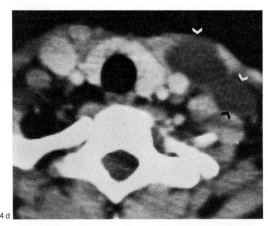

Fig. 61-4 d: **Lymphangioma.** Demonstration of cystic formation (>) in the upper thoracic aperture left with moderate displacement of adjacent organs.

Fig. 61-4 e, f: **Lipoid tumours.**
4 e: Herniation of retroperitoneal fatty tissue through the diaphragm right dorsal (>). »Lipoma of the diaphragm«.
4 f: Adipose body in the right pericardiophrenic angle simulating cardiomegaly at X-ray.

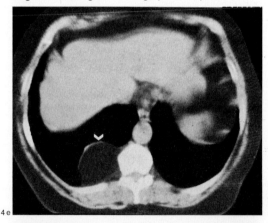

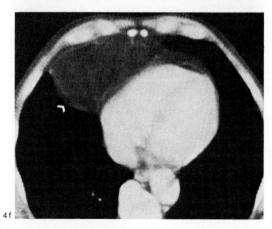

Lymphangiomas (hygromas) occur mainly in childhood. They can extend as far as the neck region, cause considerable signs of displacement and occur as cavernous or cystic tumours. Those occurring in adulthood are usually smooth, multichambered, soft masses. They are localized in the lower anterior mediastinum and, unless complicated by chylothorax, cause no symptoms.

- **CT**

Lipomas and lipomatosis can be unequivocally identified by their radiodensity (−80 to −100 HU) (271, 282). Malignancy can be suspected when a fat-containing neoplasm is found in the posterior mediastinum and the density values are distinctly increased in comparison to normal fatty tissue (265) − even if lymph node metastases cannot yet be recognized. Fibromas cannot be differentiated from other non-cystic masses and should be considered in the differential diagnosis of the more frequently occurring thymomas, teratomas and tumours of the (para-)thyroid. Phleboliths within the masses may be an indication of a haemangioma. A guided bolus injection reveals the high vascularity of this tumour. Lymphangiomas and hygromas display the criteria of a water-filled mass and can be diagnostically demarcated from gastroenteral and oesophageal cysts (61-62) by virtue of their position.

Thymomas (61-42)
Thymomas can occur at any age, but the highest incidence is in the fourth decade of life. They do not usually grow as big as teratomas. The malignant form, which is marked by high invasiveness of the adjacent tissues, is about as frequent as the benign variant (14). Subpleural metastases are usually demonstrated, while haematogenic and lymph node metastasis is very rare. A thymoma is found in 15 % of patients with myasthenia gravis, while myasthenia gravis is found in 50 % of thymoma patients. Thymomas of the posterior mediastinum have also been described (14).

- **CT**

Computerized tomography reveals a roundish, oval, smoothly bordered or lobate mass which is usually situated at the junction of the heart and the major vessels or directly in front of the ascending aorta. Regardless of the histology, punctate calcifications arranged at the border of or diffusely within the tumour can be demonstrated in some cases. The density values lie within the solid range, although they can occasionally be in the water range or higher if cystic components (thymic cysts) are present. Since the capsule of the tumour can be fused with the pericardium and pleura, absence of the fat plane which demarcates the tumour from mediastinal structures does not signify tumour invasion (273). Invasion into the superior vena cava can only be clearly identified following contrast enhancement (290). An all-round poorly defined border – particularly at the margin of the pleura (286) – must be interpreted as a criterion of malignancy. Because of the great likelihood of malignant degeneration, a tentative diagnosis of thymoma is an indication for surgery, even if no signs of malignant growth are present.

A **thymolipoma** can display distinct connective-tissue areas, so the density values ($\sim$–30 HU) are increased in comparison to pure fatty tissue (265).

Thymic hyperplasia, which occurs preferentially in adolescence, must be demarcated as regards the differential diagnosis. It expands bilaterally in the anterosuperior mediastinum and can be identified in the computed tomogram as a corresponding zone of soft-tissue density.

Thymic persistence only rarely leads to large masses, the usual finding being small, retrosternal nodular structures occasionally interspersed with fat (293). Not infrequently, the thymus is the site of origin of **Hodgkin's disease**. Moderately large cysts within the mass are not considered unusual in this constellation (679).

Teratoid blastomas (61-43)

Teratoid blastomas are about as frequent as thymomas, accounting for 11–17 % of mediastinal masses. Malignancy is found in 25–30 % of cases. Cystic tumours are usually found to be benign, solid tumours to be malignant. While teratomas contain ectodermal, mesodermal and endodermal tissue components, dermoid cysts are of epidermal origin. The disease is found most frequently in teenagers, and calcifications are found in 50 % of the tumours (39).

● **CT**

The majority of teratomas and dermoid cysts are localized in the anterior mediastinum at the origin of the major vessels of the heart. They are rarely found in the posterior mediastinum. Lobate contours and solid tissue are more an indication of malignancy, while cystic, smoothly bordered and roundish masses

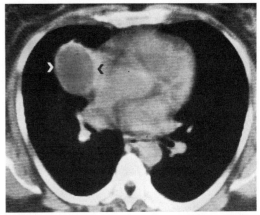

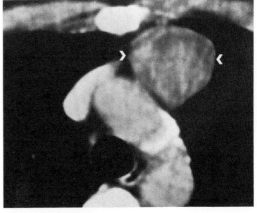

Fig. 61-4 g, h: **Thymoma.**
4 g: Cystic thymoma, the walls of which enhance clearly following contrast medium (><).
4 h: Solid thymoma. Only moderate enhancement of 20 HU following a bolus injection.

Fig. 61-**4 i: Teratoma** with calcifications and lipoid components (>) which demarcate more clearly following administration of contrast material.

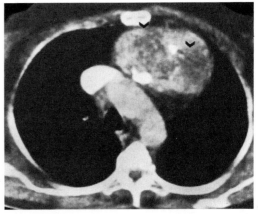

are a sign of benign growth. Both teratomas and dermoid cysts can calcify (usually shell-like). Calcium-containing appendages of the skin (bones, teeth) are pathognomonic for dermoid cysts. The signs of displacement increase with tumour growth (compression of the bronchi and superior vena cava [functional blockage]). Rapid expansion is a sign of malignancy, although haemorrhage into a cystic mass can also cause an increase of volume. Pulmonary and regional metastases are unequivocal signs of malignancy.

The **radiodensity** depends on the composition of the tumour tissue. In general, cystic components can be determined by the density value. Since haemorrhage can lead to an increase of density of the contents, contrast medium administration may be necessary to achieve unequivocal demarcation of the solid vascularized component of the tumour. Teratomas can contain fatty tissue components with negative density values which are not as low as those of pure fatty tissue (−80 to −100 HU). Dermoid cysts frequently consist of sebum-containing material with density values in the negative range. Fat-containing teratomas cannot be distinguished from thymic lipomas in the computed tomogram.

The differential diagnosis must take account of other masses of the anterior mediastinum, e.g. **thymic cysts** (61-42), **seminomas** and **choriocarcinomas** (293). A choriocarcinoma must be considered if clinical signs of feminization are present. It is marked by high invasiveness and a tendency to tumour necrosis, which can be demonstrated by computerized tomography.

Endothoracic goitre (61-44)

75–80% of endothoracic goitre originates from the lower poles of the thyroid lobes or isthmus and extends retrosternally in front of the trachea. The rest originates from the dorsal parts of the thyroid and extends behind the trachea or oesophagus, including the brachiocephalic vessels, into the posterior, usually right-sided mediastinum. The dystopic nodes are surrounded by a firm capsule and receive their blood via a cord communicating with the thyroid. **Dystopic** mediastinal goitre is rare and manifests itself early by signs of displacement. The incorporation of radionuclides in the region of the mass and an empty thyroid bed in the neck region confirm the diagnosis.

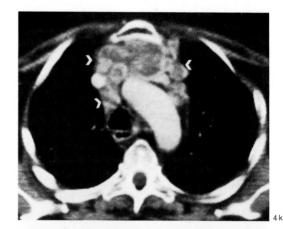

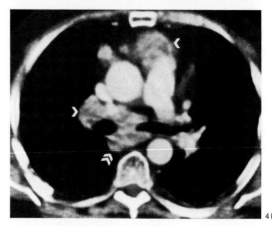

Fig. 61-**4 k, l: Teratoid blastomas.**
4 k: Metastatic teratoma with numerous mediastinal metastases displaying hypodensity due to lipoid tissue components. Demonstration of subcarinal and tracheobronchial lymphomas (k_2 ≫).

4 l: Cystic teratocarcinoma. Inhomogeneous density pattern due to solid tissue components. Displacement of the aorta and pulmonary trunk (≫) by the extensive mass.

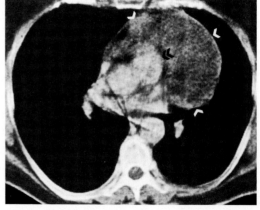

Mediastinum

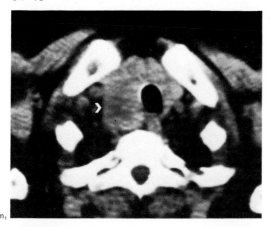

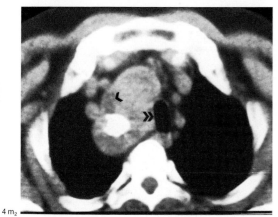

Fig. 61-4 m, n: **Tumour of the thyroid.**

4 m: Intrathoracic goitre originating from the right lobe of the thyroid (m_1 >). The goitre exhibits different components (m_2 >) and calcifications as a sign of regressive changes. Mainly paratracheal growth with impression of the trachea from the right (m_2 ≫).

4 n: Carcinoma of the thyroid with intrathoracic expansion. Retrotracheal lesion with tissue components of varying density (≫).

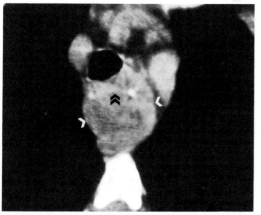

- **CT**

Depending on its seat, the thyroid mass displaces and compresses the trachea beneath the thoracic aperture. The brachiocephalic vessels are displaced sidewards. The veins can appear dilated due to compression of the superior vena cava. Regressive changes are usual, so that shell-like calcifications can frequently be demonstrated. Cystic changes are encountered less frequently. Since incorporation of radionuclides in the dystopic intrathoracic thyroid lobe takes place only in a minority, CT clarification of the relationship between the thyroid and the mass is particularly important. The diagnosis of endothoracic or cervicothoracic goitre is highly probable if a communicating cord can be demonstrated. A slightly increased tissue density ($\sim$ 75 HU) in the plain scan in comparison to the surrounding vessels is attributed to the iodine content of the thyroid tissue (272).

Parathyroid tumours (61-45)

Neoplasms of the parathyroid are usually hormonally active, so the clinically manifest hyperparathyroidism leaves no doubt as to its existence. After the thyroid region, the upper and middle anterior mediastinum is the most frequent location of the adenoma, which is a rare occurrence in comparison to the other mediastinal tumours.

- **CT**

The aim of computerized tomography is to locate a smoothly bordered, very small mass with a diameter of about 0.5–2 cm in the anterior mediastinum (277). The adenoma rarely calcifies. In our own experience, the performance of thoracotomy to locate the mass has very little chance of success where the CT finding is negative. The administration of contrast medium and the great expense of a narrow slice sequence (0.5 to 1 cm interval) are therefore warranted. In an extensive adenoma, computerized tomography determines only the size and positional relationship to the vicinity.

Primary tumours of the middle mediastinum (61-50)

Tumours of the trachea (61-51)
Myelomas and carcinomas rarely develop in the trachea. Expansion of the carcinoma takes place into the paratracheal space with invasion of the regional lymph nodes. Constriction and displacement of the trachea depend on the extent of the process. Differentiation from metastasizing bronchial carcinoma is possible with computerized tomography only in the early stage.

Bronchogenic cysts (61-52)
Most bronchogenic cysts are situated in the vicinity of the tracheobronchial angle; only a few are found in the posterior mediastinum. Even small cysts can cause signs of tracheobronchial obstruction, particularly in childhood. Larger masses with no pronounced clinical symptoms are usually found by chance.

● CT

The typical criteria of a cyst may be less distinct because of thickening of the contents (viscid, usually brownish secretion), since the density values are then above those of water. If necessary, contrast medium must therefore be administered to achieve differentiation from a solid, vascularized lesion.

Pleuropericardial (mesothelial) cysts (61-53)
Pleuropericardial cysts are usually localized in the right anterior cardiophrenic angle, but can also be found on the left side in the hilar region and the anterior mediastinum. They display a diameter of 3–8 cm and, but rarely, more than 13 cm.

● CT

The mass appears in the computed tomogram as a thin-walled cyst. The density lies within the range of that of water (spring water cyst: −5 to +25 HU [290]). An accumulation of fat, which can cause a similar radiological shadow, can be reliably demarcated by virtue of its typical density values (287). The pericardium is clearly recognizable in the majority of cases, particularly in adipose patients. Fibrous opacification within the accumulation of fat is indicative of the rare condition of pericardial liponecrosis, which progresses to fibrosis following an episode of inflammation.

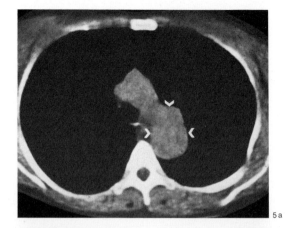

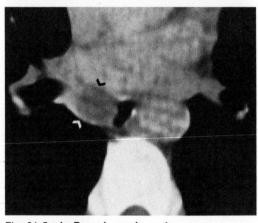

Fig. 61-5a, b: **Bronchogenic cysts.**
5a: Oval mass at the dorsal part of the aortic arch with density values of about 55 HU. No enhancement after administration of contrast medium. Histologically, gelatinoid protein-rich contents.
5b: Small hypodensity 2 cm in diameter at the level of the tracheal fork.

Fig. 61-5c: **Neurogenic cyst.** Retrocardial hypodense lesion with density values of 19 HU.

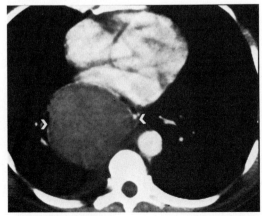

Primary tumours of the posterior mediastinum (61-60)

About 30% of tumours in the posterior mediastinal space are malignant (14). Lymphomas cf. 61-31 and 61-32.

Solid neurogenic tumours (61-61)

Ganglioneuromas and neuroblastomas (sympathicoblastomas) are forms of tumour which occur in early childhood, while neurofibromas and neurinomas are found primarily in young adults. Phaeochromocytomas and paragangliomas are extremely rare. With the exception of the paraganglioma, all neurogenic tumours are found exclusively in the posterior mediastinum. Calcifications, the overall incidence of which is very low, occur mainly in neuroblastomas and ganglioneuromas.

● **CT**

The strict paravertebral localization is readily demonstrable in the majority of cases. Dilation of the intervertebral foramina can usually only be depicted with an accurate scanning technique and is frequently more readily demonstrable in a spot X-ray film. Widening of the osseous vertebral canal suggests intraspinal genesis, which then requires further clarification. Diffuse bone destruction, which is an indication of malignancy, must be demarcated from usurption of the vertebral bodies and ribs, which can be encountered both in malignant and in benign masses.

If a mediastinal mass is accompanied by clinical signs of hypertensive crises, the very rare phaeochromocytoma should be considered (82-42).

Cystic masses (61-62)

All cystic masses are very rare and, if at all, can only be differentiated from each other by secondary signs.

Meningoceles develop from unilateral or bilateral protrusion of the leptomeninx through the intervertebral foramina. They contain cerebrospinal fluid and can also occur in multiples. Dilation of the intervertebral foramina is usual, while usurption of the bone is rare.

Neuroenteric cysts consist histologically of neural and enteral elements and are frequently associated with congenital defects of the thoracic vertebral column. The smooth or lobate mass contains an aqueous fluid and can also display air if it communicates with the gastrointestinal tract. **Gastroenteral** and

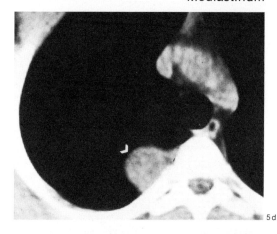

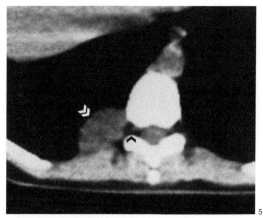

Fig. 61-5 d–f: Neurinomas.

5 d: Smoothly bordered lesion isodense with muscle tissue. Typical paravertebral localization.

5 e: Similar finding, slightly hypodense compared to muscle tissue. No dilation of the intervertebral foramen (>) or intraspinal expansion was demonstrable.

5 f: Paraganglioma of the vagus nerve. Demonstration of a smoothly bordered lesion left hilar with density values of 18 HU and no distinct enhancement.

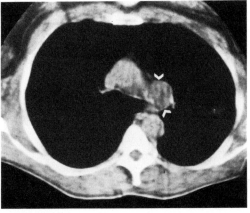

oesophageal cysts, which can only be differentiated from each other by the histology, differ from bronchogenic cysts by virtue of their tendency to be found in a paravertebral position, where **thoracic duct cysts** are also found preferentially.

● CT

In general, only the cystic nature of the mass can be determined. Changes of the vertebral column and ribs are additional diagnostic indications. Pancreatogenic pseudocysts which have erupted from the retroperitoneal cavity into the lower posterior mediastinum must be considered in the differential diagnosis (73-32).

Tumours of the oesophagus (61-63)

Oesophageal tumours can only be demonstrated following administration of a barium meal. In the case of malignant growth, a knowledge of the extent of the tumour is important for planning the therapeutic procedure. Oesophageal carcinomas spread early by invasion of the vicinity via numerous lymphatic channels or submucosally. The close topographic relationship to the bronchus, trachea, pericardium and lung results in direct, unhindered infiltration of these structures.

● CT

When it is surrounded by adequate mediastinal fatty tissue, the oesophagus is readily demonstrable in the plain computed tomogram as an air-filled annular figure of roundish soft-tissue structure with a diameter of 1–2 cm. The thickness of the oesophageal wall and any asymmetry can be demonstrated following opacification of the lumen with dilute Gastrografin solution. The relationship to the adjacent organs (bronchus, trachea, lung, pleura, pericardium and aorta) can be adequately evaluated. Unless irradiation or surgery has been performed, obliteration of the contours of the oesophagus should be interpreted as a sign of infiltration. The diagnosis can be restricted or even rendered impossible by the absence of adequate mediastinal fatty tissue, e. g. in cachectic patients. In some cases,

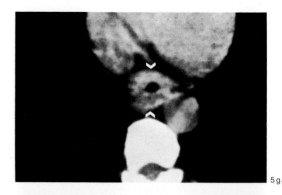

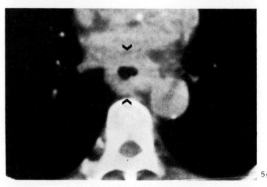

Fig. 61-**5 g, h: Oesophageal carcinoma.**
5 g: Thickened oesophageal wall with smooth delimitation from the surrounding tissue, i.e. with no signs of infiltration.

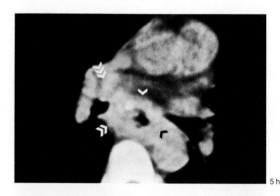

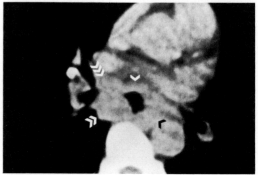

5 h: Irregularly demarcated external contours of the oesophagus (>) and filling of the azygooesophageal recess (≫) as a sign of mediastinal tumour invasion and regional lymphomas (⋙).

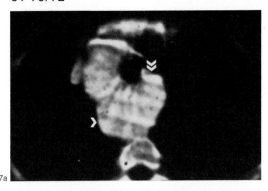

Fig. 61-7a: **Incomplete vascular ring** in dextrodescending aorta (>) and rudimentary left aortic arch (≫).

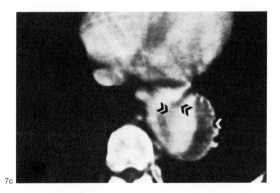

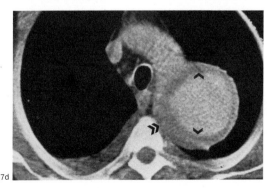

changing the position of the patient can provide information about the mobility of the oesophagus, which is abolished by infiltration of the vicinity. Special attention must be paid to regional lymph node enlargement, particularly in the retrocrural space (86-12) of the diaphragm (276).

Vascular processes (61-70)

Aorta (61-71)

A number of congenital malformations (722) of the aortic arch can be seen as masses in the standard chest film. They are usually discovered in the first year of life. The vascular ring formed from the persisting aortic arches and the left ductus arteriosus is frequently a chance finding. This anomaly can easily be confirmed by computerized tomography following contrast medium administration.

Aneurysms of the thoracic aorta (61-72)

Aneurysms can be subdivided etiologically into arteriosclerotic, syphilitic, traumatic, dissecting (following medial necrosis) and mycotic forms. Calcifications within an aneurysm are a frequent finding. Supravalvular, lamellar incorporation of calcium in the ascending region is primarily an indication of syphilitic genesis. Traumatic aneurysms usually develop in the region of the arch beyond the origin of the subclavian artery. Dissecting aneurysms are encountered mainly in patients with Marfan's syndrome (cystic degeneration of the media), in aortic coarctation, hypertension and during pregnancy.

● **CT**

The contours and the enlarged diameter of the aorta can be readily and unequivocally evaluated in the region of the ascending and descending aorta. The thrombotic parts of the aneurysm frequently contrast with the vascular lumen even in the plain scan, although administration of contrast medium leads to un-

Fig. 61-7b–d: **Aneurysms.**

7b: Dissecting aneurysm at the level of the aortic arch. Detached intima membrane (≫).

7c: Dissecting aneurysm with floating intima membrane (≫). Demonstration of thrombotic deposits at the left lateral aortic wall (>).

7d: Aneurysm (true) in the region of the aortic arch. The aneurysm and thrombotic deposits can be seen even in the plain scan (≫).

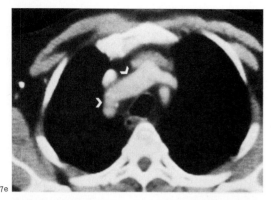

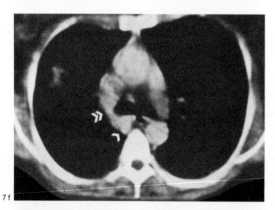

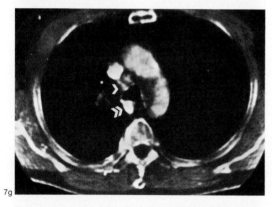

Fig. 61-7 e: **Aneurysm of the brachiocephalic trunk.** Distinct dilation of the trunk (>), causing dilation of the mediastinum in the standard chest film.

Fig. 61-7 f: **Azygos vein continuation syndrome.** Large-calibre azygos vein (>) right paravertebral and dilated azygos vein arch (≫). The intrahepatic segment of the vena cava is missing.

Fig. 61-7 g: **Collateral circulation** via the azygos vein in the superior vena cava occlusion syndrome caused by bronchial carcinoma. Drainage into the superior vena cava is only partial due to enlarged azygos vein lymph nodes (>). The reversal of flow within the dilated azygos vein (≫) can also be recognized by opacification of the retrocardial sections.

equivocal identification of the lumen. Differentiation of a solid tumour invading the aortic arch from a thrombotic aneurysm is not always possible, particularly when the tumour grows around the aortic arch like a cuff.

In the case of dissection, contrast enhancement leads to identification of the detached intima, which demarcates the false lumen as a sickle-shaped figure in the transversal plane. If the space of dissection is blocked by (partial) thrombosis, the latter opacifies at a later stage (702). The density values above the two enhanced lumina are, however, usually the same. The haemodynamics and direction of flow in the dissection space have not yet been demonstrated by computerized tomography. The left brachiocephalic vein can lie against a high aortic arch in such a way as to create the impression of a dissecting aneurysm (723). This possibility of deception can be ruled out by careful analysis of the image. (A markedly floating intimal membrane can escape CT demonstration if scanners with a scanning speed of 20 seconds are used [personal observation].)

Brachiocephalic trunk (61-73)
Right-sided dilation of the upper mediastinum is found in older patients with arteriosclerosis and hypertension. The cause is elongation with tortuosity or, but less frequently, an aneurysm of the brachiocephalic trunk. Computerized tomography can distinguish between the two in doubtful cases.

Azygous vein (61-74)
Dilation of the azygos vein, which is recognizable in the general film of the thorax, is usually the expression of increased central venous pressure before the right atrium. In occlusion of the superior and inferior vena cava and portal vein and in absent development of the inferior vena cava, the azygos vein becomes part of an extensive collateral circulation with corresponding enlargement of its calibre.

● **CT**
Frequently, computerized tomography reveals the cause of the obstruction of the superior vena cava, permits assessment of the calibre of the azygos vein at the level of the diaphragm and demonstrates the absence of the inferior vena cava or the cause of its occlusion.

Mediastinum

Inflammations of the mediastinum (61-80)

Acute mediastinitis (61-81)

Acute mediastinitis occurs most frequently as a sequel of an external trauma or following perforation of the mediastinal organs (oesophagus, trachea), and less frequently following purulent processes of the pharynx and neck, which spread caudalward in the fascial spaces. Inflammatory processes of the pleura and lung spread at a later stage directly to the mediastinum (depending on the severity of the disorder) (7). The exudation can give rise to phlegmonous permeation of the mediastinal fissures or (less frequently) develop into abscesses which can penetrate into adjacent cavities (oesophagus, bronchus, pleural cavity).

● **CT**

Mediastinal exudate appears in the computed tomogram as an increase of density of the fatty tissue planes. In the case of thin patients, attention must be paid to the distance between the vessels, which increases with increasing exudation. The incorporation of air can be a sign of a perforation or of gas-forming bacteria. Local accumulations of fluid or cystoid formations must be interpreted as abscesses in association with the serious clinical picture (radiodensity 3-53). Varying degrees of pleural effusion are present even in the early stage of mediastinitis. The administration of contrast medium facilitates demarcation of the masked mediastinal structures and can demonstrate (hypervascularized) granulation tissue, e. g. around abscesses.

Chronic mediastinitis (61-82)

The etiology of chronic mediastinitis is heterogeneous and partly unclarified. In the majority of cases it is of infectious origin (tuberculosis, mycoses, histoplasmosis, actinomycosis, syphilis) and is also known histologically as **granulomatous mediastinitis.** Tuberculous mediastinitis is accompanied by lymph node swelling which can be very pronounced in childhood and tends to produce signs of compression. Lymphomas can liquefy and penetrate the respiratory tract. A subacute clinical course is usually observed. Lymph node enlargement in adults is only moderate. In the final stage specific, non-specific inflammations (61-81) and organizing haematomas culminate in the picture of **sclerosing (fibrotic) mediastinitis.** The presence of **idiopathic fibrotic mediastinitis** can

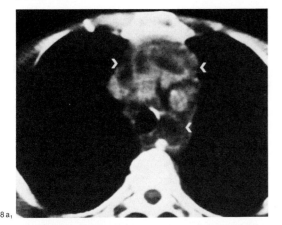
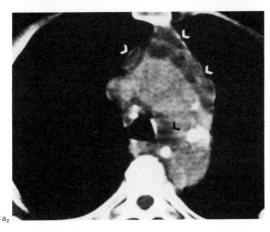

Fig. 61-**8a**: **Acute mediastinitis** due to phlegmonous expansion of a parotid abscess. Demonstration of numerous hypodense, ring-shaped zones paratracheal and in the anterior mediastinum with density values of 13–20 HU. Following administration of contrast material, enhancement of the annular figures as a sign of septation (abscess formation).

Fig. 61-**8b**: **Mediastinal abscess** consequent to phlegmon of the floor of the mouth. Lesion right paratracheal and retrotracheal with density values of 25 HU and incorporation of gas (≫).

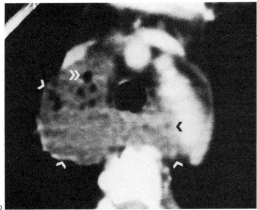

be assumed if retroperitoneal fibrosis (86-40), Riedel's struma or an orbital pseudotumour (51-64) is demonstrated at the same time. Almost without exception, the upper mediastinum — and particularly the paratracheal, carinal and hilar regions — is affected in chronic mediastinitis. Calcification is comparatively rare. The patho-anatomical appearance of sclerosing fibrosis is that of a tough connective-tissue plate walling-in the vessels, trachea and oesophagus. The vena cava occlusion syndrome has been described in more than 10 % of cases of chronic mediastinitis, but is encountered much more frequently in neoplastic processes of the mediastinum.

● CT

In chronic mediastinitis, computerized tomography reveals lymph node enlargement which cannot be differentiated from that of other etiology (61-31, 61-32). Although liquefaction appearing as hypodense, unenhanceable areas is also found in extensive metastases (86-52), it must be regarded primarily as a specific sign in younger patients. The distribution of the affected groups of lymph nodes (see above) should be considered in the diagnosis. Sclerosing mediastinitis appears as a zone of soft-tissue density surrounding the vessels, trachea and oesophagus, causing varying degrees of constriction and masking the mediastinal layers of fat. In the vena cava occlusion syndrome, the extent of the thrombosis and that of the collateral circulation via the azygos system can be assessed by computerized tomography following administration of contrast medium.

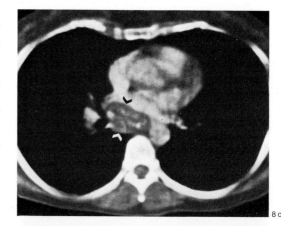

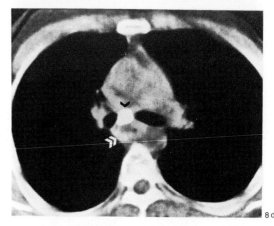

Fig. 61-8 c, d: **Chronic mediastinitis.**

8 c: Lymph node tuberculosis with enlargement mainly of the retrocardial and subcarinal lymph nodes, which demarcate clearly following contrast medium administration (>). Regression of this lesion after tuberculostatic therapy.

8 d: Sclerotic mediastinitis after tuberculosis. Demonstration of calcified lymph nodes (>) and deformation of the azygooesophageal recess by soft-tissue structures (≫). Oesophagography reveals a 7-cm long stenosis in this region with no mucosal changes.

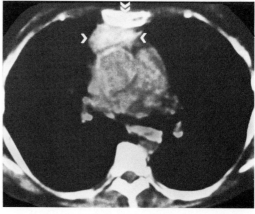

Fig. 61-9a: **Haematoma.** Retrosternal lesion, hyperdense in comparison to the muscle tissue and the heart. Status after sterneotomy for heart surgery (≫).

Injuries of the mediastinum (61-90)

Pneumomediastinum
(mediastinal emphysema) (61-91)
Air enters the mediastinum via different routes. Its pathway of entry in spontaneous mediastinal emphysema is along the peribronchial fissures (61-11) via the pulmonary root following alveolar rupture. Injuries to the **oesophagus** and **tracheobronchial tree** permit air to enter the surrounding mediastinal connective tissue directly. Retroperitoneal and intraperitoneal accumulations of air and pneumothorax can lead to pneumomediastinum via various pathways.

● CT

Computed tomography is a very sensitive method of demonstrating air in the mediastinum because the image is free from overlying shadows and because the density values of air are greatly reduced. In inflammatory processes, the bacterial production of gas, which arises within the infected tissue, must be considered in the differential diagnosis (61-81).

Mediastinal haematomas (61-92)
Haemorrhage into the mediastinum is caused mainly by blunt or perforating traumas and less frequently by spontaneous rupture of an existing aneurysm. Blunt thoracic trauma can lead to injuries to the retrosternal brachiocephalic **veins** and thus to a haematoma in the anterior mediastinum. The incidence of rupture of the thoracic **aorta** is increasing – particularly in car accidents –, and the isthmus region is involved in up to 95% of cases (19). Since this section of the vessel lies within the pericardium, fatal cardiac tamponade is not a rare event. An aneurysm can form gradually if rupture of the wall is incomplete (**chronic aneurysm**). The taut, perivascular adventitia can arrest or prevent the fatal haemorrhage in a few cases. This then gives rise to a perivascular haematoma (**spurious aneurysm**) of varying size. The localization of haematomas following iatrogenic injuries (puncture, surgery) depends on the nature of the event.

● CT

Haematomas appear in the computed tomogram as masses which displace the mediastinal structures (trachea, oesophagus, vessels) to varying degrees. The fatty tissue layers are masked in diffuse mediastinal haematoma. The radiodensity depends on the age of the haematoma (3-52). Because of the lack of enhancement, a guided bolus injection permits differentiation of a haematoma from highly vascularized neoplasms. To be able to identify perivascular haematomas, the dose of contrast medium administered should be sufficient to achieve distinct demonstration of the vascular lumina.

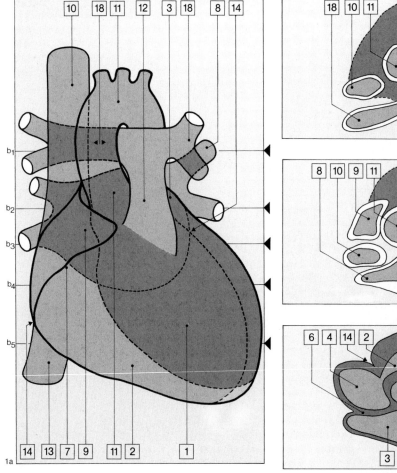
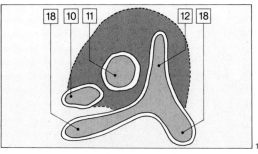
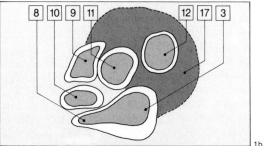
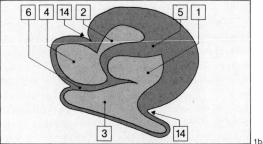
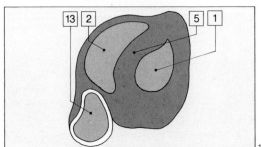

Fig. 62-1a–c Topography of the heart.

1a: Anterior view (diagram).

1b: Internal spaces and outflow tract in the transverse section. Cf. 1a for level of projection.

1c: Analogous sectional planes in the computed tomogram.

Key

1 Left ventricle
2 Right ventricle
3 Left atrium
4 Right atrium
5 Interventricular septum
6 Interatrial septum
7 Coronary sulcus
8 Pulmonary vein
9 Right auricular appendix
10 Superior vena cava
11 Ascending aorta
12 Pulmonary cone
13 Inferior vena cava
14 Atrioventricular plane
15 Mitral valve
16 Tricuspid valve
17 Transverse pericardial sinus
18 Pulmonary artery

Heart – pericardium (62-00)

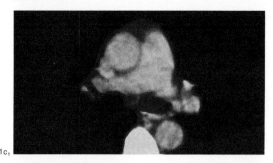

1c₁

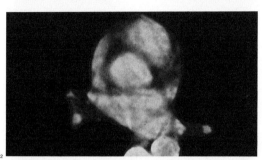

1c₂

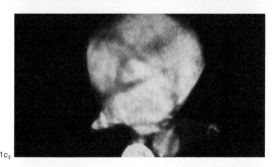

1c₃

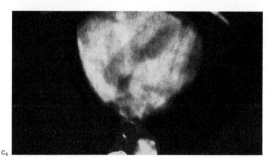

1c₄

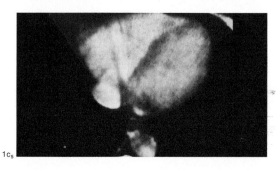

1c₅

Anatomy and imaging (62-10)

The long axis of the heart is aligned obliquely to the horizontal sectional plane. Following administration of an adequate dose of contrast medium and depending on the level of the slice, the individual ventricles of the heart can be depicted in the computed tomogram in varying size and positional relationship to each other. The right ventricle is depicted at its greatest extent in the caudal sections of the heart. The conically arched interventricular septum allows the left ventricle to be depicted at its largest diameter in a cranial direction. The wall of the left ventricle is clearly demonstrable in the computed tomogram and the papillary muscles can frequently be demarcated, while the thin walls of the right ventricle render the myocardium barely recognizable. The atria (including the right auricular appendage) can be reliably evaluated. The paraaortic sections of the coronary arteries, which run almost axially through the CT slice, can be demonstrated following adequate contrast enhancement (310, 312).

These imaging conditions obtain at scan times of 4–8 seconds. They are a result of a time-averaging process and can be improved by cardiac phase-controlled scanning (ECG triggering [311]), providing for more accurate measurement of the actual thicknesses of the myocardial wall in individual cardiac phases. Consequently, the end-systolic and end-diastolic volume and the determination of the ejection fraction also become accessible to computerized tomography. At the present time, computerized tomographic diagnosis is restricted to the following determinations: 1. the size of the heart, 2. the shape and thickness of the ventricles, 3. the relative position of the chambers and major vessels to each other and 4. the patency of the coronary arteries. These parameters permit a number of diagnoses to be made.

Examination technique (62-20)

- **Plain scan** to establish the position of the apex of the heart (or aortic root [62-50]).
- **Administration of contrast medium.**

Total dose: no more than 74 g iodine (i. e. a 200-ml bottle of Urografin 76%). Injection rate: within 30–60 seconds intravenous injection of 100 ml Urografin 76%. Subsequently about 30 ml/min depending on the density values in the monitor. Enhancement in the blood space should amount to at least 100 HU (310).

- **Scanning:** commencement 10 seconds after the start of injection with the fastest possible slice sequence. Slice interval 10 mm. Duration of examination no longer than 5 mins.

(Sequential technique with the shortest possible time intervals for demonstration of the aortocoronary bypass [62-50]).

Functional conditions of the heart (62-30)

Volume load (62-31)

Volume load on the left ventricle occurs as a result of regurgitation following valvular incompetence or a shunt. It is recognizable initially in the end-diastolic phase as ventricular enlargement which later on can also be demonstrated systolically in the presence of contractile insufficiency. Right-sided volume load is present primarily in a left-right shunt and can lead to considerable enlargement of the ventricles.

- **CT**

Depending on the extent, computerized tomography reveals distinct enlargement of the ventricles, the interventricular septum rotating to the right in left-sided volume load and to the left in right-sided volume load. The apex of the ventricle is usually rounded but, in general, there is no thickening of the ventricular walls.

Pressure load (62-32)

Pressure load on the left ventricle occurs in hypertension or cardiac abnormalities and leads to concentric hypertrophy. IHSS (idiopathic hypertrophic subvalvular aortic stenosis) is a special form in which asymmetrical hypertrophy of the septum is found. Right-sided pressure load occurs as a result of pulmonary hypertension (cor pulmonale, mitral stenosis) or as a consequence of pulmonic stenosis.

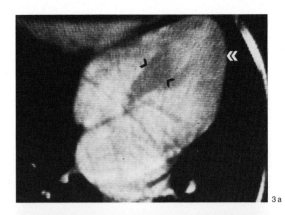

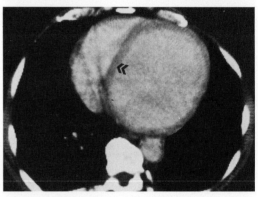

Fig. 62-3 a: **Pressure load.** Circumscribed thickening of the interventricular septum (><) is found in idiopathic hypertrophic subvalvular stenosis of the aorta. The hypertrophy of the rest of the wall of the left ventricle is seen as moderate thickening (≫).

Fig. 62-4 a: **Cardiomyopathy** (dilational form). Considerable enlargement of the left ventricle with rounding of the apex of the heart and protrusion of the interventricular septum to the right (≫).

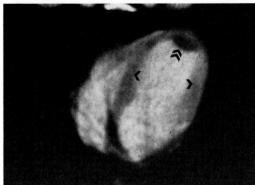

● CT

In hypertrophy of the left ventricle, computerized tomography reveals distinct thickening of the ventricular wall with greater prominence of the trabeculae. The interventricular septum can display moderate rotation to the right and a conical configuration. In IHSS it reveals a broad bulge of muscular tissue in the middle section of the interventricular septum (307). Frequently, muscular hypertrophy of the right ventricle is not clearly recognizable because of the partial volume effect and cardiac movement (310).

Cardiomyopathy (62-40)

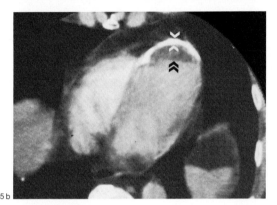

Metabolic and regressive changes usually lead to dilation of the ventricles or to thickening of the myocardium. In both cases the contractility is impaired, a condition which cannot be evaluated in the stationary computed tomogram. However, the dilation of the ventricles concerned and the thickening of the walls can be adequately demonstrated (310).

Coronary diseases (62-50)

Although computerized tomography cannot yet demonstrate a fresh **myocardial infarction** (297), it can depict its sequelae – the scar and the **aneurysm.** The signs in the computed tomogram are corresponding protrusion of the cardiac ventricle and circumscribed retraction of the wall, respectively.

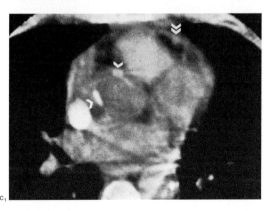

Following insertion of an **aortocoronary bypass,** its patency can be checked by computerized tomography. The transplant displays punctiform enhancement following a bolus injection, thus revealing the flow. However, the flow rate (flow volume) cannot be assessed.

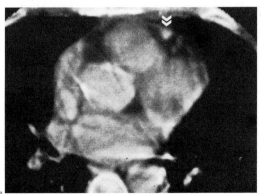

Fig. 62-5 a, b: **Aneurysms of the heart wall.**

5 a: Aneurysm of the heart wall ($\gg$) with a small thrombus at the apex of the heart, clearly visible because of its hypodensity.

5 b: Chronic aneurysm of the heart wall (apex of the heart) with calcifications ($><$) and thrombotic deposits ($\gg$).

Fig. 62-5 c: **Aortocoronary bypass.** The patency of the bypass can be demonstrated by computerized tomography following administration of contrast medium. Enhancement ($c_2 \gg$) of the transplant, which is of soft-tissue density in the plain scan ($c_1 \gg$), reveals the flow of blood. (Clips where the bypasses leave the aorta [$>$].)

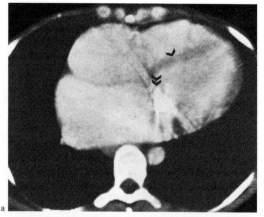

Fig. 62-**6 a**: **Stenosis of the mitral valve.** Considerable enlargement of the left atrium with a relatively small left ventricle. The interventricular septum (>) is rotated to the left. Calcifications of the mitral valve (≫).

Fig. 62-**7 a**: **Atrial thrombus** in stenosis of the mitral valve. Ventricular configuration similar to that in Fig. 6a. Opacification first of the right ventricle (a_1) and then of the left ventricle (a_2) following a bolus injection. Within the left atrium, demonstration of a hypodense, marginal, calcified (≫) filling defect corresponding to the thrombus.

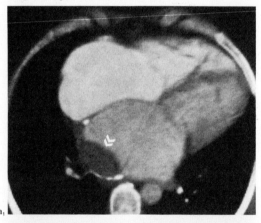

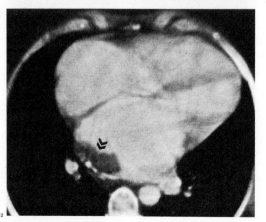

Valvular defects (62-60)

A number of congenital and acquired valvular defects can be detected by analysis of the cardiac chambers and vessels. Mitral stenosis, for example, displays a small left ventricle, enlargement of the left atrium − which then greatly compresses the right atrium from a dorsal direction − and, possibly valvular calcifications or concentric hypertrophy of the right ventricle. Even if measurement of the cardiac pressure or cardiography is essential in most cases initially, computerized tomography is highly suitable for the follow-up of valvular defects under therapy.

Intracavitary masses (62-70)

The most frequent tumour is the **myxoma**, which occurs almost exclusively in the atria (75 % in the oval fossa of the left atrium). It is encountered in all age groups, but most frequently between the ages of 20 and 60 years. Cystic components within the tumour have been described (4). **Rhabdomyomas** can develop either in isolation or in multiples in all sections of the heart. They protrude into the cardiac lumen, are rarely pedunculated, and are encountered mainly in children (tuberous sclerosis).

The group of primary **malignant tumours** includes sarcomas consisting of the most diverse kinds of tissue. They occur much less frequently than secondary neoplasms (metastases of the lung, melanomas, malignant lymphomas).

● **CT**

Computerized tomography reveals the tumour as an intraluminal filling defect, the density values of which do not permit differential diagnosis from a parietal thrombus (309).

Heart – pericardium

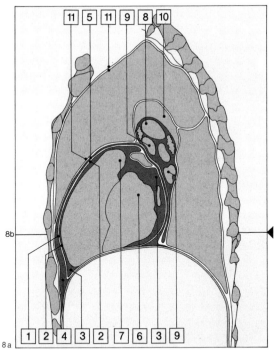

Fig. 62-**8a: Topography of the pericardium.** Left paravertebral sagital section. Varying degrees of subepicardial fatty tissue rounding off the contours of the heart. The parietal membrane of the pericardium is fused with the pleura at some points (pleuropericardial membrane), while additonal spaces filled with fatty tissue arise in other areas.

Key
1. Parietal membrane of the pericardium
2. Visceral membrane of the pericardium (epicardium)
3. Subepicardial fatty tissue
4. Adipose body
5. Pleuropericardial membrane
6. Left ventricle
7. Pulmonary outflow tract
8. Left pulmonary artery
9. Left pulmonary vein
10. Aorta
11. Pleura

Pericardium (62-80)

Anatomy and imaging (62-81)

In the computed tomogram, the subepicardial fatty tissue gives rise to a hypodense gap between the pericardium and the myocardium. Since the irregularly shaped surface of the myocardium is rounded off by subepicardial fatty tissue, the filling tissue is present to varying degrees. It is present in particularly great quantities in the region of the venous inflow and arterial outflow pathways, but to varying degrees in the paracardial region and the vicinity of the apex of the heart (Fig. 62–8a). Since the pericardium and mediastinal pleura form a common membrane only in places (pleuropericardial membrane), additional gaps filled with mediastinal fatty tissue (e.g. the epiphrenic and precardial adipose bodies) can appear.

In the computed tomogram, the hypodense, subepicardial fatty tissue can be seen tangentially as a gap in the region of the maximum circumference of the heart and is best demonstrable here. In obese patients, the pericardium can be demarcated as a linear opacity in the region of the apex of the heart. Since the pericardium extends cranialward up to the point of departure of the pulmonary trunk, the layer of subepicardial fatty tissue makes the aortic root and the pulmonary trunk readily identifiable.

Examination technique (62-82)

● Preparation of the patient is unnnecessary.

● **Scanning** with slice thicknesses of 8–10 mm and an adjacent slice sequence.

Scanning area: the entire pericardium.

● **Intravenous contrast medium administration** (facultative)

As a bolus injection (4-32) in circumscribed processes.

As an infusion (4-36) in extensive processes or for better demarcation from the myocardium.

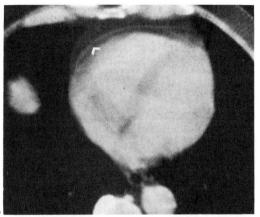

Fig. 62-**8b: The pericardium in the computed tomogram.** The best images are obtained when the pericardium is scanned axially near the base of the heart. Cf. Fig. 8a for level of section.

Pericardial accumulations of fluid (62-83)

The main clinical feature is acute, non-specific pericarditis, for which a viral etiology has been suggested. The other forms are usually concomitant inflammations. Bacterial pericarditis occurs mainly in pulmonary inflammations, while the non-infectious form occurs in cardiac infarction and heart surgery, uraemia, neoplasia and collagenoses. Acute accumulation of more than 250 ml of fluid can lead to cardiac tamponade. The possible causes include perforating trauma with haemopericardium, and bacterial, tumorous and rheumatic pericarditis. The pericarditis proceeds anatomically with serous, fibrinoserous, fibrinous, fibrinopurulent or purulent exudates which, depending on the severity of the disease, occur in the various etiological types.

● CT

The computed tomogram demonstrates the accumulation of fluid at the contours of the heart as a circular zone which is hypodense in comparison to the myocardium and separated from the subepicardial fatty tissue, which is present in varying amounts. The zone of fluid can be of varying width at the individual sections of the heart, corresponding to the pericardial pouches. The epicardium and pericardium, which are thickened by coatings of fibrin, can frequently be demarcated from the hypodense zone of fluid lying between them. If controls of the progress over a longish period of time show that the thickening of the pericardial membranes has not regressed, connective-tissue transformation must be considered. Involvement of the pericardium and any (hypodense) pericardial exudation can be clearly depicted in adjacent tumours (of the mediastinum, pleura, lung), the extent of which can be readily assessed by com-

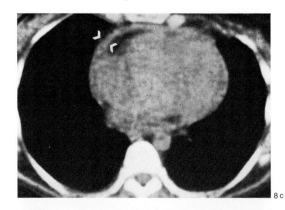

8c

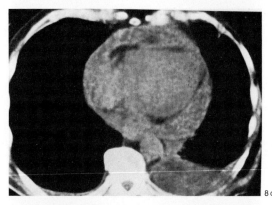

8d

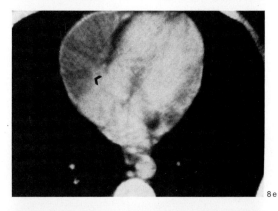

8e

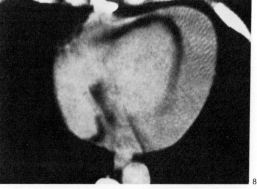

8f

Fig. 62-8 c–f: Pericardial collections of fluid.

8c: Uraemic pericarditis with haemorrhagic exudate. The density of the fluid collection (><) is 7 HU.

8d, e: Tuberculous pericarditis. Circular arrangement of the effusion (d). The pericardial membranes appear to be thickened due to fibrinous deposits and display a hint of callosity (>). Encapsulated tuberculous pericarditis (e); the density values of the exudate are 29 HU. A pleural effusion is also present in both cases.

8f: Acute non-specific pericarditis. The effusion, which displays density values of 22 HU, is encapsulated and pronounced only on the left side.

- **Acute idiopathic, non-specific** pericarditis

- **Infectious** pericarditis
  (viral, pyogenic, **tuberculous,** mycotic, parasitic, syphilitic etc.)

- Acute myocardiac infarct
  Dressler's syndrome
  Postthoracotomy syndrome
  Trauma, blunt or penetrating
  Aortic aneurysm
  (with penetration into the pericardium)

- Collagenoses

- Tumours, primary or metastatic
  (including lymphomas and leukaemia)

- Irradiation

- Uraemia

- Drugs
  (e.g. procainamide, hydralazine)

Fig. 62-**8g: Causes of pericardial effusion** (after Harrison [55]).

puterized tomography. Encapsulation of the pericardial effusion leads to asymmetrical accumulations of fluid which do not drain away on repositioning the patient.

The **radiodensity** lies slightly above that of water and can inrease to 10–40 HU depending on the protein content (fibrin) and admixture of blood (3-52). The density increases in haemopericardium to the values of blood ($\sim$ 50 HU or more) (306). Unless an adequate subepicardial fatty lamella is present, demarcation from the myocardium – the density of which is about the same – can be difficult and necessitates the administration of a guided bolus injection to differentiate the effusion from the vascularized myocardium. If the amounts of blood present in the pericardial space are small, demarcation from fibrosis (chronic constrictive pericarditis), which displays about the same density, may be impossible.

The pericardial effusion is usually demonstrable by sonography. The main indication for using computed tomography is to demonstrate dorsal (encapsulated) exudates and to evaluate complex diagnostic situations involving the pericardium and its immediate vicinity.

Chronic constrictive pericarditis (62–84)

All purulent (specific and non-specific) and serofibrinous forms of pericarditis, as well as haemopericardium, may progress into chronic constrictive pericarditis. Tuberculous pericarditis is considered to be the most frequent cause, although the etiology remains obscure in many patients. Tumour-induced pericarditis can also progress to the clinical picture of constrictive pericarditis. Calcifications are demonstrated in the standard X-ray film in about 50% of cases.

● **CT**

Computerized tomography reveals a smooth or irregular thickening of the pericardium. Connective-tissue organization can be assumed if calcifications are demonstrated. Differentiation from acute pericarditis with small amounts of fluid is difficult in the individual case, since the admixture of fibrin and blood raises the density values of the exudate far above those of water and up to the density of connective tissue. Sonographic correlations and computerized tomographic follow-ups are recommended in these cases.

Tumours (62–85)

Primary tumours – mesotheliomas and fibrosarcomas – are extremely rare. Almost without exception, tumours of the pericardium are secondary and usually originate from the mediastinum, the pleura and the lungs.

● **CT**

The role of computerized tomography is to demonstrate pericardial involvement in secondary tumours. Tumours surrounding the pericardium are frequently demarcated from the myocardium only after a guided bolus injection. The individual heart chambers and any pericardial effusions are depicted at the same time (62-83).

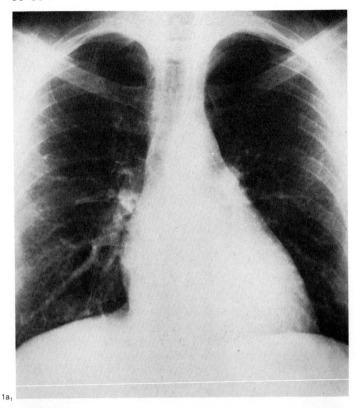

Fig. 63-1a: **X-ray film of the lung** postero-anterior and lateral.

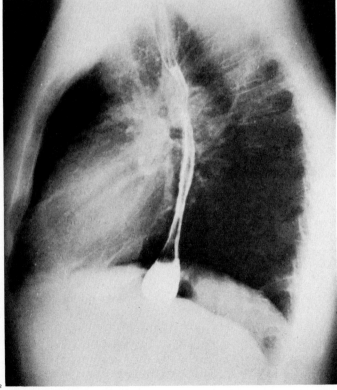

Fig. 63-1b: **The lung in the computed tomogram** of the same patient at different levels.

Lung – pleura (63-00)

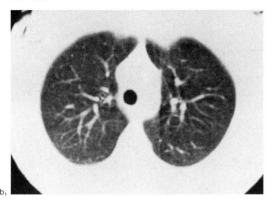

1b₁

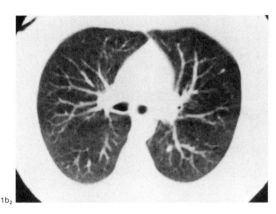

1b₂

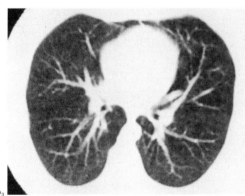

1b₃

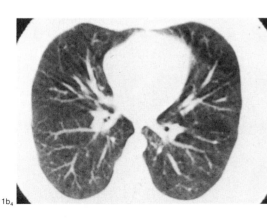

1b₄

Anatomy and imaging (63-10)

The high tissue contrast of the lung permits differentiated diagnosis of pulmonary disease with conventional radiological methods. The good spatial resolution of the X-ray film enables numerous fine details to be visualized which can be lost in computerized tomography because of the restricted resolution. The conventional tomogram also permits better spatial orientation, since structures which lie outside the sectional plane are demonstrated in a blurred manner but provide topographical information which is missing in the computed tomogram. Computerized tomography is employed in pulmonary diagnosis as a complementary method for the following reasons:

● Cavities and angles of the lung which are difficult to demonstrate by standard radiographs are depicted free from overshadowing (retrohilar space, retrosternal space, phrenic angle).
● Freedom from overlying shadows means that very small discrete (areal) opacities can be recognized.
● Computerized tomography offers a better (unblurred) picture in dense pulmonary processes and in pronounced overshadowing.
● The transitions to soft tissue (tumour, mediastinum, pleura) can be assessed exactly by varying the width of the window.
● The density values permit quantitative evaluation.

Pulmonary structure (63-11)

Apart from the lobus venae azygos and cardiacus, the main and accessory septa, i. e. the boundaries of the lobes, cannot be recognized in the computed tomogram because of their oblique course through the sectional plane (63-81). The same goes for the boundaries of the intrapulmonary segments, which are usually not aligned axially because of the hiloradial structure of the lung as a boundary surface. In analogy to the X-ray film, the structure of the normal lung in the computed tomogram is determined by the vessels. Depending on the image matrix of the scanner employed, they can be followed with their ramifications

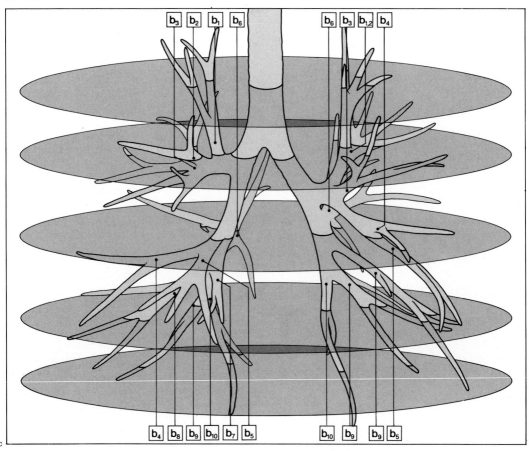

Fig. 63-1 c: Spatial arrangement of bronchial structures in transverse sections.
b_{1-10} = segmental bronchus 1–10 (nomenclature cf. 61-1 c, d).

Fig. 63-1 d: Segments of the lung in the computed tomogram.
$d_{1,2}$: the segmental borders on the pulmonary surface of the left (d_2) and right (d_1) lung.

d_3–d_{12}: the segmental borders in computed tomograms can only be expressed approximately by the course of the vessels and individual central bronchial structures. At the same time, it should be noted that the majority of pulmonary veins run intersegmentally. Cf. Fig. 61-1 c, d for identification of the pulmonary vessels in the computed tomogram.

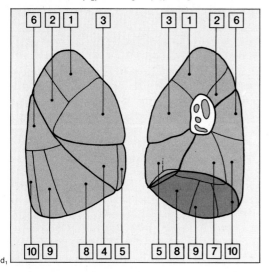
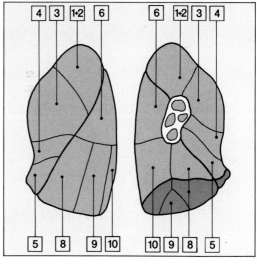

Lung – pleura

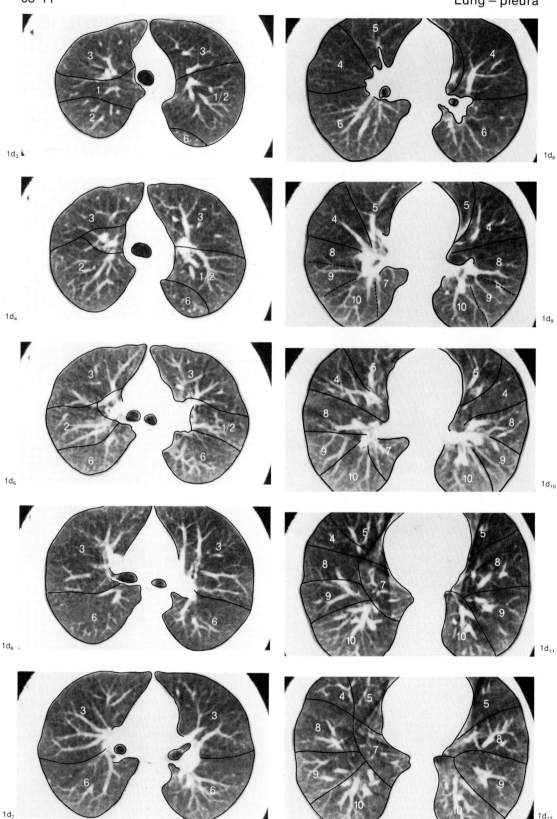

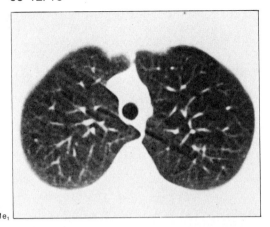

Fig. 63-1e: **Lung at maximum inspiration (e_1) and maximum expiration (e_2).**

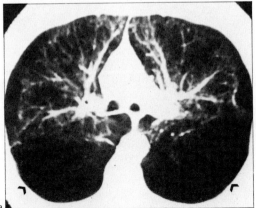

Fig. 63-3a: **Pulmonary emphysema.** Sensitive demonstration of destructive changes of the lung, particularly of the bullous emphysema dorsolateral (>).

into the subpleural space. Some vessels at the level of the hilum (3rd, 4th, 5th and 6th pulmonary segments) run horizontally through the computerized tomographic plane, while the majority run in an oblique direction. This creates the impression of an increase in calibre because of the fact that, in ramifications, only one branch is usually imaged in the horizontal section. The main bronchi are always recognizable because of their large calibre up to the ramification, while the individual segmental bronchi can only be depicted if they run axially.

Although, in principle, the **fine structure** of the pulmonary tissue is depicted in the same way as in the standard chest film, the presentation is determined to a decisive extent by the fineness of the matrix, the slice thickness and the chosen window setting. As Fig. 63-5h shows, fine nodular opacities are just as recognizable as a reticular pattern (Fig. 63-5l). Hairlines (Kerley) cannot be depicted because of their direction of travel. On the other hand, zones of minimal infiltration can be detected without difficulty even if they disappear in the blurred patterns of the conventional tomogram. In particular, their relationship to the vessels and the form of expansion can be assessed in detail as far as the subpleural space.

Pulmonary nodules (63-12)
Pulmonary nodules can be detected subpleurally in the periphery from a diameter of 3 mm. In the core of the lung they must be differentiated from intersected vessels. The contours can be assessed (round, angular, lobulated), but not fine details (fuzziness, sharpness) which are demonstrated better in the conventional tomogram. The density values within the lesion must be interpreted with caution, since even the incorporation of slight amounts of air leads to great deviations of the mean value because of the partial volume effect (3-54). Any nodular lesions which are to be measured should therefore display a diameter of at least twice the slice thickness. Moreover, the measuring accuracy of the individual scanners varies (87) and should be checked by model studies for this special problem. Plaque-like and, in particular, diffuse calcifications can be detected with great sensitivity by computerized tomography.

Density of the lung (63-13)
The density of the lung depends on the degree of inspiration. The ventrodorsal density gradient is low ($\sim$ 20 HU/10 cm stretch of lung) at

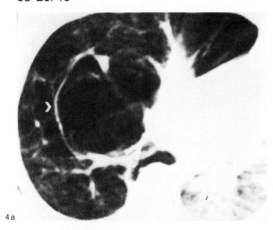

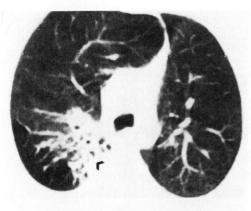

Fig. 63-4 a: **Dysgenesis** of the right lung with cystic changes and emphysematous expansion of the right lobe.

Fig. 63-4 b: **Cystic degeneration** of the superior segment of the right lower lobe. Demonstration of thick-walled, cylindrical and cystic spaces corresponding to bronchiectasias.

Fig. 63-4 c: **Bronchiectasia** of the right middle lobe. Demonstration of honeycombed, mainly central thick-walled pulmonary structures.

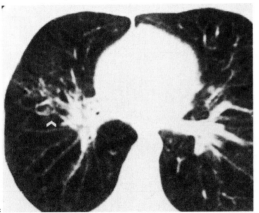

maximum inspiration (TLC) due to varying perfusion. The gradient increases with increasing expiration as a result of varying regional ventilation. This increase in density in the dependent parts of the lung is symmetrical and can readily be differentiated from infiltrations if the ordered structure of the lung is conserved.

Examination technique (63-20)
- No preparation of the patient is required.
- **Scanning** in adjacent slice sequence 10 mm, 13 mm. In local lesions and in the hilus region: if necessary, close slice sequence with thin slices (5–8 mm).

Scanning area: dependent on the extent of the lesion or the problem.

- **Administration of contrast medium** only in special cases.

Emphysema (63-30)
Emphysema is evaluated on the basis of the usual radiological criteria. Subpleural, bullous changes can be accurately depicted, as can the rarefied pulmonary structure. Dilation of the retrosternal space with narrowing of the anterior mediastinum to a fissure-like space is clearly demonstrated. The mean pulmonary density value (measured at TLC as the water-to-air ratio or in the respiratory mid-position) is reduced (114, 337).

Bronchopulmonary malformations, bronchiectasis (63-40)
The absence of an upper lobe artery is recognizable not only by a corresponding vascular anomaly, but also by reduced pulmonary density. In **arteriovenous aneurysms**, the afferent and efferent vessels can also be depicted by computerized tomography. Congenital **cystic dysplasias** of the lung and secondary (cystic) **bronchiectatic deformities** can be clearly seen in the computed tomogram and their size estimated. Their (sub)segmental boundary and secretion level are clearly depicted. Peribronchitic infiltration is reproduced with such clarity that the site of any bronchiectasis can be established (Fig. 63-4 c).

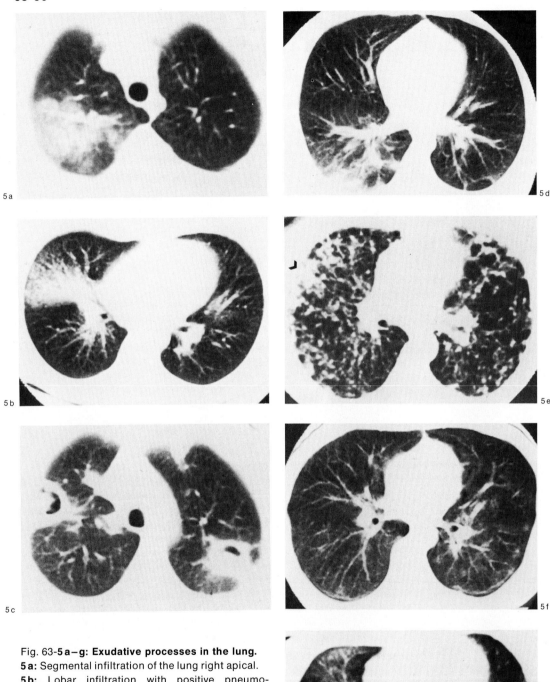

Fig. 63-5a–g: Exudative processes in the lung.

5a: Segmental infiltration of the lung right apical.

5b: Lobar infiltration with positive pneumobronchograms. The border between the upper and lower lobes is demonstrable as a straight contour.

5c: Abscessing staphylococcal pneumonia. Demonstration of dense, relatively sharply demarcated infiltrates with central liquefaction. Sensitive demonstration of the relationship to the pleura.

5d: Loose infiltrate in the right lower lobe due to pulmonary embolisms (infarction pneumonia).

5e: Coarse-miliary tuberculosis with confluent caseous foci. The subpleural space is affected particularly clearly on the right (>).

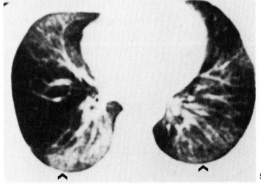

Inflammations of the lung (63-50)

Exudative processes (63-51)

Alveolar infiltration is marked by exudation in some areas of the lung or, on progression of disease, by air bronchograms within the zone of infiltration. Both processes are recognizable in the computed tomogram. Segmental boundaries of the infiltration are demonstrable (Fig. 63-5b), although less clearly than in the chest X-ray. In the case of effusions, the infiltrated lung can be demarcated from the zone of fluid and the differential diagnosis (dystelectasis, encapsulated effusion, pneumonia) can be furthered if extensive shadowing is present. A subpleural abscess displays an irregular, partly septated cavity, a wall of varying thickness and, frequently, ill-defined delimitation from the surrounding pulmonary tissue. It can be differentiated in the majority of cases from pleural empyema, which is marked by its localization, its smooth inner and outer walls and the homogeneous density values of the exudate (330).

Discrete, localized interstitial infiltrations can be demonstrated at an early stage by a weak zone of increased density. The extent – particularly in the subpleural space – and the relationship to the pulmonary vessels can be assessed (Fig. 63-5f).

These properties make the use of computerized tomography appear beneficial in discrete pulmonary changes, e.g. in fibrosing alveolitis, which usually develops symmetrically, or in patients with viral, parasitic or bacterial inflammations if doubt exists about pulmonary infiltration.

Granulomatous inflammations (sarcoidosis) (63-52)

Stage II sarcoidosis is present if pulmonary changes are visible in the standard chest X-ray. This classification is arbitrary to a certain extent, since even Stage I displays histological signs of pulmonary infiltration (14). In fact, granulomatous pulmonary changes are also recognizable in the computed tomogram when they are not (yet) visible in the general film of the thorax. A general increase in density (water-to-air ratio) of the pulmonary tissue is

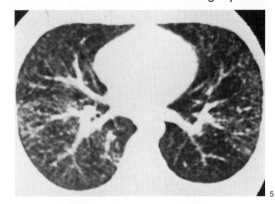

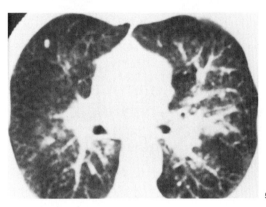

Fig. 63-5h,i: Sarcoidosis.
5h: Fine disseminated involvement of the entire lung, particularly marked in the periphery.
5i: Fine-granulomatous infiltration orienting more on the central vessels and only discretely demonstrable in the periphery.

an indication of very early interstitial involvement (337), even if no structural changes are visible in the computed tomogram.

● CT

Fine, relatively evenly distributed nodular structures (0.3–0.6 cm in diameter) are demonstrated – particularly in the subpleural space – in Stage II sarcoidosis (Fig. 63-5h). Small, subpleural or perivascular group formations are occasionally found in less pronounced cases. A pattern of increased reticulation is an indication of progression to fibrosis (Stage III, see below). Slight concomitant pleural effusions have been described (336).

Fibroses (63-53)

Diffuse interstitial fibrosis can develop insidiously and becomes clinically manifest as a result of the restrictive disturbance of ventila-

◄
5f, g: Fibrotic alveolitis. Clowdy reduction of pulmonary transparency demonstrable only by computerized tomography (f). Distinct infiltration dorsal (g >).

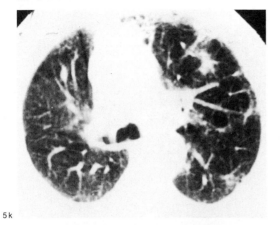

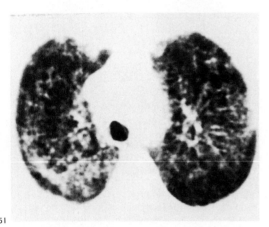

Fig. 63-5k, l: **Pulmonary fibrosis.**
5k: Wegener's granulomatosis (diffuse type). Demonstration of dense cord- and star-shaped structures corresponding to indurations of the interstice of the lung.
5l: Idiopathic pulmonary fibrosis. Demonstration of honeycombing.

tion. The exudative forms (idiopathic fibrosing alveolitis) give rise to marked pulmonary changes which culminate in a coarse reticular pattern or honeycombing of the pulmonary interstice. This pulmonary structure is the final stage of various diseases of the lung (histiocytosis X, Stage III sarcoidosis, collagenoses, pneumoconioses etc.) and is reproduced in the computed tomogram in the same way as in standard radiographs (Fig. 63-5k, l). Computerized tomographic determination of the density of pulmonary tissue (337) permits quantitative evaluation of structural changes. To what extent these data can contribute to the differential diagnosis has not yet been established.

Granulomas (63-54)

The most frequent granuloma is the tuberculoma, which usually displays a diameter of 0.5–4 cm, is sharply demarcated and, in 25% of cases, lobular. Smaller, roundish structures in the vicinity (satellites) are found in up to 80% of cases. Calcifications are frequent and usually of an amorphous type. The histoplasmoma, which is not so frequent in Europe, seldom exceeds a diameter of 3 cm, is normally sharply demarcated and displays mainly central calcification.

Nodules from the group of collagenoses (rheumatoid necrobiotic nodes, Wegener's granulomatosis) are rare and do not calcify.

Neoplasias of the lung (63-60)

Differential diagnosis of pulmonary nodules

The following data apply both to inflammatory (63-54) and to neoplastic coin lesions in the present state of computerized tomography.

The density value of an intrapulmonary nodule of soft-tissue density (50–125 HU) does not permit any conclusions as to its identity. Provided that measurement of the density is accurate (63-10), computerized tomography offers no more than the possibility of picking out the rare fat-containing and cystic shadows from the plethora of nodules. The differential-diagnostic criteria of the other nodules of soft-tissue density are based on the familiar radiological signs, although diffuse calcifications can be demonstrated with greater sensitivity by computerized tomography. Density values over 200 HU measured above the nodule in an artifact-free computed tomogram indicate that the lesion is not malignant (334).

Benign tumours (63-61)

Of the benign tumours (adenomas, hamartomas, leiomyomas, fibromas), only the rare lipoma can be unequivocally identified by its density value and diagnosed. Overall, calcifications are rare and are of virtually no assistance in the differential diagnosis (exception: hamartoma, which can display popcorn-like calcifications).

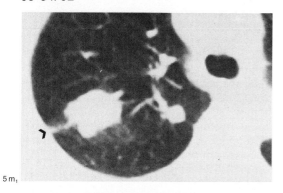
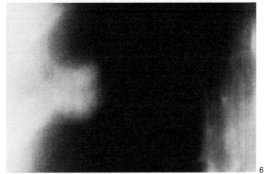
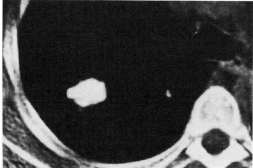
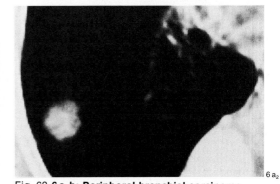

Fig. 63-**5 m, n: Tuberculosis. 5 m:** Tuberculoma. The density values, 250 HU, are distinctly increased. Demonstration of specific remains perifocal and pleural (m_1 >). **5 n:** Clarified pulmonary cavern left apical with thickened wall (><), perifocal emphysema and relationship to the pleura (≫).

Fig. 63-**6 a, b: Peripheral bronchial carcinoma.**
6 a: The tumour periphery is shown in greater detail in the conventional tomogram (a_1), while its pleural relationship is demonstrated better by CT ($a_{2,3}$≫).
6 b: Sharp (lobate) borders (a_3) indicate expansive growth, radial lines (b) infiltration.

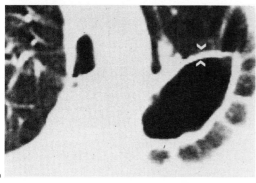
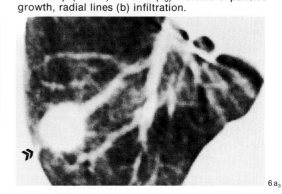
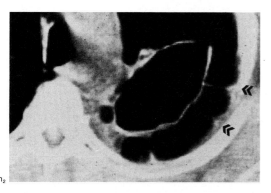
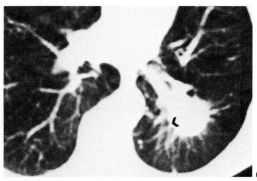

Bronchial carcinoma (63-62)

Peripheral bronchial carcinoma, which originates in the segmental bronchi and their ramifications, is found primarily in the upper lobes and appears in the computed tomogram as a round focus (with somewhat sharp, lobulated boundaries). It is more common than tuberculoma in the lower lobes. Satellite foci are rare, but pleural involvement with cord-like branches can frequently be demonstrated in the case of lesions close to the pleura. Fine radial striations, which appear in the conventional tomogram, are lost in the computed tomogram due to the lack of spatial resolution. CT differentiation from a tuberculoma (histoplasmoma) is based on the radiological criteria described earlier, of which some can be demonstrated more sensitively by CT than with conventional methods (calcifications, satellite foci, specific residues of the vicinity). The incorporation of air within the round foci, which corresponds to bronchiolograms and can be recognized densitometrically by a reduced density value, is indicative of a bronchioloalveolar carcinoma. Poorly defined relationship to the hilum is found as a sign of hilopetal growth and presents the familiar radiological picture. The extent to which a peripheral bronchial carcinoma has invaded the thoracic wall or mediastinum can be assessed in detail by computerized tomography before it becomes clinically manifest (Pancoast syndrome).

Central bronchial carcinoma, which originates from the main bronchi, can be demonstrated easier by conventional tomography than in the computed tomogram, since the spatial arrangement of the hilar vessels can be analysed better and variations in the calibre of the central bronchial tree can be visualized in detail.

Hopes of differentiating tumour tissue from poststenotic atelectatic pulmonary parenchyma or from poststenotic pneumonia in the obstructive syndrome by means of computerized tomography have not yet been fully realised, even with guided bolus injections. In contrast, computerized tomography can be relied upon to demonstrate subpleural metastases of a central bronchial carcinoma.

A distinction must also be made as regards the accessibility of hilar lymphomas. While the bronchopulmonary lymph nodes can be reliably demonstrated with conventional methods, the subcarinal, paratracheal and perivascular groups of lymph nodes can be imaged by computerized tomography above a diameter of 1 to 1.5 cm if the mediastinal contours are otherwise normal. A condition for this is a detailed examination technique which ensures unequivocal identification of the vascular structures, if necessary with administration of contrast medium. At the present time, conventional hilar tomography is regarded as being on a par with CT as regards the demonstration of enlarged bronchopulmonary and tracheobronchial lymph nodes (264). The superiority of computerized tomography (261, 322, 275) in the detection of enlarged mediastinal lymph nodes due to bronchial carcinoma has not gone undisputed (264). It should always be borne in mind that, although enlarged mediastinal lymph nodes can be sensitively demonstrated by computerized tomography, they sometimes represent nothing more than reactive inflammation in the presence of bronchial carcinoma (321). Radiation therapy can be planned better if the tumour is exactly demarcated; computerized tomography is more successful at this in 75% of cases than other methods – particulary in the presence of overlying effusions and atelectasis (322).

Fig. 63-6 c–f: **Central bronchial carcinoma.**
6c: Paramediastinal, central tumour (>) contrasting with the hypodense dystelectatic pulmonary tissue (≫). Demonstration of tumour expansion up to the right hilum and of regional lymph node enlargement (≫).
6d: Tumour at the point of departure of the upper lobe bronchus (≫), clearly demarcated from the opacified pulmonary vessel (d_1 >). Demonstration of hilar and mediastinal lymph node enlargement (d_2 >).
6e: Central bronchial carcinoma (≫) with poststenotic pneumonia of the right middle lobe. Demonstration of positive pneumobronchograms (e_1 >).
6f: Central bronchial carcinoma with total atelectasis of the right lung. The tumour and its regional metastases (>) can be largely demarcated from the pulmonary tissue. Demonstration of considerable mediastinal displacement to the right, a pleural effusion (≫) and slight residual ventilation in individual sections of the lung (f_2 ><).

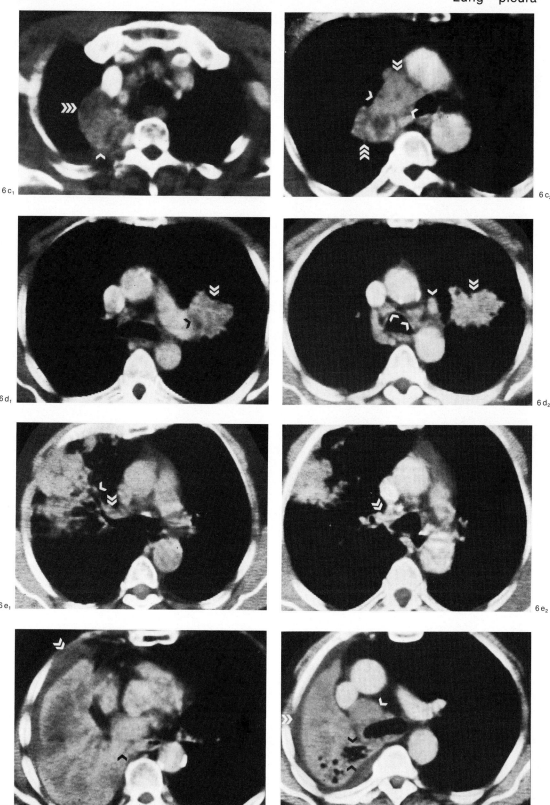

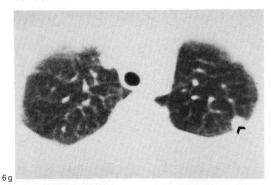

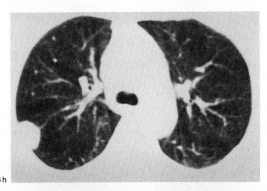

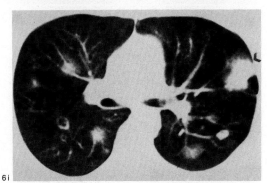

Multiple circumscribed lesions (metastases) (63-63)

Most haematogenous metastases are localized in the periphery of the lung (325). Consequently, the superior reproduction of the subpleural space leads to a higher detection rate of nodules (327, 261). In a prospective study by Schaner (333) in tumour patients, 38 (65%) of 69 nodules confirmed by computerized tomography were demonstrated by whole lung anteroposterior laminography and 21 (30%) by a standard radiograph in two planes. 66% of the lesions detected were metastases, while histology showed the others to be granulomas, the appearance of which could not be differentiated from that of malignant nodules. Computerized tomography is therefore indicated when decisive therapy must be made dependent on the demonstration of metastases in the lung.

Vascular lesions (63-70)

The computerized tomographic appearance of congestion in the minor circulation in left-heart failure is the same as that in the standard radiograph. An increase of the central and, perhaps, peripheral vessel markings is found in addition to cardiac enlargement. The ventrodorsal density gradient (63-13) increases. In over-hydrated dialysis patients, horizontal linear shadows which can regress following hemodialysis are frequently found in the dependent areas of the lung in addition to increased pulmonary tissue density (water-to-air ratio). Similar changes have been interpreted as preoedema (325). As in the X-ray film, a past pulmonary infarction must be suspected in wedge-shaped subpleural opacities. Computerized tomography detects these processes early on and sensitively and permits, where required, detailed control of the course (liquefaction, pleural involvement, pneumonia) (335).

Fig. 63-**6 g–i: Pulmonary metastases.**

6g: Demonstration of a solitary, subpleural pulmonary metastasis from an osteosarcoma (>).

6h: Solitary metastasis from a mammary carcinoma.

6i: Liquefying metastases from a melanoma. The poorly defined zones of infiltration are also caused by metastases (>).

Fig. 63-**7 a: Central congestion of the lung.** Demonstration of central hypervascularity. General increased density of the lung and its periphery.

Pleura (63-80)

Anatomy and imaging (63-81)

The visceral leaf of the pleura covers all the pulmonary lobes, while the parietal leaf lines the outer walls of the pleural cavity. The thin layers can only be depicted when they run axially in the computerized tomographic slice, in which case they completely fill a volume element and achieve adequate contrast with the adjacent structure. Consequently, the apical pleura, the diaphragmatic pleura and the main and accessory septa of a healthy person cannot usually be demonstrated by computerized tomography. The costoparietal and mediastinal pleurae and, occasionally, septa of accessory lobes can be depicted. In pleural thickening and accumulations of fluid which are encapsulated, structures running horizontally and semi-axially can be demonstrated, depending on the degree of deformity and increase in volume.

The sum of the two pleural leaves and the endothoracic fascia are depicted in the computed tomogram as a linear soft-tissue structure. In some, the great increase in contrast at the boundary surface to the lung leads to edge enhancement, which can simulate calcifications. These artifacts can be identified with some experience because of their tangential nature.

Examination technique (63-82)

- **Preparation of the patient** is unnecessary.
- **Scanning** with an adjacent slice sequence of 10 mm (13 mm).

In extensive processes slice intervals of 20 mm.

Scanning area dependent on the extent and position of the process to be examined.

- **Intravenous contrast medium administration** in special cases, usually as a bolus injection (4-32).

Pleural effusion (63-83)

Accumulations of fluid in the pleural cavity are a non-specific radiological sign which can be found in a broad spectrum of different diseases. The most common causes are transudation due to cardiac decompensation and inflammatory and malignant infiltrations originating from lung disease. The etiology of pleural exudates unaccompanied by any other thoracic disease is presented in Fig. 63-8a.

Following pneumectomy, the empty pleural cavity fills with fibrinous exudate within 14

Cause	Transudate	Serous	Purulent	Serofibrinous	Serosanguinous	Other disease in the thorax	Extrathoracic disease
● frequent ◐ occasional ○ rare			Exudate				
Infectious							
Bacteria							
Klebsiella – Enterobacter – serrata genera			●			●	
Pseudomonas, salmonella			●			●	
E. coli, A. actinobacter			●			●	
Haemophilus, M. mallei			●				
Anaerobic organism, C. perfringens			●			●	
Str. pneumoniae, F. tularensis		●				●	
Str. aureus		◐	●		◐	●	
Str. pyogenes		●	●			●	
M. tuberculosis		●	●			◐	
Pancreatitis, subphr. abscess		●					●
Fungi							
Actinomyces, Israelii Nocardia			●			●	
Blastomyces, Cryptococcus		●				●	
Histoplasma, Aspergillus		●				●	
Virus (incl. mycoplasma)		●				◐	
Parasites							
Entamoeba histolytica			○	●		●	
Echinococcus granulosus				●		●	
Immunologic							
Systemic lupus eryth.		●				◐	
Rheumatoid disease		●				◐	
Wegener's granulomatosis		●				●	
Neoplastic							
Bronchial carcinoma		●			◐	●	
Alveolar cell carcinoma		●			●	●	
Malignant lymphoma					●	◐	●
Metastatic carcinoma		●			●	◐	●
Mesothelioma					●	●	
Multiple myeloma					●	●	
Thromboembolic						●	◐
Cardiovascular							
Cardiac insufficiency	●					●	
Constrictive pericarditis	●					●	
Obstruction of superior vena cava or azygos vein	●					●	
Traumatic							
Closed chest trauma					●	●	
Following abdominal surgery		●					●
Incidental causes (rare)							
Asbestosis		●				○	◐
Sarcoidosis		●					●
Nephr. syndrome, cirrhosis	●						●
Myxoedema, Hydronephrosis	●						●
Fam. recurrent polyserositis				●			●
Uremic pleuritis	●			○			●

Fig. 63-**8a**: **Causes of pleural effusion** (from Fraser-Paré [14]).

days and decreases slightly in size. Connective-tissue organization of the fibrin-containing exudate takes place slowly over the following months (cf. 63-84).

● **CT**
Acute dry pleurisy cannot usually be depicted. In analogy to the lateral decubitus position, 15–50 ml fluid can be demonstrated in the computed tomogram. Since, for technical reasons, the density values particularly in narrow fluid spaces are subject to considerable inaccuracy, it is advisable to reposition the patient on the side to achieve diagnostic demarcation of a callosity or encapsulation. Amounts of free fluid collect at the deepest point of the pleural cavity in the shape of a halfmoon. In the case of encapsulation, the exudate may be localized ventrally and laterally and a connective-tissue capsule can frequently be demonstrated.

The density values permit unequivocal differentiation between a sanguinolent and a serous exudate only in the case of marked admixture of blood. The creamy pus of an empyema displays the same density value as an abscess (∼ 30 HU), although it can vary depending on its age and consistency. The reduction of density caused by the lipoid content of 2–3 % chyle (39) is not sufficient to permit unequivocal diagnosis. Consequently, the diagnosis of haemothorax, pyothorax, serothorax and chylothorax cannot be made simply on the basis of the density value, which should be interpreted in a clinical context. Concomitant findings of the lung, thoracic wall and epigastrium can be of great assistance in the differential diagnosis (Fig. 63-8a).

Pleural thickening (63-84)
Pleural thickening is usually consequent on a past inflammation which has healed leaving fibrous tissue, and usually occurs basally in the region of the costophrenic recess. Pleural thickening at the apices is usually non-specific rather than due to tuberculosis(14). A broad, circular fibrous layer (fibrothorax) is usually caused by connective-tissue organization of a haemothorax or pyothorax. In the later stages of the process, coarse, partly plaque-like and areal calcifications develop on the inner as-

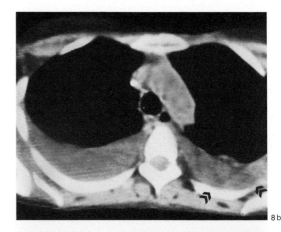

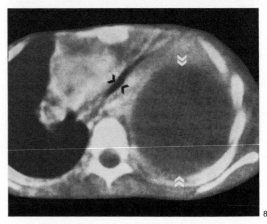

Fig. 63-**8 b–d: Pleural accumulation of fluid.**
8b: Bilateral pleural effusion. Demonstration of sickle-shaped shadows on the dorsal side of both lungs. The density values of 15 HU indicate fluid, but artifacts (≫) frequently make them inaccurate even with rapid scanners.
8c: Pleural empyema. Large cystoid hypodensity in the region of the left thorax. Within the collapsed lung, only the main bronchus (><) is recognizable as an air-containing structure. Displacement of the mediastinum to the right.

8d: Status after pneumectomy. Clearly thickened pleural wall as a sign of coating with fibrin (><). Incorporation of air (≫) within the fibrin-containing secretion from the wound. The secretion cannot change its position to any great extent.

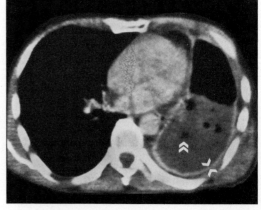

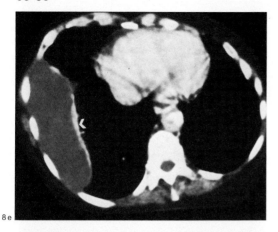

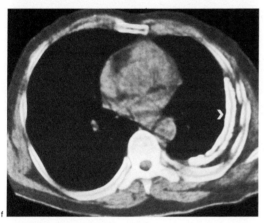

Fig. 63-8 e–g: **Pleural callosity.**

8e: In status after tuberculosis, demonstration of a broad pleural scar. At 45 HU, the density of the callosity approximates that of soft tissue. Calcareous incrustations (>) stand out clearly from the soft-tissue mass.

8f: Calcareous pleuritis following thoracic trauma. A double, sickle-shaped calcareous structure situated on a soft-tissue zone of the pleura.

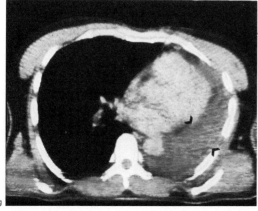

pect of the peel. Pneumectomy constitutes a special case in which the affected half of the thorax is filled with fibrin organized by connective tissue.

● **CT**

Computerized tomography normally reveals a circular, shell-like soft-tissue zone covered in some cases by calcareous encrustations. Tuberculosis can be assumed with a high degree of probability when indurative pulmonary changes are seen. Extensive fibrous pleuritis is also found in uraemia.

Asbestosis, talcosis (63-85)

Asbestosis does not normally become manifest until after 20 years or is discovered during routine examination. Pleural change is found in about 90% of cases and isolated involvement of the pulmonary parenchyma in only 10%. The guiding symptom is localized thickening of the pleura consisting of fibrotic, hyaline tissue. It is encountered most frequently above the intercostal spaces of the 6th – 9th rib and less frequently on the phrenic domes and on the mediastinal or pericardial pleura. The thickening, which generally occurs in the parietal membrane of the pleura, adheres with the visceral pleura only in exceptional cases. Calcifications develop about 20 years after exposure to dust and can be demonstrated histologically in 87% of cases; their radiological detection succeeds much less frequently (in 20 to a maximum of 70% of cases in different studies and regions). They are found relatively frequently on the phrenic dome and can surround the entire circumference of the lower lung. In studies to date, no pleural plaques have been demonstrated in the phrenicocostal angles or interlobar septa. Pleural effusions can be related to asbestosis only when other causes of serous pleurisy, e.g. tuberculosis, have been reliably ruled out. The incidence of mesothelioma is considerably increased in patients suffering from asbestosis (35).

● **CT**

Pleural plaques stand out typically as sharply demarcated elevations about 1–5 mm (maximum 10 mm) thick which may be local or spread over several centimeters. Symmetrical

8g: Fibrothorax following pneumectomy left. At 20/35 HU, the density values of the thoracic space, which is filled with soft tissue, are below those of muscle tissue.

involvement of the pleural cavities is the usual finding. Calcifications penetrating the plaques to different depths are found in varying degrees. Pleural calcifications in the paravertebral region of the pleura and even further caudalward can be demonstrated more frequently by computerized tomography than in the standard radiographs (324). Reticular pulmonary changes, particular those occurring subpleurally in the vicinity of the pleural plaques, are indicative of the simultaneous pulmonary manifestation of asbestosis. Both honeycombing and fine nodules have been described by Kreel (324).

Primary neoplasias of the pleura (63-86)
The most important benign tumour is the **local mesothelioma,** which is usually found after the age of 40 but sometimes earlier (14). It is pedunculated in 30–50 % of cases, originates from the visceral pleura in the majority of cases, displays a smooth or lobate surface and is found more frequently in the lower half of the thorax. Concomitant hypertrophic osteoarthropathy is found relatively frequently, while tumour calcifications are the exception. Multifocal nodular hyaline thickening of the parietal pleura is found in **pleural hyaloserositis** (Zuckerguß). The calcifications not infrequently observed in this condition are usually shell-like and roundish, and not lamellar as in asbestosis. A **lipoma** originating from the subpleural parietal fatty tissue and not infrequently leading to invasion of the ribs is a fairly frequent finding in addition to the rare, roundish to oval **fibrin bodies,** which usually display a diameter of 3–4 cm and can regress spontaneously, and multiple fibromas.

● **CT**
The good demonstration of the pleurae usually permits unequivocal allocation of a circumscribed mass to this space. The nature of a lipoma can be diagnosed simply by analysing the density values. Fibrin bodies and fibromas usually occur in multiples, while the benign mesothelioma occurs in isolation. If necessary, the administration of contrast material can aid the differential diagnosis, since the benign mesothelioma is highly vascularized.

Diffuse mesothelioma (63-87)
The diffuse mesothelioma is a highly invasive, malignant tumour which occurs five times more frequently in men than in women. Exposure to asbestosis is found in 10–40 % of cases or more. The typical patho-anatomical ap-

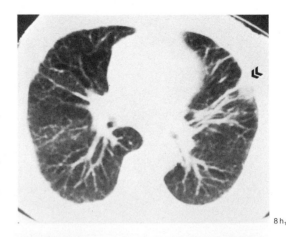

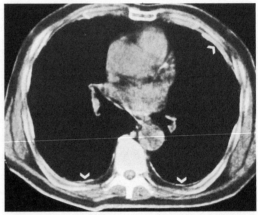

Fig. 63-**8h: Asbestosis.** Demonstration of delicate pleural calcification left and right dorsal, plaque-shaped left ventrolateral (>). A lung scan reveals fibrotic zones extending to the plaque regions (≫).

Fig. 63–**8i: Mesothelioma.** Capsular soft-tissue structure right dorsolateral in the region of the pleural membranes, which are surrounding fluid. Cords radiate into the pulmonary tissue. Demonstration of a broad soft-tissue zone right ventral (≫). Plaque-shaped thickening of the pleura right dorsal (>). These zones enhance distinctly following administration of contrast medium.

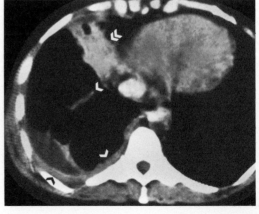

pearance is of a partly tuberous, partly areal neoplasm which permeates the entire pleural cavity and embraces the lung. Flat, usually multiple tumours have also been described which are frequently accompanied or covered by an effusion which is sanguinolent in 50 % of cases. The thoracic wall and the pericardium are invaded and destroyed in the course of this rapidly progressive, unfavourable disease. Not infrequently, even the histological differentiation of the mesothelioma from fibrothorax or metastatic adenoid carcinomas presents great difficulties.

● **CT**

Computed tomography does not help in the differential diagnosis of mesothelioma from fibrothorax because circular, partly lamellar thickening of the pleura is a feature of both conditions. Unilateral involvement is also common in both mesothelioma and fibrothorax. The concomitant effusions can be surrounded by a broad, partly tuberous layer of solid tumour tissue which displays distinct enhancement following contrast medium administration (Fig. 63-8 i, k). Localized linear calcifications, particularly on the opposite side, are an indication of past or concomitant asbestosis (63-85). Infiltration of the subpleural sections of the lung in the sense of lymphangiosis is the first sign of invasive spread. This becomes clearer during the course of the disease with infiltration of the thoracic wall with destruction of the ribs and regional lymphadenopathy.

Secondary tumours of the pleura (63-88)

Bronchial carcinoma is the primary tumour in 40–50 % of pleural metastases, followed by mammary carcinoma, malignant lymphomas, ovarian tumours and gastrointestinal tumours. The effusion present in 50 % of cases only becomes noticeable on progression of the disease. The pleural exudate displays a high protein content.

● **CT**

Only the pleural effusion without solid components can be demonstrated in most cases. Concomitant disease of the lung and chest can, unless previously diagnosed, provide differential-diagnostic aspects.

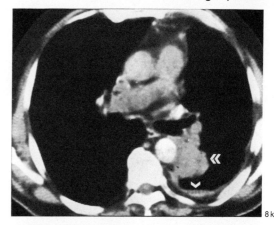

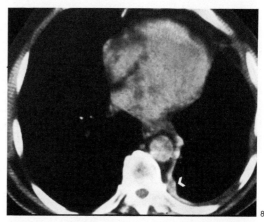

Fig. 63-8k: **Mesothelioma.** Polycyclic soft-tissue structure lying against the descending aorta (≫). Plaque-shaped pleural thickening left dorsal (>). Distinct enhancement of the tumour after contrast medium administration. No demonstration of costal destruction.

Fig. 63-8l: **Malignant lymphoma** of the chest wall and pleura. Irregularly demarcated thickening of the pleura, particularly right dorsal (>). At the same time, infiltration of the dorsal muscles and the lung right (≫).

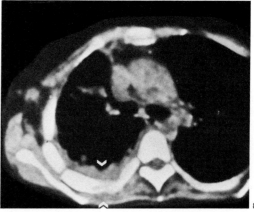

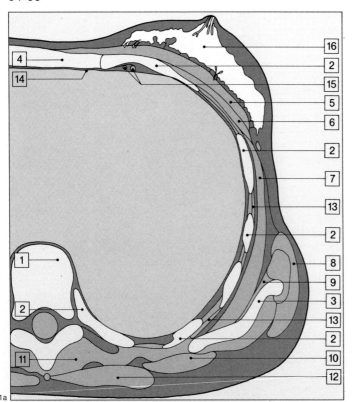

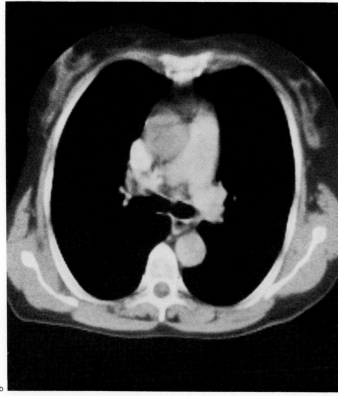

Fig. 64-**1a,b: Topography of the chest wall.**

1a: Transverse section (diagram)
1b: Computed tomogram

Key
1 Third thoracic vertebra
2 Rib, sternum
3 Scapula
4 Sternum
5 M. pectoralis major
6 M. pectoralis minor
7 M. serratus anterior superior
8 M. teres major
9 M. subscapularis
10 M. rhomboideus major
11 M. erector trunci
12 M. trapezius
13 Mm. intercostales
14 Membrana endothoracica
15 A. V. thoracica interna
16 Mamma

The chest wall (64-00)

Anatomy and imaging (64-10)

As a cylindrical structure, the thoracic wall is a good scanning object for computerized tomography. The internal surface, which is invested by the costoparietal pleura, can be evaluated in detail. The ribs, which run obliquely through the slice, are difficult to assess on the computed tomogram. The cortical substance appears as streaks and creates the impression of an open medullary space (Fig. 64-1 b). The heads of the ribs can be scanned at such an angle as to create the impression of "destruction". On the other hand, the anterior and posterior boundary surface of the sternum including the sternoclavicular joints can be clearly depicted.

The thoracic muscles can be adequately differentiated in a healthy person if there is adequate interposition of fat (2-00). The soft tissues of the axillae, the course of the brachial vessels and the scapula together with its surrounding muscles are clearly depicted in the upper section of the thoracic wall.

Vertebral column cf. 93-51.

Examination technique (64-20)

- No preparation of the patient is required.
- **Scanning** with an adjacent slice sequence of 10 mm (13 mm).

Scanning area dependent on the extent and position of the process to be investigated.

- **Contrast medium administration** in special cases (see below).

Tumours (64-30)

Primary neoplasias are rare and originate primarily from the bone, the incidence of benign and malignant variants being about equal. **Chondrogenic** tumours, such as (osteo-)chondromas, chondro-(myxoid-)sarcomas and enchondromas, are most common with 40% of cases. By comparison, the **osteogenic** variants, e.g. the osteoblastoma, endostoma and osteogenic sarcoma, are rare. Second in order of frequency come neoplasms of the **haematopoietic** and **reticuloendothelial** system, a group which is dominated by malignant forms such as myeloma, Hodgkin's disease, Ewing's sarcoma and reticulum cell sarcoma. Benign variants are, overall, less frequent and are represented mainly by fibrous dysplasia and Paget's disease, while haeman-

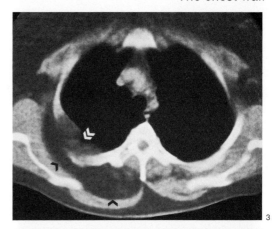

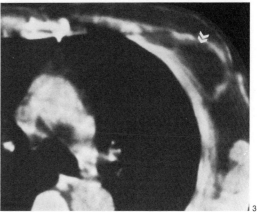

Fig. 64-**3 a, b: Lipomas.**

3 a: Lipoma of the right dorsal thoracic wall in general obesity. Demonstration of a fat-equidense mass beneath the M. rhomboideus and serratus anterior. Slight prolapse of the fatty tissue into the thoracic cavity, simulating a pleural tumour (≫).

3 b: Lipoma of the ventrolateral thoracic wall beneath the M. pectoralis major (≫).

Fig. 64-**3 c: Chondrosarcoma** of the back. Demonstration of a lesion which is hypodense compared to muscle tissue, with destruction of the left root of the arch of thoracic vertebra 10 and of the head of the rib (≫).

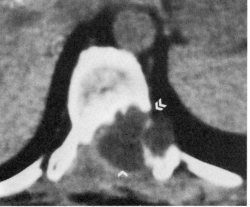

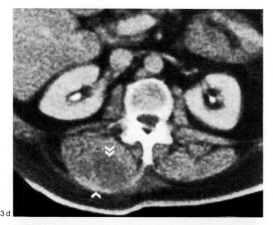

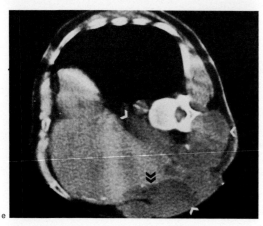

Fig. 64-3 d, e: **Chondromyxoid sarcoma.**

3 d: The mass is smoothly bordered and displays expansive growth without infiltration of the adjacent layers of muscle. Demonstration of hypodense (myxoid) areas (≫) following contrast medium administration.

3 e: Extensive chondromyxoid sarcoma of the chest wall. Infiltration of the entire muscles of the wall and also of the liver (≫).

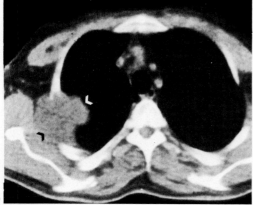

giomas, eosinophilic granulomas and aneurysmal bone cysts are found only occasionally. Primary soft-tissue tumours, e. g. (benign) lipomas and fibrosarcomas, are rarities.

Secondary neoplasias, which occur more frequently than the primary forms, develop within the osseous structures – particularly in the ribs and the sternum. Primary tumours are found in the breasts, lungs, prostate, kidneys, thyroid and stomach. Infiltration of the thoracic wall usually takes place in the late stage of mediastinal malignant growths and in mammary carcinoma, but relatively early in diffuse mesotheliomas.

● **CT**

Since the overwhelming majority of primary and secondary neoplasias originate from cartilaginous and osseous tissue and from tissue of the medullary space, the indications arising for the thoracic wall are similar to those in other regions of the skeleton (93-40). The deformation and destruction of the bone can be adequately described and differentially diagnosed with spot X-ray films. Evaluation of the soft-tissue component is, however, easier in the computed tomogram, particularly in regions in which the costal cartilage has not calcified. With the exception of lipomas (258), it is not usually possible to diagnose the nature of the lesion. This task can, however, be accomplished by puncture, which is easy to perform in this region.

Tumour invasion appears in the computed tomogram pectorally and dorsally as masking of the layers of muscle, which are separated by fatty tissue. Distention of the thoracic wall and protrusion of the tumour into the thoracic cavity can be accurately depicted. A guided bolus injection is recommended in doubtful cases for better demarcation of the tumour tissue from the surrounding soft tissue. Regional lymphadenopathy, particularly of the retrosternal chain of lymph nodes, can be demonstrated above the size of one centimeter in diameter (61-15) (259).

Fig. 64-3 f: **Eruptive cancer** of the lung. Demonstration of a soft-tissue mass which is slightly hypodense compared to muscle tissue, with destruction of the third rib right dorsolateral.

Inflammations (64-40)

Inflammations rarely develop in the thoracic wall itself. Primary osteomyelitis of the ribs and sternum, for example, can spread to the surrounding soft tissue. More frequently, inflammations of the lung and pleura — usually as a feature of tuberculosis or mycosis — also affect the thoracic wall, producing osteomyelitis.

● **CT**

Computerized tomography cannot demonstrate the structural changes of the ribs in osteomyelitis as well as the spot X-ray film. Inflammatory soft tissue infiltration manifests itself as masking of the layers of muscle, which are separated by fatty tissue, and as regional distention of the thoracic wall. The demonstration of hypodense zones which demarcate clearly following contrast medium administration is a sign of (incipient) abscess formation.

Even if the skeleton is intact, malignant infiltration must always be considered in the absence of external signs of inflammation.

Trauma (64-50)

Initially, thoracic injuries caused by an external event affect the thoracic wall. Fractured ribs, local haematomas and soft-tissue emphysemas can be adequately clarified by X-ray examination. Computerized tomography can be the least aggressive and most comprehensive examination technique in complex trauma with suspected mediastinal, pleural or pulmonary involvement.

● **CT**

Haematomas appear in the computed tomogram as homogeneous, perhaps slightly hyperdense zones with attenuation values close to soft-tissue density. They mask the muscular structures and lead to distention of the thoracic wall (64-30 and 64-40). Fractures of the ribs and sternum can only be unequivocally identified when dislocation is also present.

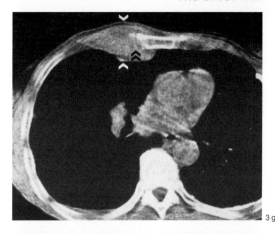

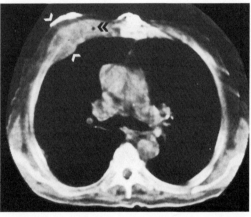

Fig. 64-**3 g: Chest wall metastasis** from a small-cell bronchial carcinoma. The muscle layers can no longer be demarcated because of the infiltrative process, the sternum is eroded (≫).

Fig. 64-**4 a: Abscess.** Swelling of the right ventrolateral chest wall and masking of the muscles by the inflammatory infiltration. Demonstration of a minute gas bubble (≫) as a sign of infection.

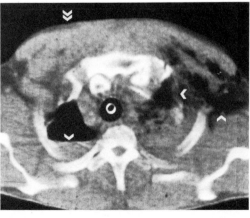

Fig. 64-**5 a: Severe thoracic trauma.** Presternal haematoma of the chest wall with masking of the pectoral muscles (≫). Also, demonstration of soft-tissue emphysema, pleural effusions, pulmonary contusion and rib fractures.

Abdomen, peritoneal space

(70-00)

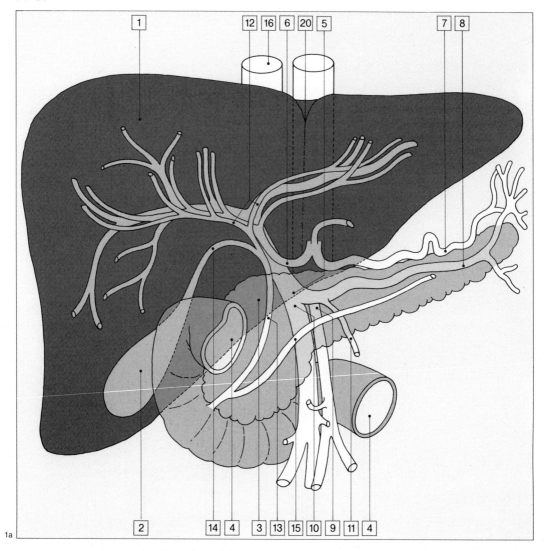

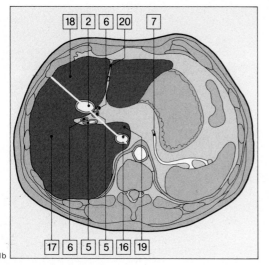

Fig. 71-**1 a–c: Topography of the porta hepatis.**

Key
1 Liver
2 Gallbladder
3 Pancreas
4 Duodenum
5 Portal vein
6 Hepatic artery
7 Splenic artery
8 Splenic vein
9 Superior mesenteric artery
10 Superior mesenteric vein
11 Inferior mesenteric vein
12 Hepatic duct
13 Common bile duct
14 Cystic duct
15 Pancreatic duct
16 Inferior vena cava
17 Right lobe
18 Quadrate lobe
19 Caudate lobe
20 Falciform ligament (longitudinal fissure)

Fig. 71-**1 b: Border between the right and left hepatic lobes** (cf. text).

Liver (71-00)

Anatomy and imaging (71-10)

The liver, which takes up most of the upper abdomen, weighs 1,350–1,500 g in the adult and appears in the computed tomogram as an areal soft-tissue zone. It is divided in the sagittal plane right-paramedially by a peritoneal fold, the **falciform ligament,** at the anterior surface and by the insertion of the **ligamentum teres hepatis** or **ligamentum venosum**, and a more or less deep fissure filled with fatty tissue may be present. It proceeds in an approximate right angle into a frontally aligned recess – the **porta hepatis** (Fig. 71-1 b, c), which contains the portal structures. The inferior vena cava lies against the liver from a dorsal direction or is surrounded by liver tissue. A line of communication from the inferior vena cava to the gallbladder represents the approximate boundary to the right hepatic lobe (Fig. 71-1 b). Left of this line, the **caudate lobe** can be localized dorsal to the porta hepatis, while the **quadrate lobe** may lie in front of the porta hepatis up to the longitudinal fissure. The left hepatic lobe is of variable shape and usually extends on the left as far as the medioclavicular line without reaching the anterior pole of the spleen. The right hepatic lobe fills the entire right subphrenic space. Caudalward, it provides space for the renal bed by virtue of a lateroconvex excavation. The **gallbladder** (72-10) lies against the medial contour of the right hepatic lobe beneath the porta hepatis and, depending on its size, can extend as far as the abdominal wall.

At 65 ± 5 HU, the **radiodensity** of normal liver tissue is higher than that of all other epigastric organs and of muscle tissue. Consequently, the blood- and bile-containing structures are demarcated as hypodense zones. The inferior vena cava, which runs axially through the caudate lobe, can usually be identified as a hypodense, smoothly bordered zone. The **portal vein** and its branches are accompanied by the **hepatic artery** (left lateral) and **the bile ducts** (right lateral) (Fig. 71-1 a). The bifurcation of the portal vein is usually recognizable. Its further ramifications, which pass through the CT slice in various directions (Fig. 71-1 c), offer good scanning conditions only if their course is axial. Consequently, they can be identified to varying extents depending on their calibre and direction (72-10). A hint of a circular arrangement of the portal structures can frequently be seen in the cross section of the central right hepatic lobe (Fig. 71-1 c). The **hepatic veins**, which open into the inferior vena cava beneath the diaphragm (Fig. 71-1 f), appear to converge like a star in the transverse section (Fig. 71-1 g). The vessels stand out as hyperdense structures following contrast medium administration or after fatty degeneration of the liver. It is then usually possible to make a better assessment of their spatial arrangements and to compose a mental picture of it from the individual slices.

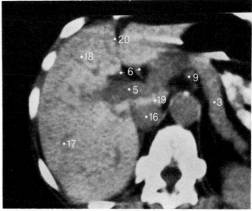

Fig. 71-1 c: **Portal structures.** The falciform ligament forms an almost perfect right-angle with the porta hepatis, which is filled with hypodense portal structures. The ramifying portal structures (branches of the portal vein, hepatic artery and biliary tract) appear hypodense within the liver tissue (c_1). They can frequently be more readily identified as hyperdense structures (c_2) following a bolus injection.

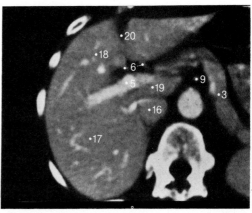

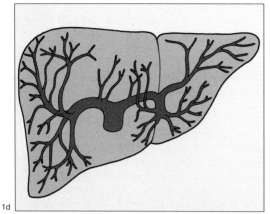

Fig. 71-1 d, e: **Ramification of the portal vein.** The branches can be followed particularly well in the fatty liver parenchyma (e).

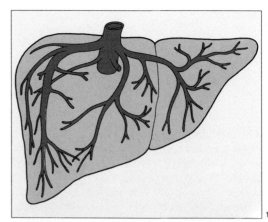

Fig. 71-1 f, g: **Confluence of the branches of the hepatic vein.** The branches frequently appear star-shaped in cranial slice planes of the liver (g).

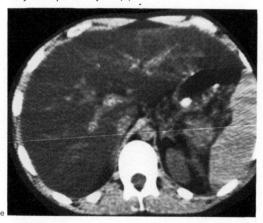

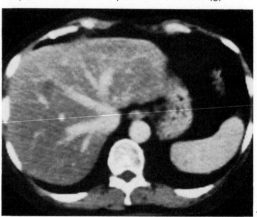

The **adjacent structures** can usually be reliably identified. Narrow horizontal or vaulted fissures at the lower or upper surface of the liver and particularly in the region of the porta hepatis are difficult to survey or are poorly defined if larger slice thicknesses (10–13 mm) are used. Caution is advised in the interpretation of such cases. An undilated subphrenic space can be assessed only at the lateral circumference of the liver.

Gallbladder, biliary tract cf. 72-10.
Subhepatic, subphrenic space cf. 75-10.

Examination technique (71-20)

● **Spasmolytics** (scopolamine-N-butyl-bromide 30–45 mg i. v. or glucagon 1–2 mg i. v.) immediately before the examination in the case of 20-second scanners, as required in the case of shorter scanning times.

● **Scanning** with slice thicknesses of 8–10 mm in an adjacent slice sequence. If necessary, slice thicknesses of 4–5 mm in the region of the porta hepatis.

Scanning area: from the dome of the diaphragm to beneath the right hepatic lobe.

● **Intravenous contrast medium administration** (following a plain scan)

Guided bolus injection (4-32) in localized lesions (for further differentiation, vascular anatomy etc.). As the **multiple bolus technique** in extensive processes, including the search for metastases.

Infusion (4-36) (in extensive processes, mechanical occlusion etc.).

Cystic diseases of the liver (71–30)

Dysontogenetic cysts (71-31)
Dysontogenetic cysts are a form of hamartomatosis which frequently occurs in combination with cystic pancreas or cystic kidneys. The liver is permeated by multiple (epithelialized) cysts of varying size containing a clear fluid.

- **CT**

The computed tomogram reveals zones of reduced density (water range) with soft, smooth and thin walls and arranged in a cluster or rosette pattern. They do not enhance after administration of contrast material (Fig. 71-3a).

Solitary hepatic cysts (71-32)
Solitary hepatic cysts are found mainly in women aged 30–50 years. The cysts, which can achieve a diameter of 20 cm and contain serous material, display epithelium, a solid fibrous capsule and a highly vascular layer of tissue towards the liver parenchyma. They are considered to be caused by malformation and retention.

- **CT**

The computed tomogram shows the usual criteria of a benign cyst (3-51) (Fig. 71-3b, c).

Echinococcus granulosus (71-33)
Echinococcosis is caused by the larval forms of E. alveolaris (multilocularis) and E. granulosus (cysticus, unilocularis), which display a differing morphological picture. The main site of manifestation of this parasitic disease is the liver, followed in order of frequency by the lungs, brain, spleen and other parenchymatous organs.

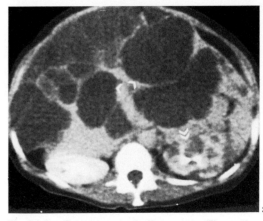

Fig. 71-**3a: Dysontogenetic liver cysts.** The entire liver parenchyma is permeated by thin-walled hypodense zones with smooth borders (>). Renal cysts are also demonstrable (≫).

Fig. 71-**3b,c: Large solitary liver cyst** (b). A faint hyperdense margin of compressed liver tissue is occasionally found in the plain scan at the edge of the cyst in fatty degeneration of the liver (c >).

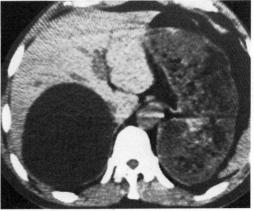

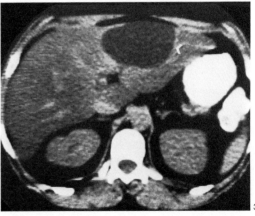

E. granulosus (cysticus, unilocularis) – endemic in Mediterranean countries, Russia and Australia – gives rise to large cysts, the histology of which reveals a typical 3-layer structure (germinal layer, hyaline endocyst and ectocyst; the latter is highly vascular and forms granulation tissue). Consequently, angiography frequently reveals the rim sign in the capillary and early venous phase. Daughter cysts develop both in the cyst itself and as adjacent cysts as a result of evagination of the germinal layer. Shell-like and polycyclic calcifications are the result of parietal calcifications of the masses, which can occasionally also accumulate calcium amorphously due to thickening of the cystic content.

● **CT**

The computed tomogram demonstrates the typical formation of a multilocular cyst, the daughter cysts of which can usually be demarcated by virtue of their spherical or ellipsoid configuration and the fact that the septa are of varying thickness. The wall of the cyst contrasts sharply with the liver tissue and can appear denser than the latter even in the plain scan (416). Partial or total parietal calcifications are regarded as characteristic, but are not a constant feature. A solitary, non-calcified echinococcus cyst can rarely be reliably distinguished from a non-parasitic cyst. The densitiy values are in the range of those of water and somewhat higher (up to 30-45 HU) (416). A ring-shaped increase of density in the region of the cystic wall can frequently be demonstrated as a sign of the perifocal granulation tissue following administration of contrast material (387).

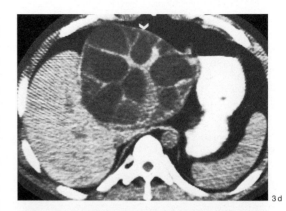

3 d

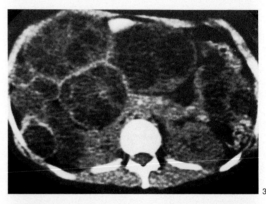

3 e

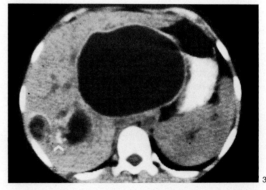

3 f

Fig. 71-3 d–g: **Echinococcus cysts.**

3 d: Echinococcus cyst with typical septation.

3 e: Hydatid disease of the epigastrium. All cysts in the liver and vicinity display typical septation.

3 f: Large, smoothly bordered solitary cyst with well demarcated, slightly hyperdense walls. Marginal calcareous encrustations of the smaller cysts (>).

3 g: Calcified echinococcus cyst consequent on infection 17 years prior to the examination.

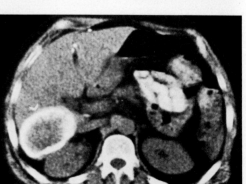

3 g

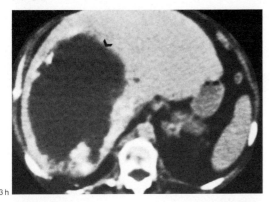

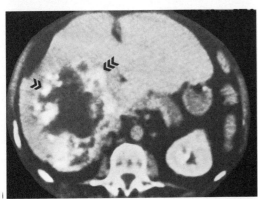

Echinococcus alveolaris (71-34)

E. alveolaris (endemic in Middle and Southern Europe, South America, Australia and South-East Asia) is acquired in childhood and is restricted almost exclusively to the right hepatic lobe. The infected liver tissue is largely necrotic. Macroscopically, it is spongy and permeated by small cysts which are frequently yellow in colour as a result of xanthematous, perifocal inflammation (58).

● CT

The disease, which has usually affected the right hepatic lobe, appears in the computed tomogram as a poorly defined, hypodense zone (14–38 HU) (416). Small nodular to expansive perifocal amorphous calcifications can be seen in 80–90 % of cases. The high degree of vascularity resulting from the concomitant inflammation frequently leads to perifocal enhancement or an inhomogeneous increase of density within the lesion. A lesion devoid of calcification or necrosis is almost impossible to differentiate from a malignant tumour (as in angiography) (387). The clinical finding and serology in particular determine the further procedure.

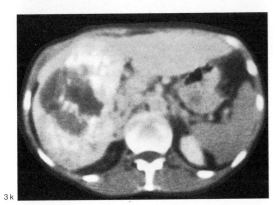

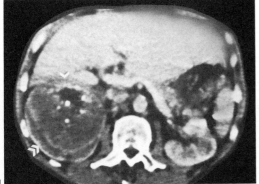

Fig. 71-3 h–l: Alveolar echinococcus.

3 h–k: Large, irregularly demarcated zones of reduced density (necrotic zones >) in the right hepatic lobe with marginal amorphous calcifications (≫). Peripheral enhancement of the lesion following administration of contrast medium (≫) (387).

3 l: Alveolar echinoccocus of the kidney. Similar aspect with peripheral enhancement (≫), liquefying necrosis central and amorphous calcifications (387).

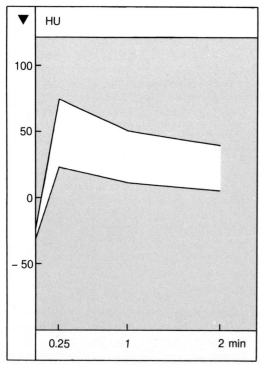

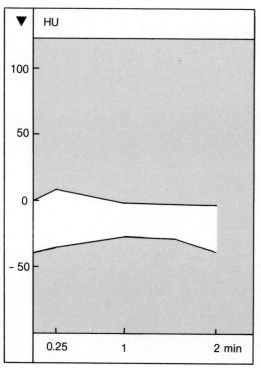

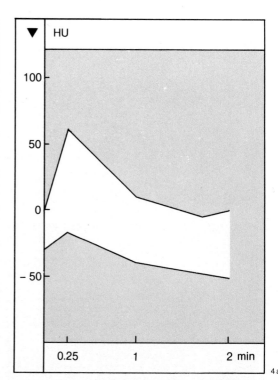

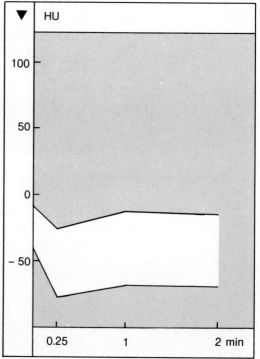

Fig. 71-4 a: **Varying density between tumour tissue and liver parenchyma** after a bolus injection (after Araki) (375).

a_1: Type I: Predominantly in haemanigomas.

a_2: Type II: Predominantly in hepatocellular carcinoma, carcinoma of colon, carcinoid, abscess.

a_3: Type III: In carcinoma of the colon, hepatocellular carcinoma, cholangiocarcinoma.

a_4: Type IV: In carcinoma of the pancreas, stomach, colon, breast or ovary and in squamous cell and hepatocellular carcinoma.

Solid tumours of the liver (71-40)

The computerized tomographic demonstration of hepatic tumours, which is achieved in the plain scan in about 85 % of cases (406), is determined by the difference in density between the tumour and liver tissue. Regardless of the fine-tissue differences, a reduction in the protein concentration, an increased water content and mucoid or fatty degeneration lead to a reduction of density in comparison to the protein-rich liver tissue. Reduced density is usually also present with increased vascularization of a tumour. Following intravenous administration of contrast medium, the increase of density – which represents the intravascular space during the first arteriovenous passage – superimposes on the plain scan. However, the special vascular supply of the liver leads to different phases of opacification. Arterial filling (hepatic artery) takes place 20–30 seconds after contrast medium administration, to be followed 35–50 seconds after the injection by portal opacification (portal vein). The liver receives a quarter of its blood volume from the hepatic artery and three quarters from the portal vein. The two vascular systems determine the degree of opacification in the same proportion. The fact that the tumours are fed almost without exception by branches of the hepatic artery is of diagnostic importance.

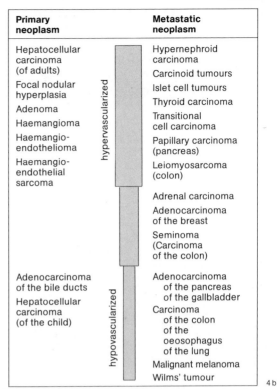

Fig. 71-**4b**: **Vascularity** of liver tumours (angiographic criteria [56]).

Angiography classifies tumours according to their degree of vascularity in comparison to the unchanged branches of the hepatic artery into hypervascular, hypovascular and isovascular tumours (Fig. 71-4b).

● **Hypervascularized regions** display positive enhancement in the arterial phase. This enhancement is usually abrogated in the portovenous phase by the relatively intense opacification of the surrounding liver tissue (temporally opposed opacification). Positive enhancement persists during portal opacification only in particularly pronounced vascularization, above all in large blood spaces (pooling).

● **Hypovascularized regions,** which constitute the largest group of non-cystic masses of the liver, lead to relative enhancement of the surrounding liver tissue even in the arterial phase. The enhancement intensifies in the portovenous phase (synonymous, maximum opacification).

● **Isovascularized regions** do not participate in enhancement in the arterial phase. The enhancement is therefore determined by portovenous opacification alone (portovenous opacification).

Scanners with brief scanning times (2–4 seconds) depict the arterial and portovenous phases separately if brief intravenous injection times (2–5 seconds) are chosen. Thus, in analogy to selective angiography, hypervascularized regions can usually be imaged in the arterial phase as hyperdense hepatic lesions. The individual waves of contrast material become superimposed on each other when the infusion technique or longer injection times are used. Enhancement is then determined by the greater portovenous supply of blood: hypovascularized and isovascularized regions stand out more clearly from the opacified liver parenchyma, while the additional arterial enhancement of hypervascularized lesions attenuates or abrogates the contrast to the surrounding tissue. A guided bolus injection with visualization of the arterial phase is therefore particularly suitable for hypervascularized lesions of the liver (4-32). If the attenuation differences between the liver parenchyma and the lesion are plotted over the time, three types

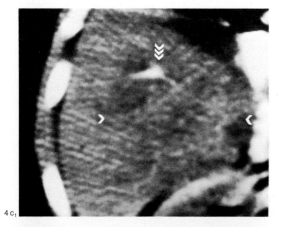

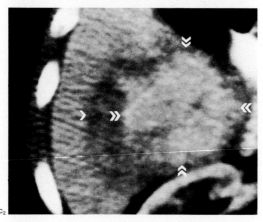

Fig. 71-4c: **Focal nodular hyperplasia.** The hypervascularized tumour appears slightly hypodense (>) in the plain scan. After contrast medium administration, a central feeding vessel (≫) can be seen in the early phase which causes centrifugal opacification of the tumour (≫) after 20 seconds (c_2).

Fig. 71-4d: **Mesenchymal hamartoma** of the liver in a 63-year old woman. Cystoid and myxomatous regions appear as irregular hypodense zones within the right hepatic lobe.

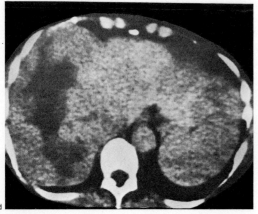

— apart from haemangiomas (71-43) — can be distinguished by the degree of vascularization (375 [Fig. 71-4a]).

Adenomas and focal nodular hyperplasia (71-41)

Adenomas of the liver are rare and originate from the liver cells (hepatoadenoma) or from the bile ducts (bile duct adenoma). Bile duct adenomas are very rare and are important in differential diagnostics only when they display cystic components (cystadenoma of the liver).

The **hepatoadenoma,** which can occur in children and men, has a solid consistency. There is also an increased incidence of adenomas in women who have taken mestranol-containing contraceptives for more than 5 years. In two thirds of these cases there is a tendency towards necrosis and infarction, in which case the normally hypervascularized tumours — which can occur either alone or in multiples — display avascular regions.

Focal nodular hyperplasia, which is encountered primarily in women aged 20–60 years, can produce nodular masses up to 8 cm in diameter. They differ histologically from adenomas because they contain bile ducts. They are mainly situated at the periphery of the liver and may be multifocal.

Adenomatous hyperplasia develops on the basis of postnecrotic cirrhosis or dystrophy of the liver (4) and differs from hepatoadenoma by virtue of its vascular supply, which runs from the periphery to the centre. The extent of the nodular hyperplasia depends on the loss of tissue due to necrosis.

Only 25% of hepatoadenomas and 50% of focal nodular hyperplasias can be detected — as storage defects — by scintigraphy.

● **CT**

Hepatoadenomas and focal nodular hyperplasia appear in the computed tomogram as hypodense or isodense zones. When the density contrasts, they are sharply demarcated from the liver. Since they are usually hypervascularized, the administration of a bolus of contrast medium leads to short-lasting hyperdensity of tumour areas. A centrally fed type can be assumed if the opacification begins in the centre of the tumour (Fig. 71-4c). Infusions of contrast material frequently mask the hypervascularized tumour, but lead to clearer demonstration of necrotic zones in the computed tomogram.

Mesenchymal hamartomas (71-42)

Mesenchymal hamartomas are malformations of the hepatic connective tissue, which forms myxomatous regions and cystic spaces (Fig. 71-4d). Their growth tends to be rapid in childhood due to the formation of cystic, avascular spaces. Progression from haemangioma to cystic degeneration has been described in older patients.

Haemangioma (71-43)

The haemangioendothelioma of childhood can be demarcated from the usual cavernous haemangioma **(cavernoma).** Cavernomas are vascular malformations and are encountered to an increased extent in older (multiparous) women. They tend to develop thrombosis, hyalinization and calcification, which displays a radial structure. Symptoms occur only when the tumours have grown to such an extent that the adjacent organs are displaced. **Haemangioendotheliomas** of childhood are not infrequently accompanied by involvement of other organs. Other features are calcification in the amorphous type, wide nutritive arteries, a. v. shunts and a multicentric arrangement.

Angiography of the cavernoma reveals early filling and delayed clearance of the blood spaces.

● **CT**

Computerized tomography of larger cavernomas reveals a hypodense zone which displays ring-shaped hyperdensity at the periphery of the mass 1–2 minutes after contrast medium administration (376). After 7–12 minutes the density at the centre of the lesion equals that of the surrounding liver tissue, but can exceed it depending on the dosage of contrast material (Fig. 71-4e). This kinetic behaviour can be explained by accumulation of the contrast material in the cavernous spaces due to decelerated flow with successive mixing. These processes cannot usually be depicted in the case of small haemangiomas with a diameter of 1–2 cm, since their blood spaces are not large enough and they appear isodense in the majority of cases. Regressive changes (thromboses) within the haemangiomas do not enhance.

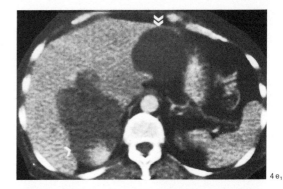

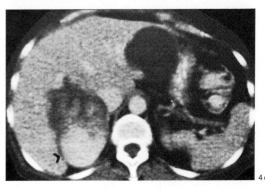

Fig. 71-4 e, f: Cavernous haemangioma.
4 e: Hypodense lobulated zone of reduced density (16 HU) which opacifies more intensely than the liver tissue ($e_2 >$) 10 minutes after a rapid infusion. The ventral cyst does not enhance (≫).

4 f: Hypodense zone (12 HU) which displays first of all peripheral hyperdensity ($f_2 >$) following a bolus injection.

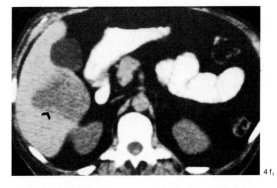

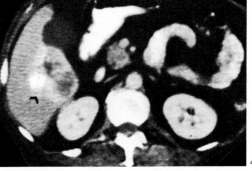

Benign mesodermal tumours (71-44)

Hepatic lipomas

Benign mesodermal tumours are very rare, and only the hepatic lipoma has so far been described (389). It is marked by reduced density values and smooth demarcation from the liver tissue.

Hepatocellular carcinoma (71-45)

Hepatocellular carcinoma is found in 1% of autopsies. Since it develops from cirrhosis in 75% of cases, the number of cases has also been observed to increase with the increasing incidence of hepatitis. The age at manifestation ranges from 40–70, and men are affected three times more frequently than women.

Hepatocellular carcinoma can be divided into three categories:
1. The multicentric form, in which intrahepatic metastasis due to venous invasion has been suggested.
2. A large solitary mass (20–40% of cases).
3. Diffuse involvement of the liver (relatively rare).

Large tumour lesions may be surrounded by a capsule or undergo necrotic degeneration. Calcifications are rarely demonstrated (400). Thromboses of the portal vein and a. v. shunts are regarded as typical.

Clinical examination usually reveals signs of cirrhosis in addition to hepatomegaly. The angiographic findings are of hypervascularized tumours with typical vascular changes suggestive of malignancy. In the diffuse form, the overshadowing signs of liver cirrhosis can present diagnostic difficulties.

Poorly vascularized hepatocellular carcinomas of the anaplastic type occur in childhood.

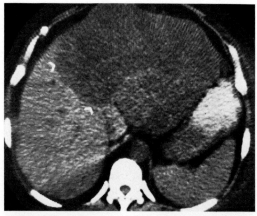

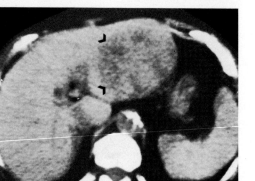

Fig. 71-4g,h: **Hepatocellular carcinoma.** Large hypodense mass of the entire left hepatic lobe in the plain scan (g). Capsule-like demarcation of the carcinoma, which appears slightly hypodense in the plain scan (h).

Fig. 71-4i: **Anaplastic carcinoma** (in a 17-year old girl). Hypodense mass in the porta hepatis which displays only a few discrete tumour vessels on angiography.

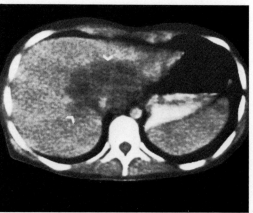

● CT

The plain computed tomogram reveals unifocal or multifocal lesions. These are often extensive hypodense areas which are either distinctly or poorly demarcated from the liver parenchyma. The liver is usually enlarged. The difference in density – usually only 15–20 HU (400, 392) – is marked only in necrotic tumours, so artifact-free computed tomograms are essential if great accuracy is to be achieved.

The administration of contrast material (as an infusion) frequently leads to better delineation of the lesion (383). In some cases, however, the tumour is masked after intravenous contrast medium due to hypervascularization of the neoplasm (71–40) (392, 400). A guided bolus injection (with demonstration of the arterial phase) (402) appears to improve accuracy – particularly in the diffuse forms developing on the basis of liver cirrhosis, which have previously escaped CT detection in individual cases. The guided bolus technique enhances the vascular structures of the liver to such an extent that extensive thromboses of the portal vein can be recognized (400). Tumour invasion of the inferior vena cava can be suggested with the aid of the infusion technique (425).

Regional (portal and paraaortic) lymph node enlargement can occasionally be demonstrated. Signs of liver cirrhosis with portal hypertension (71-53) frequently overshadow the CT image of the carcinoma.

Cholangiocarcinoma (71-46)

Cholangiocarcinoma occurs very much less frequently than hepatocellular carcinoma and affects women twice as frequently as men (age at manifestation 40–70 years.). Histologically, the fibrous component is particularly striking. On angiography, the tumour is found to be poorly vascularized; thus the vascular changes are discrete and displacement of vessels is one of the most important signs.

● CT

The tumour stands out in the computed tomogram as a poorly defined, (slightly) hypodense, usually unilocular zone which is well demarcated following administration of contrast material.

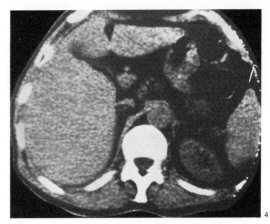

Fig. 71-4 k: **Multicentric hepatocellular carcinoma resulting from cirrhosis of the liver.** Despite administration of contrast medium (infusion), no demarcation of the tumour zone.

Fig. 71-4 l, m: **Cholangiocarcinoma.** Enlargement of the left hepatic lobe with slightly different density to the normal liver tissue.

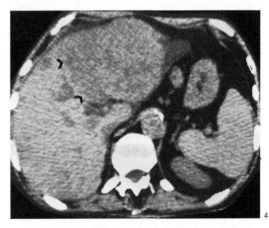

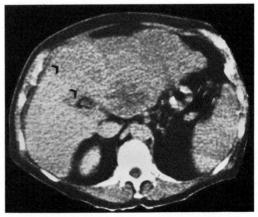

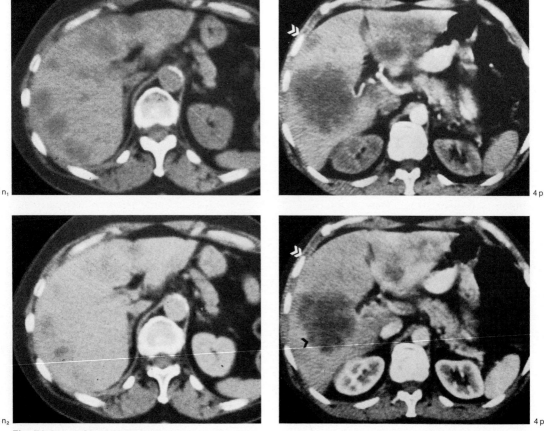

Fig. 71-4 n–q: Liver metastases.

4 n: Liver metastases from mammary carcinoma. Multiple hypodense zones in the plain scan (n_1) which display concentric diminution following contrast medium administration or become masked (n_2).

4 p: The septations of the metastases from carcinoma of the colon become clearer after a bolus injection ($p_2 >$). Masking of individual tumour zones ($\gg$).

4 o: Metastases from a carcinoma of unknown origin. The different density values of the individual hypodense zones correspond to the varying degrees of liquefaction of the tumour tissue.

4 q: Metastases from a testicular teratocarcinoma. The absence of enhancement and density values of 17 HU indicate advanced liquefaction.

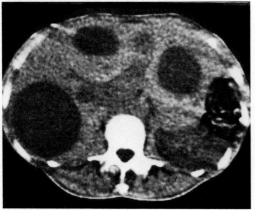
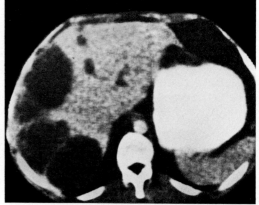

Secondary tumours of the liver
(liver metastases) (71-47)

The liver is the predilection site for metastases from tumours of the gastrointestinal tract (primarily colonic cancer), mammary and bronchial carcinomas, hypernephromas and uterine tumours. A solitary focus is found in 10% of clinical observations. Metastases are demonstrated with equal frequency in cirrhotic and healthy livers.

The pathological anatomy of the metastatic tissue resembles that of the primary tumour. Thus the metastases may be mucinous in carcinoma of the colon and stomach, and small, circumscribed and disseminated in mammary carcinoma. The search for and identification of liver tumours is aided by the fact that the metastases display frequently the same pattern and degree of vascularization as their primary tumour (Fig. 71-4b).

● **CT**

Metastases are recognizable in the plain computed tomogram as hypodense, poorly defined areas in the liver parenchyma. Multiplicity is an indication of metastases, although some primary liver tumours are also multicentric (71-45). Highly vascularized metastases (Fig. 71-4b) are also usually hypodense in the plain scan and can assume the density of healthy liver tissue, i. e. become isodense following administration of contrast material (as an infusion). Consequently, homogeneous liver density following enhancement does not rule out metastases.

Regressive changes of the metastases frequently lead to necrosis with an appearance similar to a cyst or an abscess (Fig. 71-4o,q). Hyalinization and calcifications are other forms of tumour degeneration which produce hyperdense areas in the lesion (Fig. 71-7a). Metastases with regressive changes or necrosis can also display highly vascularized regions at their margin – as known from angiography – which, following contrast medium administration (as an infusion), lead to diminution of the hypodense zones seen in the plain scan (Fig. 71-4s). The parts of the tumour which have undergone regressive change can then be clearly seen. A ring-shaped hyperdense zone appears in some cases (421), such as has been described in abscesses due to granulation tissue. This picture is found relatively frequently in the arterial phase following a guided bolus injection (402).

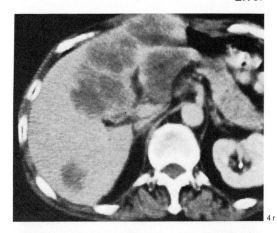

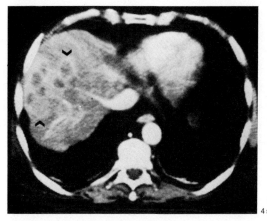

Fig. 71-4 r–t: Liver metastases.

4 r: Metastases from a rectal carcinoma with septum-like cystoid structure and density values of 48 HU in the plain scan.

4 s: Metastases from a malignant mediastinal teratoma. Note the ring-shaped enhancement.

4 t: Metastases from carcinoma of the colon. In addition to an intrahepatic metastasis (≫), demonstration of carcinomatous peritonitis with solid components (>) in the subphrenic space.

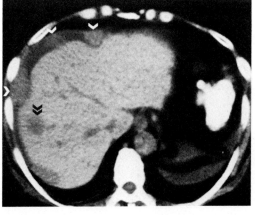

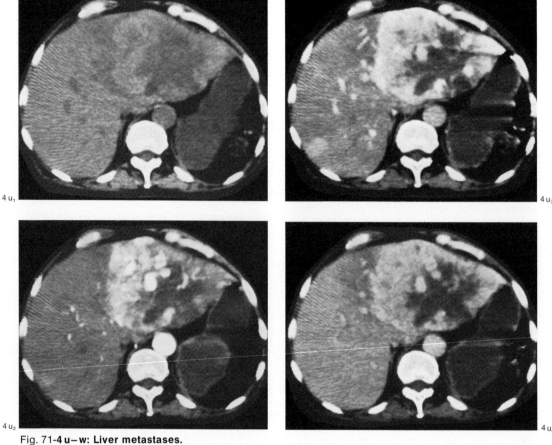

Fig. 71-4 u–w: Liver metastases.

4 u: Metastases from a hypernephroma. Marked enhancement with transient hyperdensity of the tumour zone following a bolus injection (u_1 = plain scan, u_2 = 12 seconds p. i., u_3 = 22 seconds p. i., u_4 = 60 seconds p. i.).

4 v: Metastasis from carcinoma of the colon. Demonstration of regressive changes (calcifications in the centre of the tumour zone [>]) in the plain scan.

4 w: Extensive metastatic disease from carcima of the colon in the upper right hepatic lobe (>) with central calcifications.

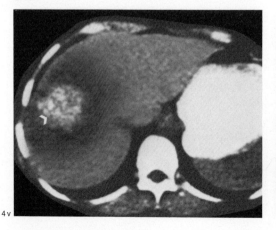

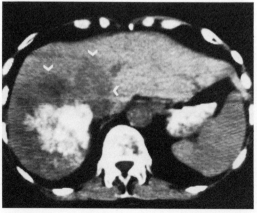

Inflammatory changes of the liver
(71-50)

Fatty degeneration of the liver (71-51)
Incorporation of fat into the liver cell takes place in such conditions as chronic alcoholism, diabetes mellitus, hyperalimentation, malnutrition (protein deficiency, kwashiorkor), chronic infections (e. g. severe pulmonary TB, chronic diarrhoea) and porphyria tarda. It is usually accompanied by an increase in size of the organ.

● **CT**

In the majority of cases the computed tomogram reveals a diffuse reduction of density of the liver tissue. In the plain scan, the vessels are frequently more dense than the parenchyma (contrast reversal). Determination of the degree of fatty degeneration depends on the measuring accuracy of the scanner (117) (3-54). Since fat is not incorporated into neoplasias (metastases, focal nodular hyperplasia, haemangiomas etc.), they appear in the plain scan as hyperdense zones (418). Fatty degeneration of the liver can leave segmental sections of the liver parenchyma unaffected.

Hepatitis (71-52)
In **non-purulent hepatitis** (following virus infection, intoxication and Weil's disease) hepatomegaly occurs only in the acute stage and is moderate in the majority of cases. Acute dystrophy of the liver usually leads to shrinkage of the organ. Concomitant hepatitis in granulomatous diseases (tuberculosis, sarcoidosis, brucellosis, tularaemia, syphilis and lupus erythematodes) does not alter the size and contour of the liver to any particular extent. Fine, disseminated calcifications of diagnostic interest can occur in tuberculosis, brucellosis and, but rarely, in sarcoidosis as well. **Purulent (bacterial) hepatitis** can consist histologically of disseminated, microscopically fine purulent foci which lie beneath the limit of resolution of computerized tomography. It can, however, be diagnosed when the foci fuse to form larger lesions (abscesses 71-55).

● **CT**

Hepatitis is **not an indication** for computerized tomography, since there are no specific diagnostic signs on CT. However, CT can reveal calcifications which are not visible in the general film.

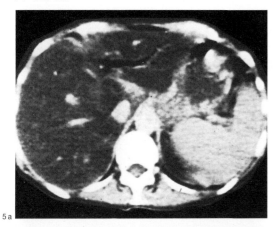

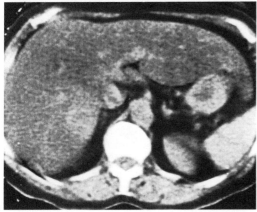

Fig. 71-**5a,b: Varying degrees of fatty degeneration of the liver.** The density values of −32 HU (a) and +16 HU (b) indicate degeneration of ∼65% and ∼35%, respectively.

Fig. 71-**5c: Fatty hepatitis due to alcohol abuse.** Diffuse reduction of density of the liver parenchyma with the exception of central areas in the left hepatic lobe (>).

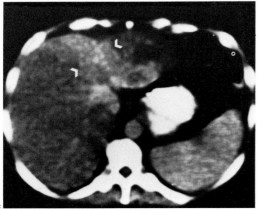

Cirrhosis (71-53)

Cirrhosis of the liver is found in 8% of all post-mortem examinations. Most frequent is the **septal** form (57% of cases), followed by the **cholangitic** (biliary) form with 20% and the **postnecrotic** (postdystrophic) form. Septal cirrhosis (Laennec) usually develops from fatty degeneration of the liver, which assumes a honeycomb structure as a result of connective-tissue septation. The size of the usually enlarged organ diminishes evenly and congruously with increasing incorporation of connective tissue. In contrast, the liver is normally enlarged in biliary cirrhosis. Bulbous regeneration nodes of varying size are found in the postnecrotic type (e. g. following hepatitis) depending on the extent of tissue loss. The signs of portal hypertension with splenomegaly, collateral circulation and ascites are determined by the degree of intrahepatic resistance.

● CT

Computerized tomography can demonstrate the shape and size of the liver, but not the extent of tissue reorganization, since the density of the regeneration nodes rarely differs from that of the cirrhotic liver tissue. Protrusion of the individual lobes – particularly of the caudate lobe in the direction of the porta hepatis, which then appears to be split-shaped and constricted – is considered to be relatively typical, but not conclusive. In most cases, the portal structures within the liver tissue are less easy to identify than in normal tissue – an observation which has been attributed to increased tortuosity of the vessels (398). The shape of the cirrhotically shrunken liver is frequently incongruous. The computerized tomographic aspect is rounded off by the demonstration of ascites, splenic enlargement, prominent splenic vessels and collaterals (reopened umbilical vein). Oesophageal varices are usually recognizable only in pronounced cases (391). A specific search should be made for malignant growth, particularly in hepatomegaly (71-45).

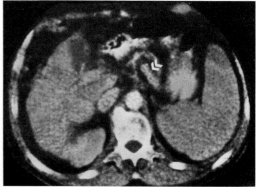

5 d

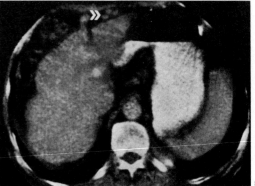

5 e

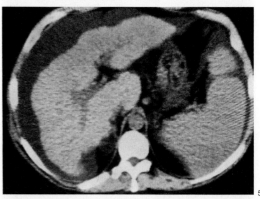

5 f

Fig. 71-5 d–g: Cirrhosis of the liver.

5d, e: Cirrhosis of the liver with a small liver and signs of portal hypertension (splenomegaly, 2 cm wide splenic vein [d] and collateral vessels via the umbilical vein [e]).

5f: Liver of normal size with humped surface, homogeneous parenchymal density (63 HU), enlarged caudate lobe and cleft-shaped porta hepatis. Splenomegaly and ascites.

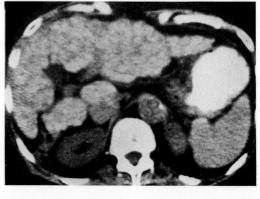

5 g

Haemochromatosis (71-54)

Haemochromatosis, an idiopathic condition, is marked by increased, pathogenetically unclarified intestinal absorption of iron, which is then deposited in parenchymatous organs (liver, pancreas, myocardium). The liver cell contains 1–10 mg iron in 100 g tissue, i. e. 5–50 times the normal value. The parenchymatous organs react to the deposition with cirrhotic reorganization. In secondary **haemosiderosis,** the increased absorption of iron is caused by chronic anaemia (thalassaemia), congenital transferin deficiency and (rarely) by (alcohol-induced) cirrhosis. Where organ function is impaired, the condition is known as secondary haemochromatosis, which deposits considerably less iron than the primary form (4).

● **CT**

In the computed tomogram, the increased iron content (and the cirrhosis) causes a distinct increase in the density of the liver tissue. At 100–140 HU it is frequently twice the normal density value (404). The portal structures and, not infrequently, the signs of portal hypertension stand out well (71-53).

Abscesses (71-55)

The **pyogenic abscess** develops as a result of ascending infection due to obstructed flow in the biliary tract and also as a result of haematogenous dissemination in systemic, septic infections (endocarditis, pneumonia) or in purulent inflammations in the drainage area of the portal vein (appendicitis, diverticulitis, colitis). Less frequent causes are the spread of bacterial inflammation from the immediate vicinity of the liver (e. g. the gallbladder) and direct infection from injuries. The abscess is cryptogenic in about 50 % of cases. E. coli is demonstrated most frequently as the pathogenic organism, and aerobes are involved in 50 % of cases. Pyogenic abscesses develop as unilocular and multilocular lesions. They are encountered to an increased extent in older patients and are promoted by diabetes mellitus, cardiac insufficiency and cirrhosis of the liver.

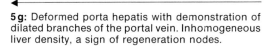

5g: Deformed porta hepatis with demonstration of dilated branches of the portal vein. Inhomogeneous liver density, a sign of regeneration nodes.

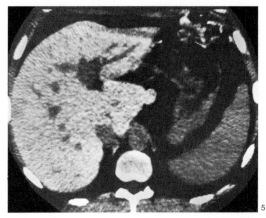

Fig. 71-**5h: Haemochromatosis.** Increased density values (98 HU) and signs of cirrhosis of the liver (splenomegaly, enlarged caudate lobe).

Fig. 71-**5i: Incipient pyogenic abscess formation.** Poorly defined hypodensity in the plain scan. The zone decreases in size after administration of contrast medium (i_2) and displays a perifocal increase of density. Faint septation within the abscess formation. Complete regression of the findings under antibiotic therapy.

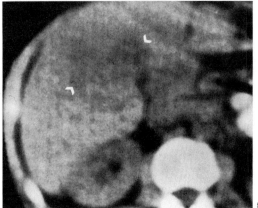

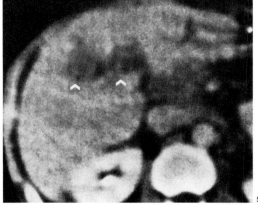

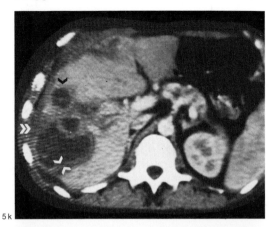

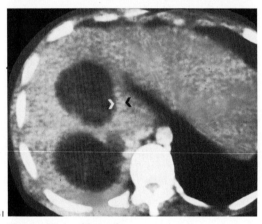

Fig. 71-5k–m: Liver abscesses.

5k: Pyogenic liver abscess. Smoothly bordered zones of reduced density (27 HU) in the right hepatic lobe (>). Demonstration of sharply demarcated ring-shaped enhancement as a sign of extensive granulation tissue (><). Subcapsular spread of the abscess (≫).

5l: Amoebic abscess. A hyperdense ring (><) can be seen around the hypodense zone (16–35 HU).

5m: Tuberculous abscesses. Demonstration of multiple, well-demarcated hypodense zones (10–20 HU).

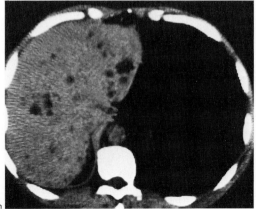

The **amoebic abscess** is found mainly in South and Middle America, Anterior Asia and parts of Africa. The pathogen, the protozoon entamoeba histolytica, enters the liver via the portal circulation and causes necroses from consistent material. This is followed later by the formation of cavities filled with a brownish fluid (anchovy sauce). The thick wall of the abscess is irregularly demarcated and permeated by necrotic material and copious granulation tissue. The condition can be complicated by thrombophlebitis of individual branches of the hepatic vessels. Superinfection by pyogenic pathogens occurs in 20 % of cases.

● **CT**

A zone of **reduced density** which is relatively well delineated from the surrounding liver tissue is demonstrated in a ripe abscess with an abscess membrane. Contrast enhancement frequently reveals a ring-shaped **hyperdense margin** – which represents granulation tissue. This is produced in particularly great quantities in the amoebic abscess as opposed to other types (71-47). The density value depends on the age of the abscess (3-53). Fresh abscesses are only moderately hypodense. The density values fall – in the case of the amoebic abscess to about those of water – with increasing liquefaction of necrotic areas and as a result of absorption processes. The mean density is usually 30 HU. The hypodense zone does not enhance following contrast medium administration – a phenomenon of value in the differential diagnosis from solid processes. A hypodense zone displaying distinct enhancement can be demonstrated in fresh inflammatory infiltrates without any actual abscess formation, a finding which makes differentiation from a tumour impossible (26). Necrotic metastases can occasionally also create the impression of abscesses (Fig. 71-4 o, q), and in these cases the clinical picture and case history are frequently the decisive factor in the differential diagnosis. Orientation of the lesions to the biliary tract is occasionally found in cholangitic abscesses.

Computerized tomography is particularly suitable for monitoring the course of therapy.

Trauma (71-60)

Abdominal trauma – usually blunt and occurring in particular after car accidents – is the most frequent cause of hepatic injury. Rupture of the parenchyma with the formation of intraparenchymal and subcapsular haematomas can lead to life-threatening haemorrhage in the abdominal cavity as a result of concomitant or subsequently occurring capsular rupture. In the case of gunshot and stab wounds the haematoma forms along the path of the perforation.

● **CT**

The computed tomogram reveals the **haematoma** as a consequence of the trauma. When fresh, its density does not always differ from that of liver tissue and it is then necessary to administer contrast material to make the liver parenchyma stand out from the haematoma. Later, 4–9 days after the trauma, the haematoma usually appears as a hypodense zone. The subcapsular arrangement is seen as a hypodense concomitant margin. Since it cannot always be differentiated from an **intraperitoneal** accumulation of fluid (blood), the relationship of the hepatic capsule to the parenchyma as well as the other fissures (75-10) of the peritoneal cavity must be carefully analysed.

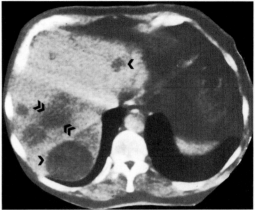

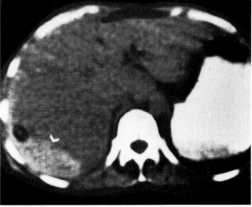

Fig. 71-**6a,b: Liver haematoma.**

6a: Demonstration of an irregularly demarcated zone of reduced density (≫) following rupture of the liver parenchyma. The sharply contrasted round hypodense areas correspond to dysontogenetic cysts (>).

6b: Intrahepatic haematoma after insertion of a drain. Hyperdense zone (>) next to the drain.

Infections
Echinococcus cysticus Echinococcus alveolaris **Abscess,** particularly amoebic abscess (Disseminated) granulomas in – tuberculosis – brucellosis – histoplasmosis (coccidioidomycosis, toxoplasmosis, sarcoidosis, gummas)
Tumours
Cysts (non-parasitic) Hepatocellular carcinoma Hepatoblastoma **Haemangioma** Cholangiocarcinoma **Metastatic:** Mucinous carcinoma **(Chest, colon, ovary, stomach)** Melanoma Insulinoma Neuroblastoma
Other disease
Intrahepatic gallstones Aneurysm of the hepatic artery Haemochromatosis Phleboliths

Fig. 71-**7a: Calcifications of the liver** (after 27, 28 [modified]).

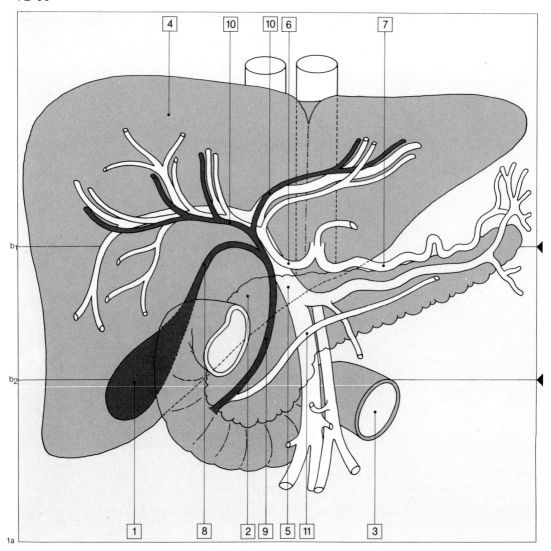
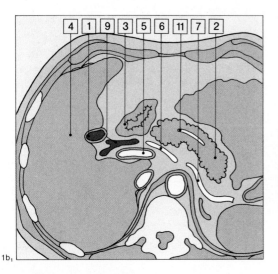
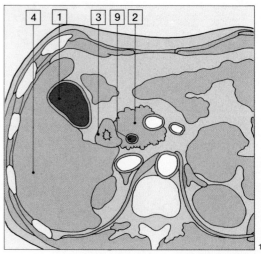

Biliary system (72-00)

Anatomy and imaging (72-10)

The **gallbladder** has a variable shape and position related to its function. In the computed tomogram it can be seen at the medial contour of the right hepatic lobe beneath the porta hepatis. The density of the lumen is slightly above that of water (zero) but density values of up to 25 HU may be found depending on the viscosity of the bile. Since, however, there is no surrounding fatty tissue in most cases, the walls of the gallbladder at the maximum circumference are rarely visible. The gallbladder then assumes the appearance of a benign cyst.

The **common bile duct** traverses the duodenum in the hepatoduodenal ligament and then runs almost vertically in a caudal direction through the head of the pancreas. The inclination of this section of the duct determines whether it is visible on the computed tomogram. If its course is virtually axial and the pancreatic tissue is opacified with a urographic agent (contrast lumen/pancreatic tissue: $\sim$ 50 HU), the common bile duct can be visualized from a calibre of 3 mm (430). If the calibre of the tubular lumen is small, deviation from the axial course of 30° from the vertical (in the sectional plane) reduces its ability to be visualized because of the partial volume effect. From a calibre of 10 mm, the common bile duct can generally be delineated in the prepapillary region – regardless of its course – if thin slices (5–8 mm) and parenchymal opacification of the pancreatic tissue are chosen.

The **intrahepatic** (hypodense) **bile ducts** lie in front of the points of departure of the portal branches (Fig. 72-1 a) and, since they are not involved in intravascular enhancement, can only be distinguished from the latter following intravenous administration of a urographic agent. They are subject to the same laws of imaging mentioned above. Moderate dilations of about 3–5 mm can be visualized only exceptionally when they pass axially through the sectional plain.

Examination technique (72-20)

● **Reduction of intestinal gas** by low residue diet 48 hours before the examination.

● **Partial opacification of the bowel.** Oral administration of 500 ml of a diluted Gastrografin solution 20 minutes before the examination.

● **Spasmolytics** (scopolamine-N-butyl-bromide 30–45 mg i.v. or glucagon 1–2 mg i.v.) immediately before the examination in the case of 20-second scanners, as required in the case of shorter scan times.

● **Scanning** at intervals of 5 mm in the gallbladder and 8 mm in the region of the head of the pancreas. Corresponding selection of slice thicknesses, overlapping slice technique in the case of non-availability.

Scanning area: the entire porta hepatis up to and including the head of the pancreas. In addition, individual peripheral liver slices in a cranial direction if dilatation of the bile ducts is suspected.

Cholecystomegaly (72-30)

The size of the gallbladder is related to its function and is not a specific sign. After fasting, in diabetes mellitus and acromegaly the gallbladder is distinctly enlarged and responds adequately to a fatty meal. However, a negative cholecystogram puts a different face on the matter. If no gallstones are demonstrated in such a case, acute cholecystitis is the first consideration as regards differential diagnosis.

● **CT**
In computerized tomography the gallbladder is considered to be enlarged when the horizontal diameter exceeds 5 cm (434). The longitudinal extention should, however, also be considered, attention being paid to the number of slices required to demonstrate the gallbladder. The wall of the gallbladder is not usually thickened in functional enlargement.

Fig. 72-1 a, b: Topography of the biliary system.
1 a: Anterior view.
1 b: Transverse section. Level of slice cf. 1 a.

Key
1 Gallbladder
2 Pancreas
3 Duodenum
4 Liver
5 Portal vein
6 Hepatic artery
7 Splenic artery
8 Cystic duct
9 Common bile duct
10 Hepatic duct
11 Pancreatic duct

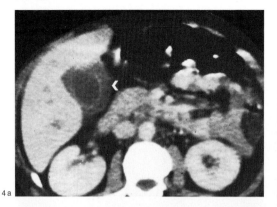

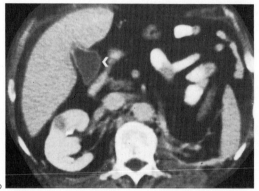

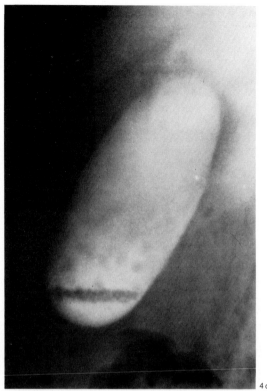

Fig. 72-4 a: **Acute cholecystitis in typhus.** Demonstration of a 1 to 2 cm wide hypodense zone (>) corresponding to the oedematous swelling of the gallbladder wall around the thin-walled inner contours of the wall.

Fig. 72-4 b: **Chronic cholecystitis.** Thickening and deformation of the gallbladder wall (>).

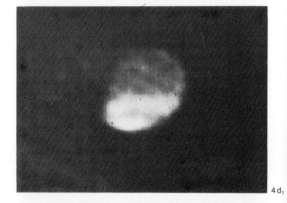

Fig. 72-4 c, d: **Cholecystolithiasis** with non-opaque concrements. In analogy to oral cholegraphy (c), stratification phenomena from cholesterol stones can also be demonstrated in the computed tomogram (d_1). The lower limit of resolution of small concrements depends on the contrast with the bile and on equipment factors.

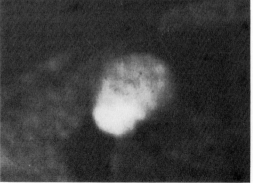

Inflammatory changes of the gallbladder (72-40)

Cholecystitis (72-41)
Chronic cholecystitis occurs almost invariably together with gallstones and results in a wall interspersed with connective tissue and, usually, fused to the surrounding tissue. Acute episodes of inflammation can cause oedematous infiltration and also thickening of the gallbladder wall. **Acute** cholecystitis without stones caused by congestion of the bile is a rare finding, but it is also marked by considerable thickening of the wall of up to 10 mm. The lumen may be enlarged to a greater extent than in chronic cholecystitis. In emphysematous cholecystitis – a very rare condition caused by anaerobic bacteria – gas is found not only in the lumen, but also discretely in the wall itself.

● **CT**
The main sign in the computed tomogram is thickening of the wall. This usually amounts to 3–5 mm, although it can exceed 10 mm. The status of the inflammation can be assessed by the vascularity: in acute inflammations, a rapid infusion or a guided bolus injection leads to distinct enhancement of the walls; a deeply opacified inner layer can frequently be demarcated from a hypodense – corresponding to subserous oedema – outer layer (60). Perforation and pericholecystitic abscesses in the vicinity of the gallbladder appear as hyopodense, encapsulated zones. Chronic indurative mural processes eventually lead to fine deposits of calcium which may progress into shell-like encrustations (porcelain gallbladder).
The differential diagnosis must include carcinoma of the gallbladder (72-50).

Cholelithiasis (72-42)
Oral cholegraphy and ultrasound are the methods of choice for the demonstration of gallstones. A **relative indication for computerized tomography** exists if cholegraphy is negative and ultrasound repeatedly unsuccessful. Over 90% of all gallstones contain

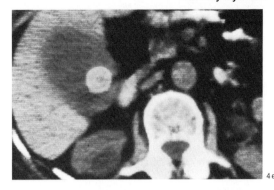
4e

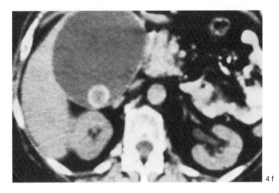
4f

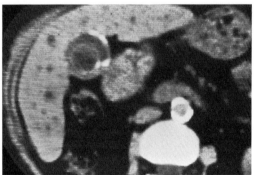
4g

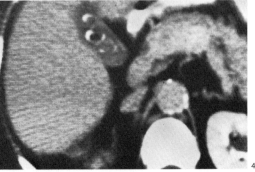
4h

Fig. 72-4 e–h: **Radiopaque gallstones** are demonstrated more sensitively than in conventional radiography, although the appearance is, in principle, similar. The concentric stratification (e–h), vacuum phenomena (h) and calcifications of the gallbladder wall (g) are usually demonstrable in the computed tomogram.

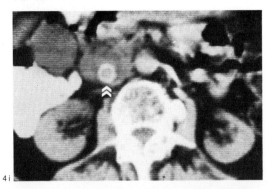

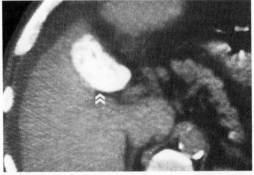

Fig. 72-4 i, k: **Cholelithiasis.** Choledochal stones (i) and lime milk bile (k).

Fig. 72-4 l: **Gallbladder hydrops.** Considerably enlarged, thinwalled gallbladder. The density values of the bile are 8 HU.

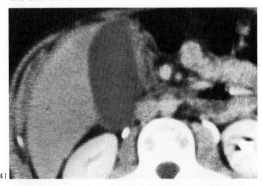

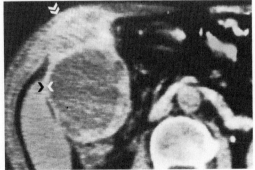

varying amounts of calcium. However, in only 20–25% of cases is it present at concentrations high enough to produce distinct contrast in the plain cholegram (16a).

● **CT**

When stones are sought specifically, a higher percentage of (calcareous) gallstones is detected in the plain computed tomogram than in the plain cholegram or in negative cholecystography. A condition for this is, however, detailed imaging with thin (5–8 mm) and contiguous slices to minimize the partial volume effect. The typical radiological pattern of calcification of the stones can be recognized in the case of larger concrements (Fig. 72-4 e, k), although not with the plethora of detail provided by the conventional film (Fig. 72-4 c). If calcifications are present, it is advisable to reposition the patient to permit discrimination of calcareous incrustations of the wall from sedimented stones. Since, depending on the viscosity, the radiodensity of the bile ranges from 0–25 with an absolute maximum of 80 HU, the contrast with the gallstones also varies, which means that isodensity can occur. In in-vitro studies (439), pure cholesterol stones display radiodensity of about minus 60 to minus 80 HU, which can clearly exceed the density of water depending on the proportion of calcium. Vacuum phenomena considerably reduce the radiodensity to 375 HU (439). In some cases, therefore, calcium-free gallstones are recognizable in the computed tomogram because of their negative density values even within non-opacified bile if a specific search is made for them.

Havrilla (433, 434) reports an overall success rate of 80% for gallbladder stones without opacification of the bile.

Hydrops and empyema of the gallbladder (72-43)

Occlusion of the cystic duct can lead to distinct enlargement of the gallbladder via a valvular mechanism (hydrops). The condition is further complicated by chronic inflammation with shrinkage of the gallbladder and by infection of the congested bile (empyema).

Fig. 72-4 m: **Empyema of the gallbladder with abscess of the abdominal wall.** Thickened gallbladder wall, the layers of which appear irregular following administration of contrast medium (density of the bile 31 HU). Masking of the muscle layers by exudation (≫).

● **CT**

The CT sign of hydrops is an enlarged gallbladder. High radiodensity of up to 80 HU (429) due to thickening of the bile is not, however, a constant feature (Fig. 72-4I). In empyema the CT image also reveals distinct thickening of the gallbladder wall. The density values of the infected bile are likewise increased (density value of pus approx. 30 HU). If the stone in the gallbladder neck or cystic duct cannot be identified, the computed tomogram offers the same picture as in acute cholecystitis.

Tumours of the gallbladder (including hyperplastic cholecystoses) (72-50)

"Cholesterol papillomas" measuring 3–5 mm with a maximum of 10 mm and usually occurring in multiples are the second most frequent filling defect in the cholecystogram after gallstones. **Cholesterosis** of varying severity is found in 23 % of cases of gallbladder surgery. **Adenomyomatosis** is segmental or general hyperplasia of the gallbladder wall. It is regarded as a hamartoma and is found in 5 % of histologically examined organ preparations. Genuine **papillomas**, which usually measure less than 5 mm and occur either alone or in multiples and with peduncles, and **adenomas**, which generally occur alone and with a larger diameter (0.5–4 cm), are rare in comparison to hyperplastic cholecystoses (0.5–1 % of cholecystectomies). Choristomas, fibromas, carcinoids and neurinomas are rarely encountered. The high coincidence of all the above-mentioned diseases with cholecystolithiasis is remarkable, ranging from 75 % in the case of adenomyomatosis to 38 % in the case of adenomas.

Carcinoma – in 95 % of cases an adenocarcinoma – is the most frequent malignant tumour of the gallbladder. Since it accounts for 3 % of the malignomas of the gastrointestinal tract it is not a rare condition. Gallstones are also found in 75 % of cases and women – particularly the over-sixties – are affected much more frequently than men. The tumour spreads in the gallbladder bed – usually before the appearance of clinical symptoms – and infiltrates the hepatoduodenal ligament, the liver and the regional lymph nodes. The prognosis is consequently unfavourable in most cases. Sarcomas of different kinds of tissue are extremely rare. Metastatic spread into the gallbladder usually originates from a melanoma.

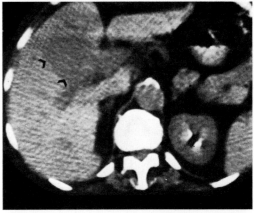

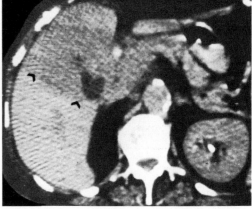

Fig. 72-5 a–c: **Carcinoma of the gallbladder.** The tumour is invading the right hepatic lobe. The contours of the gallbladder wall are poorly defined in this region (≫). Higher slices reveal hypodense tumour tissue within the liver (>).

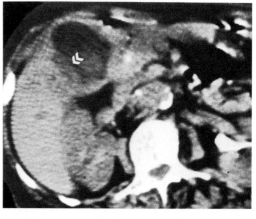

CT

Adenomyomatosis manifests itself as thickening of the gallbladder wall. However, the minute protusions of the dilated Rokitansky-Aschoff sinus, which are of importance for the differential diagnosis, are below the limits of resolution of computerized tomography. Similarly, very small polyps in **cholesterosis** and **papillomas** with a diameter of less than 5 mm are hardly recognizable even after enhancement of the gallbladder lumen with a cholegraphic agent. Only parietal filling defects from a size of 0.7–1 cm can be reliably demonstrated, although – as with conventional cholegraphy – the nature cannot be diagnosed even by means of the density value.

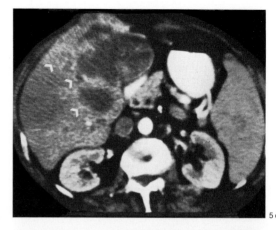

5d

Since cholecystography is rarely positive in the case of **carcinoma**, computerized tomography can provide important information. A frequent finding is a more or less inhomogeneous solid mass in the gallbladder space with poorly defined boundaries to the surrounding liver parenchyma (massive type after Itai [437]). Further CT signs of a gallbladder carcinoma are (irregular) thickening of the wall and intraluminal masses (437). A guided bolus injection leads to better demarcation from the liver parenchyma and, usually, to distinct enhancement of the thickened wall or intraluminal tumour (60, 437). Dilated intrahepatic bile ducts are another, not infrequent finding and are an indication of obstruction of the biliary tract by lymphomas or tumour invasion in the region of the porta hepatis.

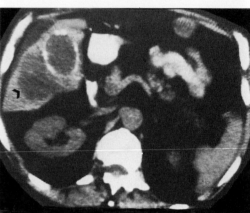

5e

Infiltration in the direction of the pancreas and duodenum can be assessed only after adequate oral opacification of the bowel. Enlarged portal and hepatoduodenal lymph nodes can be demonstrated only if sufficient fat is interposed and usually – because of the complex anatomical situation – only above a diameter of 2 cm. As with liposarcomas, a tentative diagnosis of the nature of the neoplasm based on the density values can be made only in exceptional cases (428). The site of origin of the neoplasm cannot be unequivocally determined by computerized tomography if extensive infiltration into the liver tissue has taken place (invasive carcinoma of the gallbladder or expansion of a malignant liver tumour into the porta hepatis).

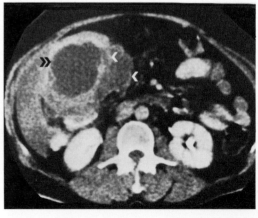

5f

Inflammations of the biliary tract (72-60)

Obstruction caused by stones, stricture or tumour forms the basis for pyogenic infection of the biliary tract. Reflux of intestinal juice following surgery (choledochoduodenostomy) is another cause. Periductal abscesses, particularly in the liver region, are a serious complication of cholangitis. Their protracted existence or frequent recurrence leads to strictures of the peripheral bile ducts which are not usually as severe as those in sclerosing cholangitis. Stenosing papillitis is regarded as a concomitant symptom of neighbouring inflammatory processes (cholangitis, cholecystitis, duodenitis) and leads to dilatation of the common bile duct.

● CT

The computed tomogram shows only circumscribed or general dilation of the biliary tract and, but rarely, thickening of the wall of the common bile duct. The hypodense zone around the intrahepatic bile ducts can be interpreted as oedema or incipient abscess formation and requires further investigation (liver abscesses 71-55). Air in the biliary tract is clearly demonstrable.

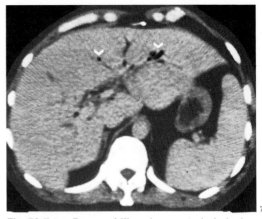

Fig. 72-**7a**: **Pneumobilia.** In post-choledocho-duodenostomy status, demonstration of air in the biliary tract, a condition readily detectable by computerized tomography.

Fig. 72-**7b, c: Dilation of the biliary tract.** The dilated bile ducts appear as hypodense structures orienting on the portal system. They do not enhance following contrast medium administration and are therefore clearly identifiable (portal branches ≫).

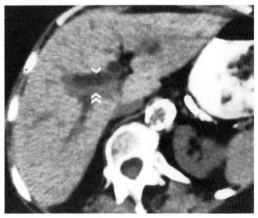

Fig. 72-**5d–f: Carcinoma of the gallbladder.**

5d: Hypodense zones in the right hepatic lobe displaying marginal enhancement. The contours of the gallbladder can no longer be clearly demarcated within the tumour mass.

5e: The gallbladder is still recognizable due to calcareous encrustations. The tumour is expanding as a hypodense zone into and below the right hepatic lobe.

5f: Following bolus injection, demonstration of a concentric hyperdensity within the tumour mass (>) around the deformed centrally situated gallbladder (≫).

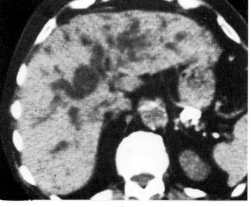

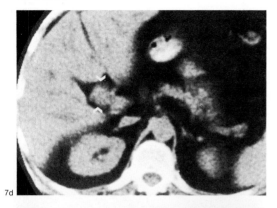

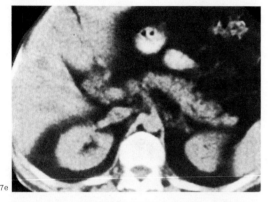

Fig. 72-7 d, e: **Bile duct adenoma** at the level of the hepatic bifurcation. Only moderate, central dilation of the bile duct, barely discernible in the computed tomogram, with no enlargement of the gallbladder. The tumour, 1.5 cm in size, can just be recognized in the porta hepatis (>), but cannot be unequivocally differentiated from the portal branches without contrast medium administration.

Fig. 72-7f: **Choledochal cyst.** Demonstration of a cystic mass in the region of the porta hepatis. Substratification and sedimentation phenomena (>) can be seen within the surgically confirmed, thick-walled choledochal cyst after intravenous cholegraphy.

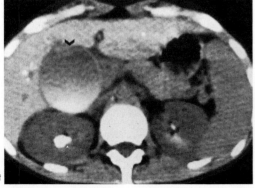

Tumours of the biliary tract (72-70)

Tumours of the bile ducts occur 2–3 times less frequently than gallbladder carcinomas and 8 times less frequently than pancreatic carcinomas. Benign neoplasms are rare (< 10% of cases). Most biliary tract tumours are adenocarcinomas, the growth patterns of which display cirrhous infiltration, circular stenosis or polyps. The main ducts affected in order of frequency are the common bile duct, the ampulla of Vater, the proximal hepatic duct close to the bifurcation and, finally, the cystic duct and the hepatic ducts. Experience shows that, at surgery, 30% of cases already have regional metastases (portal and peripancreatic lymph nodes) which occasionally invade the portal vein, thus leading to remote metastases (liver, lung).

● CT

Computerized tomography shows dilation of the intra- and extrahepatic bile ducts due to congestion. Higher tumours do not cause congestion of the distal bile ducts (common bile duct, gallbladder) (Fig. 72-7 b, c). A space-occupying lesion is demonstrated when the tumour is greater than 2 cm in diameter or when infiltration of the surrounding tissue (including regional lymph nodes) has taken place. The region of the porta hepatis should be investigated using the same slice technique as for tumours of the gallbladder (72-20, 72-50).

Differential diagnosis must take into account:
1. Biliary stones (72-42).
2. Tumours of other types in the region of the porta hepatis: metastatic lymph nodes (stomach, pancreas), malignant lymphomas (86-50).
3. Carcinoma of the head of the pancreas which has invaded the common bile duct (73-42).

Computerized tomography is unable to distinguish an extensive carcinoma of the distal biliary tract from primary carcinoma of the head of the pancreas.

Choledochal cyst (72-71)

The choledochal cyst constitutes idiopathic dilation of the common bile duct — usually of the supraduodenal portion. The wall of the cyst is thickened due to conversion to connective tissue. The mass is discovered in childhood or adolescence as a result of symptoms of compression and displacement (transient jaundice).

● **CT**
The computerized tomogram reveals the criteria of a cyst which displays a thick wall and which enhances on intravenous cholegraphy. Choledochal cysts can achieve a size of 10 cm.

Caroli syndrome (72-72)

The Caroli syndrome is a congenital malformation which usually occurs together with cystic changes of the kidneys (medullary sponge kidney). It constitutes communicating cavernous ectasia of the biliary tract in which the sac-like dilation frequently leads to intrahepatic gallstones or cholangitis. Another form, which is accompanied by cirrhosis and portal hypertension, displays proliferation of the dilated terminal bile ducts, but no dilation of the central bile ducts, cholelithiasis or cholangitis. The clinical symptoms appear in childhood or adolesence.

● **CT**
The saccular dilations of the biliary tract are seen as sharply delimited polycyclic or spindle-shaped hypodense areas with a usually segmental border. The demonstration of hyperdense (possibly calcium-containing) structures within these zones is an indication of cholelithiasis. The administration of a cholegraphic agent in doubtful cases will clarify whether the biliary system is involved by opacification of the hypodense zone. Bile ducts which are dilated due to obstruction taper off towards the periphery and differ in this respect from congenital cavernous ectasia. The Caroli syndrome should be considered if children or adolescents presenting with cirrhosis accompanied by portal hypertension (71-53) also display cystic kidney disease (438).

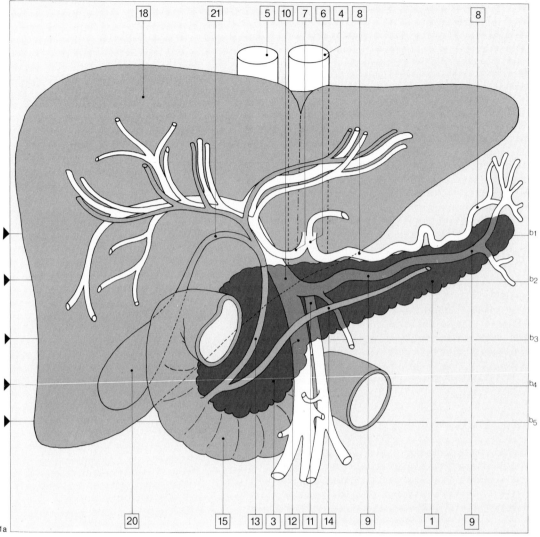

Fig. 73-**1 a, b: Topography of the pancreas.**

Fig. 73-**1 c: Pancreatic parenchyma after contrast medium administration.** Homogeneous enhancement following a bolus injection (40 secs. p. i.).

Key
1 Tail of the pancreas
2 Body of the pancreas
3 Head of the pancreas (uncinate process)
4 Abdominal aorta
5 Inferior vena cava
6 Coeliac trunk
7 Hepatic artery
8 Splenic artery
9 Splenic vein
10 Portal vein
11 Superior mesenteric artery
12 Superior mesenteric vein
13 Common bile duct
14 Pancreatic duct
15 Duodenum
16 Stomach
17 Spleen
18 Liver
19 Small bowel, large bowel
20 Gallbladder
21 Cystic (hepatic) duct
22 Kidney
23 Renal artery
24 Renal vein
25 Adrenal

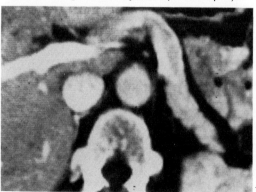

Pancreas (73-00)

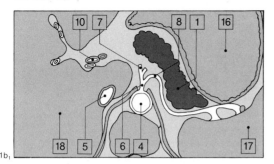
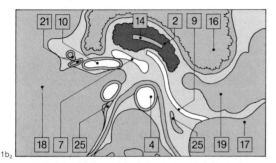
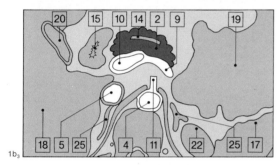
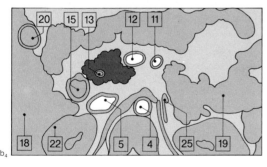
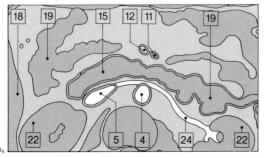

Anatomy and imaging (73-10)

The pancreas, which – in adults – weighs 60–100 g and displays a length of 12–15 cm (4), can almost invariably be depicted in the computed tomogram if a specific technique is employed. It runs almost horizontally or obliquely craniocaudally from the splenic hilum above the abdominal aorta and inferior vena cava to the right side and, consequently, can be demonstrated only in sections due to the horizontal projection of computerized tomography. The course taken by the pancreas determines the number of slices required to scan the organ completely.

The **organ boundary** appears smooth or – particularly in adipose patients – lobular in the computed tomogram. There is a lack of demarcating fatty tissue in thin patients and children, making delimitation difficult unless contrast material is used (see below). The **shape** is variable. The diameter usually decreases gradually from the head towards the tail. Slight variations in the diameter must be regarded as normal and can be simulated by the intersection of a curved organ at different levels. Distinct narrowing of the pancreas (collum) in front of the superior mesenteric artery is seen relatively frequently in healthy patients, giving rise to an hour-glass figure. The uncinate process appears at the lower pole of the head of the pancreas and passes as a narrow, transverse-oval parenchymal spur behind the superior mesenteric vein (Fig. 73-1b) without displacing it.

The **main pancreatic duct** (Wirsung) runs centrally in the body and tail region. Together with the secondary duct (Santorini), it exhibits a number of variants in the head of the pancreas and usually joins the common bile duct before reaching the duodenum. Its diameter measures between 2 and 4 mm in the retrograde pancreatogram (ERP) and tends to increase with age (3). In analogy to the organ itself, the dilated pancreatic duct is demonstrable only in sections unless the pancreas lies horizontally. As with the common bile duct (72-10), the diameter and direction of the duct, its contrast with the surrounding pancreatic parenchyma and the choice of slice thickness determine the demonstrability of the pancreatic duct. The use of narrow slice thicknesses (4–8 mm) – which reduce the partial volume effect – and enhancement of the contrast (parenchyma-lumen) by intravenous injection of contrast material permit recognition of the duct from a diameter of 5 mm when a guided technique is employed. Regardless of the state of contrast of the pancreas, the main duct is usually demonstrable from a calibre of 8 mm if the slice thickness chosen is not too great. The fatty lamella between the splenic vein and parenchymal capsule (see below) and a parallel course of the splenic artery and vein can give rise to a band-shaped zone of reduced density which can simulate a duct. Interpretations of this kind can be avoided by conversancy with the anatomy of the vessels.

Reliable diagnosis depends to a considerable extent on the analysis of the **adjacent structures** of the pancreas. Even in thin patients, the **superior mesenteric artery** serves as an important landmark for the localization of the body of the pancreas, which lies **in front** of this vessel. The **splenic vein** passes along the posterior boundary of the organ (Fig. 73-1 b) to the splenic hilum, but it can also be enveloped by pancreatic tissue. Depending on the morphology and constitution, it is demarcated and identifiable by a fatty tissue lamella. Despite its variable course, the splenic vein makes a major contribution to the shape of the pancreas in the computed tomogram. Dorsal displacement of the splenic vein is indicative of an intrapancreatic lesion, while ventral displacement suggests a retropancreatic (adrenal, renal, paraaortic) process (460). The **splenic artery**, which runs a greatly tortuous course at the upper circumference of the pancreas, is seldom recognizable in the plain scan – and even then only in sections. Neither the **superior mesenteric vein** nor the **portal vein** is isolated from the pancreatic parenchyma by an enveloping layer of fat and, consequently, cannot be reliably identified in the plain computed tomogram. However, the large intrapancreatic vessels stand out clearly in pancreatic lipomatosis. The **duodenum**, which envelops the lateral and caudal contours of the head of the pancreas (Fig. 73-1 a), requires oral opacification. Only then can the uncinate process be demarcated from the pars inferior duodeni, which passes **behind** the superior mesenteric artery and vein. Without oral contrast medium administration, it is frequently impossible to achieve unequivocal demarcation of the tail of the pancreas from the proximal **jejunal** convolutions.

The **size of the pancreas** can be estimated from the transverse diameter, which is measured perpendicular to the long axis of the organ in the individual sections (Fig. 73-1 d). It can be overestimated slightly in the plain scan in the region of the body and tail where the splenic vein cannot always be differentiated from the pancreas. In addition to the absolute measurements (462), relative values for estimating the size have also been reported which refer to the maximum frontal diameter of the simultaneously demonstrated vertebral body (459). According to these values, the head of the pancreas must be regarded as enlarged if its diameter exceeds that of the vertebral body. The body and tail region of the pancreas should not exceed two thirds of the diameter of the vertebral body. Another rule of thumb has been provided by Ferrucci, who states that any thickness of the organ perpendicular to its long axis in excess of 3 cm should be regarded as substantial or suspect (26).

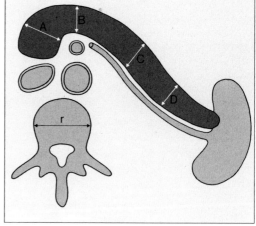

A	25 ± 3.0 mm	A/r	< 1
B	19 ± 2.5 mm	C/r	$< 2/3$
C	20 ± 3.0 mm		
D	15 ± 2.5 mm		

Reference structure: transverse diameter of the vertebral body (r).

The **administration of contrast medium** – particularly as a guided bolus injection – results in distinct opacification of the intra- and peripancreatic vascular structures. It leads to homogeneous enhancement of the parenchyma and also permits demarcation of the intrapancreatic duct system (see above).

Examination technique (73-20)

- **Reduction of intestinal gas** by means of a low residue diet, if possible 48 hours before the examination (particularly in the case of 20-second scanners).
- **Partial intestinal opacification.** Oral administration of 500 ml of a diluted Gastrografin solution 20 minutes before the examination (4-23). The patient should fast for about 4 hours before the examination.
- **Spasmolytics** (scopolamine-N-butylbromide 30–45 mg i. v. or glucagon 1–2 mg i. v.) immediately before the examination in the case of 20-second scanners, as required in the case of shorter scanning times.
- **Scanning** at a slice interval of 8–10 mm in an adjacent slice sequence. (Slice thicknesses of 4–5 mm to demonstrate the pancreatic duct.)

Scanning area: the entire pancreatic bed from the splenic hilum up to and including the pars inferior duodeni.

Right-lateral position if the tail of the pancreas is overshadowed by the fundus of the stomach, if the duodenum is inadequately contrasted or if demarcation of the head of the pancreas is indistinct. Scanning area see above.

- **Intravenous administration of contrast medium** for additional differentiation of pathological processes (dilated bile duct, tumour, inflammation, thrombosis). Guided bolus technique (4-32) in circumscribed lesions, and infusion (4-36) in extensive lesions. Intravenous cholegraphy (4-40) in status following Billroth II (partial gastrectomy) for opacification of the duodenum.

Cystic diseases of the pancreas (73-30)

Dysontogenetic cysts (73-31)
Dysontogenetic cysts constitute hamartomatosis, which occurs frequently together with cystic kidneys and cystic liver and occasionally together with cerebellar angioma and encephalocele.

- **CT**
Computerized tomography reveals several water-filled spaces with soft walls and of varying size which fulfil the usual CT criteria of benign cysts (3-51).

Retention and pseudocysts (73-32)
A retention or pseudocyst is found in 15–25 % of cases of inflammatory disease of the pancreas, by far the most frequent of which is chronic pancreatitis (37, 16).

Retention cysts develop in stenosis or as a result of occlusion of the pancreatic duct and are therefore situated initially within the pancreas.

Pseudocysts form following necrosis of the parenchyma, which is initially surrounded by granulation tissue. A firm wall fused with the surrounding tissue forms after some time as a result of fibrosis. The contents of the cyst can assume a liquid or gelatinous consistency and show brown discolouration following admixture of blood. Pseudocysts develop partly as a result of direct exudation through the peritoneum into the lesser sac. These fluid collections are not pseudocysts in the narrow sense, since they fill a preformed (encapsulated) space (487).

Pseudocysts are encountered more frequently in the head than in the region of the tail and, on enlargement, extend into the lesser sac. Expansion into the porta hepatis (487), the perirenal space and the mediastinum (289) has been reported. In acute pancreatitis, pseudocysts can develop in the region of the exudation (necrotic roads). A feared complication is eruption into the peritoneal cavity or infection (abscess) (16).

◄

Fig. 73-1 d: **Standard values** for a pancreas of normal size according to Haertel and Kreel (462) and Haaga (460). The diameter is the maximum distance vertical to the longitudinal axis of the gland (A = head, B = neck, C = body, D = tail).

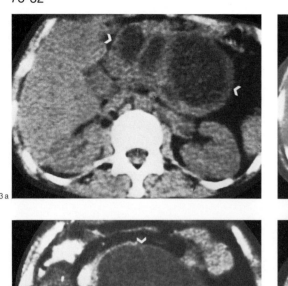
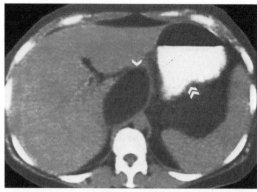
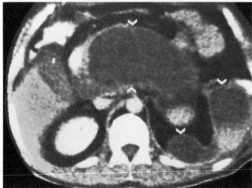

Fig. 73-3 a–f: Pseudocysts of the pancreas.

3 a: Multi-chambered pseudocyst in the body of the pancreas.

3 b: Multiple pseudocysts occurring in subacute pancreatitis in the body of the pancreas, the spleen and the posterior pararenal space.

3 d: Pseudocysts in the region of the upper recess of the lesser sac with compression of the fundus of the stomach (≫).

3 e: Pseudocyst of the pancreas with haemorrhagic infiltration recognizable by slight central hyperdensity (>).

Density of the cystic contents: a: 0–5 HU, b: 15–20 HU, c: 12–14 HU, d: 9–11 HU, e: 30–46 HU, f: 15–17 HU.

3 c: Demonstration of a pseudocyst in the head of the pancreas displaying distinct enhancement of its walls (≫) after administration of contrast medium. Concomitant ascites (>).

3 f: Small pseudocyst with delicate wall in the body of the pancreas with good demarcation following contrast medium administration.

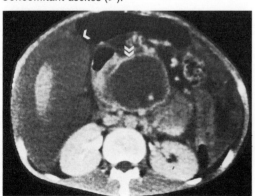
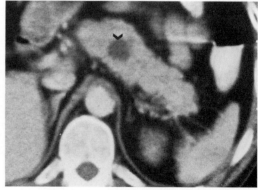

CT

The computed tomogram reveals the picture of a hypodense, relatively smoothly bordered mass which closely resembles that of a cyst. However, the wall is usually thickened (up to a maximum of a few centimeters). The cystic contents can assume the same density as that of water but can also be considerably higher in the case of fresh necroses or if admixed with blood, making the zone of liquefaction barely distinguishable from the parenchyma. The administration of contrast medium (bolus injection) can be of assistance in such cases, the object being to achieve unequivocal demarcation of the necrotic zone and the vascularized pancreatic or granulation tissue. In many cases, the differential diagnosis from necrotic zones of neoplastic masses can be narrowed down even further by demonstration of the highly vascularized granulation tissue.

The **traumatic pseudocyst** develops from an intrapancreatic haematoma – frequently in the presence of pancreatitis. In the fresh stage it stands out as an isodense mass, the density values of which are determined by its age (73-60, 3-52).

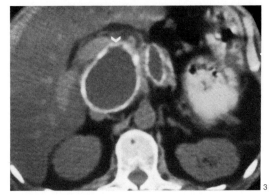

Fig. 73-**3 g: Calcified pseudocysts.** In the head of the pancreas displaying plaque-like but uniform calcifications of their walls (>).

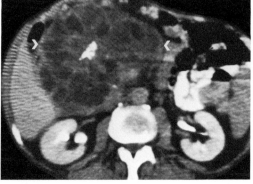

Fig. 73-**4 a, b: Cystadenoma of the pancreas.** Enlargement of the head of the pancreas. The mass displays hypodense (21 and 24 HU), smoothly bordered, septate zones of reduced density. The septation in case b is less pronounced. Calcifications (≫).

Solid tumours of the pancreas (73-40)

Cystadenoma (73-41)

The cystadenoma is the most frequent benign neoplasm of the exocrine pancreas. It occurs in women in 90 % of cases. The tumour usually becomes clinically manifest between the ages of 40 and 60 years and can achieve considerable proportions (3-15 cm in diameter). The mass is permeated by epithelialized cysts of varying size and containing mucous secretion. Peripheral and radial calcifications are found in about 10 % of cases.

CT

Computerized tomography reveals a localized mass with hypodense zones which, because of the protein content, display higher density than water (484, 474). The organoid and cystic structures become more clearly recognizable following administration of contrast medium – if possible as a guided bolus injection –, since the solid component of the tumour is usually highly vascularized. A pseudocyst (73-32) and cystadenocarcinoma (73-43) must be considered in the differential diagnosis.

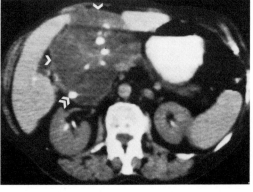

Adenocarcinoma (including anaplastic carcinoma) (73-42)

The incidence of carcinoma of the pancreas is on the increase and currently accounts for 4-5% of all carcinomas in man. Since the overwhelming majority of pancreatic carcinomas (50-70%) are found in the head of the pancreas, the clinical symptoms are determined by bile duct obstruction. Those localized in the region of the tail (20% of cases) are usually discovered too late. Histology usually reveals a hypovascularized adenocarcinoma of varying differentiation with adenoid and cirrhotic growth forms, and less frequently an anaplastic carcinoma. Regional dissemination takes place early via the perineural and peripancreatic lymphatic channels into the periaortic, peritoneal, gastric, portal and, later, pleural and pulmonary groups of lymph nodes. Haematogenous dissemination takes place into the liver, lungs, bones and adrenals. Direct invasion of adjacent organs (stomach, colon, spleen and kidney) is found in advanced stages.

● **CT**

Primary signs

The **localized solid mass** is the salient diagnostic feature. The overall appearance of the pancreas must be considered in addition to the normal dimensions of the organ (73-10). An abrupt alteration of width and an irregular organ configuration are uncertain signs which must be analysed.

Infiltration of the adjacent regions manifests itself as obliteration of the fat planes surrounding the retroperitoneal organs and possibly leading to masking of the inferior vena cava, the abdominal aorta and the superior mesenteric artery (recognition of this sign may not be so easy in emaciated patients without interposition of retroperitoneal fat). A circumscribed deformation at the pancreatic contours may indicate tumour growth and should not be neglected. In particular, the uncinate process, which usually lies immediately lateral to the superior mesenteric vein and appears as a transverse oval shape in the section, should be evaluated in detail. The initial signs of retroperitoneal infiltration are club-like bulging of the uncinate process, its position behind the superior mesenteric vein or displacement of the latter (Fig. 73-4d, k). Invasion of the duodenum can frequently be demonstrated better with hypotonic duodenography than with computerized tomography. Retraction phenomena are occasionally found in cirrhotic forms (Fig. 73-4i). Placing the patient in the right lateral position is frequently of assistance in assessing the mobility of the pancreas in relation to the adjacent organs.

The **radiodensity** of the tumour tissue in the plain scan is usually the same as that of healthy pancreatic parenchyma. Hypodense zones corresponding to intratumoral necroses are an indication of anaplastic carcinoma, although their demonstration is relatively infrequent. The liquefaction can present the picture of a pseudocyst (467). Structural inhomogeneities and hypodense areas are indications of concomitant pancreatitis, which is present in 10% of cases. In pancreatic lipomatosis, the tumour can be recognized as a solid mass within the hypodense (fatty) pancreatic tissue (463).

In analogy to angiography, a guided **bolus injection** can produce a hypodense zone of the hypovascularized tumour tissue, which is initially isodense with the pancreatic tissue (475). Further diagnostic measures are then necessary even if the shape and contours of the organ appear to be normal.

Fig. 73-4c: **Carcinoma of the pancreas.** Incidence of individual CT findings in 75 confirmed cases (Haertel [463]).

CT-features	%
Mass (Increase of volume, deformation of contours [463])	95
Peripancreatic infiltration	84
Localized decrease of density (Defect of density [463])	41
Structural inhomogeneity	56
Regional lymph node enlargement	65
Biliary obstruction	61
Liver metastases	56
Ascites	13

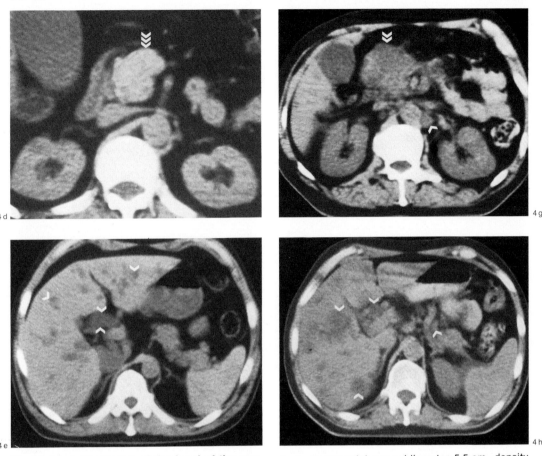

Fig. 73-4d–i: Carcinoma of the head of the pancreas.

4d–f: Polycyclic enlargement of the uncinate process (≫). Congestion of the biliary tract (>) leading to enlargement of the gallbladder (≫). No demonstration of regional lymphomas.

4g,h: Substantial mass (diameter 5.5 cm, density 35 HU) in the head of the pancreas with regional lymph nodes (g >) and liver metastases (h >).

4i: Carcinoma of the head and body of the pancreas. Diffuse infiltration (>) of the retropancreatic space leading to masking of the large vessels.

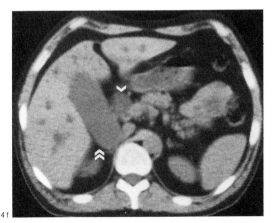
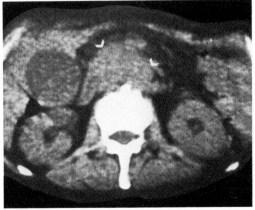

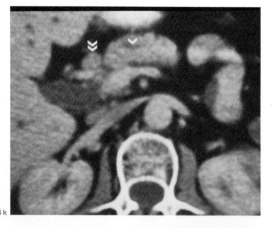

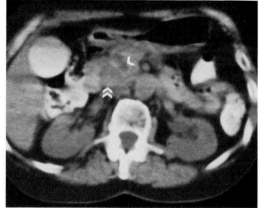

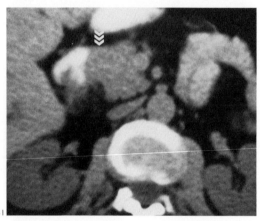

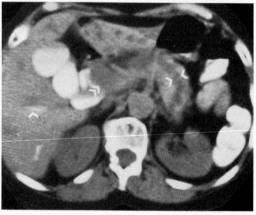

Fig. 73-4 k–p: Carcinoma of the pancreas.

4 k, l: Carcinoma of the head of the pancreas with deformation of the head (≫) und dilation of the pancreatic duct (>). Lymphoma at the hepatoduodenal ligament (≫).

4 n, o: Carcinoma of the head of the pancreas. Considerable dilation of the pancreatic duct and intrahepatic bile ducts (>) and of the common bile duct (≫). Opacification (with stratification) of the biliary system after administration of cholegraphic contrast medium.

4 m: Carcinoma of the head of the pancreas (anaplastic carcinoma). Large, almost homogeneous mass in the head of the pancreas. Incipient infiltration of the retropancreatic space (≫).

4 p: Carcinoma of the body of the pancreas with enlargement of the body and regional lymph node enlargements (>).

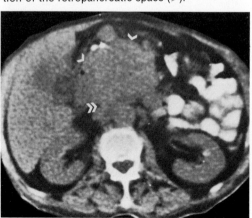

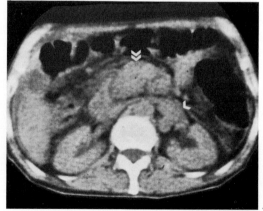

Secondary signs

Secondary signs narrow down the diagnosis of malignant growth to a great extent and signify inoperability in most cases (with the exception of 1.).

Secondary signs are:

1. Dilation of the **bile ducts** or **pancreatic duct** due to tumour obstruction.
2. **Regional metastases**.
3. **Liver metastases** (71-47).
4. **(Malignant) ascites.**

Metastases from other tumours (e. g. seminomas) or malignant lymphomas must be considered in localized enlargement of the pancreas with regional lymph node enlargement. A conglomerate mass of lymph nodes can lie at the head of the pancreas in such a way as to simulate a mass (Fig. 73-4 v). Following intravenous administration of contrast medium, dilation of the bile ducts within the liver becomes more clearly recognizable and a dilated pancreatic duct stands out better from the surrounding pancreatic parenchyma (73-10).

Cystadenocarcinoma (73-43)

The predilection site of the rare cystadenocarcinoma is the head of the pancreas. Its macroscopic appearance is similar to that of its benign variant, the cystadenoma. The malignancy manifests itself as metastases and infiltration into the surrounding area. Unless metastases can be demonstrated, even angiographic differentiation from a cystadenoma rarely succeeds.

● **CT**

The computed tomogram should be evaluated for secondary signs of malignancy (73-42) in addition to the signs described in 73-41. The mucinous cystadenocarcinoma has been described as being poorly vascularized in solid regions.

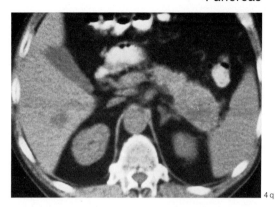

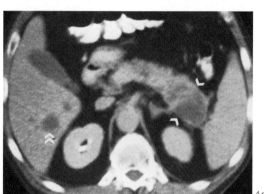

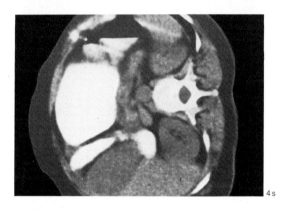

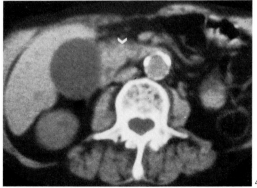

Fig. 73-4 **q, r: Metastasising carcinoma of the tail of the pancreas.** Enlargement of the tail with irregularly defined hypodense zones (>) which demarcate clearly after contrast medium administration (r). Liver metastases (≫).

Fig. 73-4 **s, t: Carcinoma of the head of the pancreas** with no sign of a mass.

4 s: Pancreas on the small side (in the right lateral position). Large gallbladder as an indirect sign of the obstructed bile flow. No demonstration of enlarged lymph nodes.

4 t: Similar case to 4 s. At the most slight deformation of the head of the pancreas.

Islet cell tumours (73-44)

Islet cell tumours originate from the B cells in 80% of cases (insulinomas) and are encountered in the body/tail region in 80%. The other neoplasms of the insular apparatus are localized in the head/body region and can produce glucagon (A cells), gastrin (Zollinger-Ellison syndrome) and serotonin (Verner-Morrison syndrome). Three quarters of all islet cell tumours are hormonally active. The disease becomes clinically manifest between the ages of 20 and 60 years. The tumours are encountered in multiples in 10–15% of cases and usually display a size of 1–2 cm, although they can attain a diameter of up to 10 cm. While insulinomas turn to malignancy in about 10% of cases, malignant degeneration of gastrinomas is considerably more frequent – in about 60% of cases. Carcinomas are usually larger and metastasize into the regional lymph nodes and the liver. Invasive growth into adjacent tissues is a more reliable sign of malignancy than the histology. With few exceptions, all islet cell tumours, regardless of their hormonal activity and malignancy, are highly vascularized.

● CT

On exceeding a diameter of 2 cm, islet cell tumours usually appear in the computed tomogram as isodense masses. The criteria presented under 73–42 apply to carcinomas.

The necessity to identify even small adenomas as hyperdense regions was recognized early on (457). There has so far been very few reports of successful experience, since islet cell tumours enhance only briefly in the early arterial phase. A sequential scanning technique with short intervals should therefore be used.

Secondary tumours (73-45)

Not infrequently, malignant lymphomas invade the pancreas. Remote metastases originating from tumours of the lung, breasts, thyroid, kidney, ovary and testes and from malignant melanomas are occasionally observed in the pancreas. Advanced tumours of the adjacent organs (stomach, colon, kidney) usually invade the pancreas.

● CT

As isolated masses, secondary tumours of the pancreas cannot be differentiated from primary neoplasms in the plain scan. They become demarcated after a guided bolus injection (Fig. 73-4v) because of their poor vascularity. Together with other clinical parameters, epigastric tumours and metastases frequently clarify the diagnostic situation.

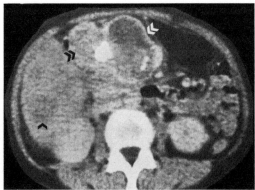

Fig. 73-4 u: **Malignant gastrinoma** of the head of the pancreas. Encapsulated areas in the region of the head of the pancreas with irregularly demarcated hyponse zones (≫). Demonstration of liver metastases (>) which appear hypervascularized in the angiogram.

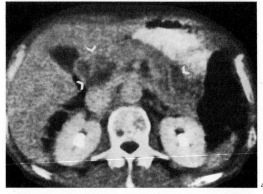

Fig. 73-4 v: **Malignant lymphomas** in the region of the pancreas. The initially isodense tumour regions of the pancreas become hypodense following a bolus injection (>).

Fig. 73-4 w: **Insulinoma.** Demonstration of a 20-mm insulinoma (><) of the tail, confirmed by angiography and surgery. Only brief, early enhancement following bolus injection (courtesy of Priv. Doz. Dr. med. H. Hauser, Hôpital Cantonale Universitaire de Genève).

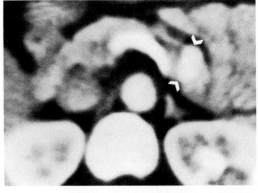

Pancreatitis (73-50)

Acute pancreatitis (73-51)

Acute pancreatitis is found in 1 % of patients. The cause is reported to be biliary disease in 38 % of cases and chronic alcoholism in 27 %, while the etiology cannot be established in 24 % of cases (2). A distinction is made between acute and acute relapsing forms, both of which heal without any loss of function.

There are also two forms from a pathoanatomical point of view – oedematous (interstitial) and haemorrhagic necrotizing pancreatitis. The severity of the condition depends on the extent of the necroses, which can permeate either the greatly enlarged organ like a mantle or whole sections of it. Both forms are accompanied by varying degrees of exudation which can penetrate into the retroperitoneal space or become encapsulated. The condition can be complicated by infection of the necrosis or exudate (abscess formation). Serous or haemorrhagic ascites is found to varying degrees.

● CT

The characteristic sign of acute pancreatitis is excessive enlargement of the organ. The pancreas is usually surrounded by an isodense or slightly hypodense exudate which can spread into the anterior or posterior pararenal space. The predilection site is the paracolic retroperitoneal space (86-14), which is readily accessible to computerized tomography. Expansion into the root of mesentery with masking of the preaortic vessels can likewise be recognized. Even slight concomitant ascites can be identified early as a narrow margin at the lower pole of the right hepatic lobe.

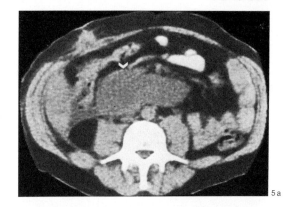

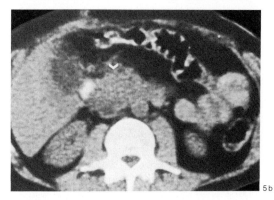

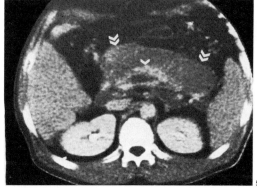

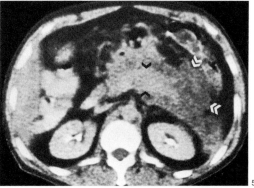

Fig. 73-5 a, b: **Acute oedematous pancreatitis.** Diffuse enlargement of the pancreas, which is sharply demarcated from adjacent tissue (>). Moderate, diffuse reduction of the tissue density. Distinct diminution of the size of the gland after 3 weeks of conservative therapy (b).

Fig. 73-5 c, d: **Haemorrhagic necrotic pancreatitis.**
5c: Enlarged gland, in the centre of which the tissue displays both vessels and blood circulation after contrast medium administration (>). Mild clinical course.
5d: A different patient under conservative therapy. Only slight tendency for the masses caused by exudation or sequestration and surrounding the (opacified) pancreatic parenchyma (>) to regress.

Oedematous pancreatitis, which has a favourable prognosis, is marked by moderate, local or general enlargement of the organ. The contours of the pancreas can usually be demarcated and are frequently poorly defined because of the slight, surrounding exudation. There is only slight if any reduction of the tissue density of the pancreas, but there is no encapsulation as in the case of a pseudocyst. A tendency to regress rapidly is typical of the oedematous form.

Acute **haemorrhagic necrotic** pancreatitis leads to considerable swelling of the organ, the borders of which merge with the surrounding exudative or necrotic masses. Since purely **haemorrhagic** forms without macroscopic necrosis can also occur, particular attention should be paid to the homogeneity of the tissue density. There have so far been no reports of a general, significant increase of density as in the case of a fresh haematoma (3-52) — probably because of the concomitant oedema –, although (hyperdense) haemorrhage (482) into (hypodense) necrotic zones has been described (Fig. 73-5g). **Necrosis** must be considered if any inhomogeneity of the parenchymal density is seen. The intravenous administration of contrast medium can demarcate the highly vascularized organ tissue from the necrosis or exudative margin (Fig. 73-5c, d). The necrotic zones can become demarcated or liquefy in the further course of the disease, leading to the formation of a pancreatic pseudocyst.

Expansion of exudative masses or necrosis into the pararenal spaces (necrotic roads) can be readily identified by computerized tomography (Fig. 73-5e, f). In the majority of cases observed by us the fascias of the perirenal space have not been penetrated. Incipient mantle-like penetration through the renal fascia into the adipose capsule of the kidney is regarded as a sign of fermental activity of the exudate (449, 461). According to Meyers (32), involvement of the posterior pararenal space can be explained by caudal encirclement of the fascial cone of the kidney (86-14). The demonstration over weeks to months of soft-tissue zones in the retroperitoneal space which are not absorbed by the border surfaces of the fascial space is an indication of a pancreatic sequestra (Fig. 73-5d).

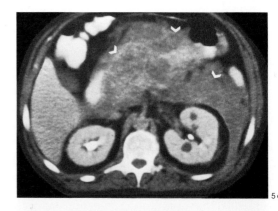

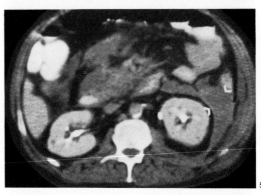

Fig. 73-5e, f: **Haemorrhagic necrotic pancreatitis** with extensive exudation into the root of the mesentery (e >) and the anterior paracolic space (f >). Greatly inhomogeneous density pattern due to irregular haemorrhagic saturation of the retroperitoneum.

Fig. 73-5g: **Acute haemorrhagic pancreatitis** with haematoma-like haemorrhagic permeation of the head of the pancreas (≫). Demonstration of accompanying ascites (>).

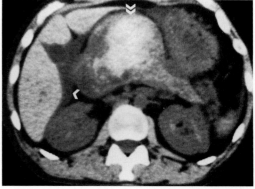

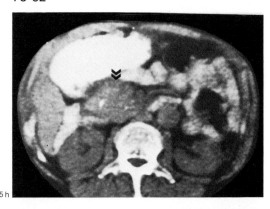

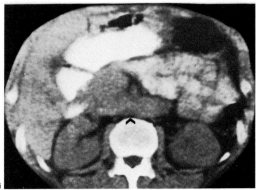

Fig. 73-5 h, i: **Chronic pancreatitis** (hypertrophic form). Demonstration of considerable enlargement of the head with isolated calcifications. The pancreatic tissue extends behind the superior mesenteric artery to the aorta, creating the impression of malignant growth (>).

Fig. 73-5 k: **Chronic pancreatitis.** Incidence of individual CT findings in 50 surgically confirmed cases of chronic pancreatitis (after Ferrucci [453]).

CT-features	%
Enlargement/mass	36
Pseudocyst/abscess	30
Calcifications	36
Atrophy	14
Duct dilatation	4
Normal gland contours	16

Abscess formation is a serious complication (supurative pancreatitis), the demonstrable CT signs of which are encapsulated, cystic structures in the region of the pancreas and the pararenal pathways of spread (487). Since no reliable distinction can be made between a pseudocyst and an abscess on the basis of the density, resort must be made to the clinical findings for the differential diagnosis. Only the incorporation of gas is regarded as pathognomonic for an infection (476).

Chronic pancreatitis (73-52)

Chronic pancreatitis is encountered in 0.07 % of patients and, at 0.2 %, is found at autopsy about as frequently as acute pancreatitis. As regards the etiology, alcoholism predominates with 37 % of cases, followed by biliary causes in 27 %. Chronic pancreatitis is accompanied by calcification in 32 % of cases (chronic calcifying pancreatitis). A distinction is made clinically between a chronic relapsing form and a progressive (and insidious) form.

Patho-anatomical evaluation reveals multifocal inflammatory foci which need not necessarily alter the external appearance of the pancreas even when the disease is clinically apparent. On progression of the disease, connective-tissue organization leads primarily to perilobular fibrosis. General or circumscribed **enlargement** of the organ due to sclerolipomatosis and/or dilation of the ducts (36) is found in the further course. **Atrophy** of the organ is quite frequently found in late stages (e. g. at autopsy). **Dilation of the ducts** can be caused by stenosis of the pancreatic duct or by distraction of the parenchyma as it shrinks due to scarring. **Calcifications** are more frequent in alcohol-induced chronic relapsing pancreatitis (about 40 % of cases) than in the biliary form (22 % of cases), and are localized mainly in the ductal system. Some authors discriminate between calcifications and genuine **lithiasis**, in which isolated, larger stones are demonstrated for the greater part in the distal section of the main duct. Statistical reviews and the clinical course suggest that chronic pancreatitis is a pathogenetic factor in the development of carcinoma of the pancreas (in 2–3 % of cases of chronic calcifying pancreatitis). In this connection it must also be considered that pancreatitis can be induced by a carcinoma, e. g. due to obstruction of the ducts (concomitant pancreatitis in 10 % of carcinoma patients).

● CT

Calcifications are a guiding diagnostic sign. They are frequently found in a linear arrangement corresponding to the course of the pancreatic duct.

If **enlargement** of the pancreas is present, it usually affects the entire organ. An isolated mass is more likely to be encountered in the region of the head (pancreatitis of the head of the pancreas), although the rest of the organ is then usually also found to be enlarged. The contours can generally be sharply demarcated in the computed tomogram, although they can sometimes merge with the adjacent fatty tissue (oedema during an episode of inflammation [453]).

Atrophy, the final stage of chronic pancreatitis, has so far been observed – in surgically confirmed cases (453) – less frequently than enlargement of the organ. It is recognizable in the computed tomogram as narrowing of the entire organ with sharp, usually smooth contours. In some cases, the pancreas appears only as a fibrous sheath for the splenic vessels. Partial atrophy of the tail and body is frequently the result of ductal occlusion and, consequently, is usually an indication of a malignant process in the head of the pancreas (73-42). Atrophy of the organ can, however, also take place by fatty-tissue replacement of the gland lobules, in which the interlobar connective tissue is increased (sclerolipomatosis). The transitions to pancreatic lipomatosis are fluent.

Dilation of the ducts in chronic pancreatitis, which is more easily discernible in the computed tomogram following contrast medium administration, is caused by obstruction (calcified and non-calcified concrements) or by shrinkage of the organ and should be evaluated diagnostically in association with the other signs. Chronic pancreatitis is the most probable diagnosis in general atrophy of the organ (including the head region), extensive parenchymatous calcifications and dilation of the ducts.

Enlargement of the lymph nodes is observed only in exceptional cases.

Pseudocysts are a complication of chronic pancreatitis (73-32).

Pancreatic abscess (73-53)
The pancreatic abscess usually develops as a result of infection of a pseudocyst (as a feature of acute or chronic pancreatitis). The spread of an infection from adjacent organs (kidney,

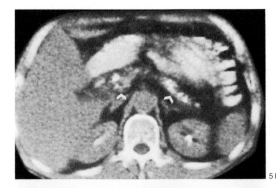

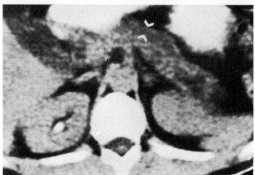

Fig. 73-5l–o: **Chronic pancreatitis. 5l:** Diffuse calcification in a generally shrunken gland.
5m, n: Small gland with dilated main pancreatic duct (><) and discrete calcifications in the head region (>).
5o: Pseudocysts (>) in chronic pancreatitis following resection of the tail.

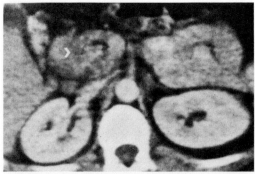

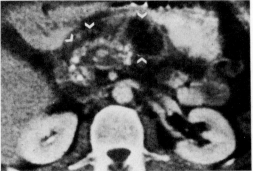

Trauma of the pancreas (73-60)

Abdominal trauma – usually blunt – tends to involve the region of the body of the gland and usually occurs in combination with other internal injuries. There are different forms of trauma – contusion, incomplete rupture (without rupture of the capsule) and complete rupture (parenchymal and capsular rupture with or without rupture of the pancreatic duct).
A (traumatic) pseudocyst frequently develops in incomplete rupture. Complete ruptures can lead to separation of the tail, pseudocysts and fistulae into the lesser sac. Pancreatitis is induced depending on the extent of the contusion.

● CT

Computerized tomography reveals a haematoma as a consequence of the trauma (171). It appears as an isodense (later hypodense) mass, the extent and expansion of which can be evaluated in the retroperitoneal space. Computerized tomography cannot distinguish between a traumatic pseudocyst and a primarily inflammatory pseudocyst (73-32). Signs of oedematous pancreatitis: 73-51.

Lipomatosis and atrophy (73-70)

Lipomatosis is one of the features of general adiposity. Another cause is occlusion of the pancreatic duct, in which the parts of the parenchyma situated in the region of the occlusion undergo atrophy and individual gland lobules are replaced by fatty tissue. Lipomatous permeation of the glands likewise occurs in the final stage of chronic pancreatitis, and is known as sclerolipomatosis because of the concomitant fibrosis. Lipomatous atrophy of the pancreas, for which a viral genesis has been suggested, is a rare disease of the infantile pancreas.

● CT

In adipose patients, computerized tomography usually reveals a lobular structure of the pancreatic parenchyma. The individual gland lobules are forced apart depending on the extent of fatty tissue invasion. A loose connective tissue matrix which still permits recognition of the original contours of the organ is found in the final stage of lipomatous atrophy. The splenic vessels are particularly prominent.

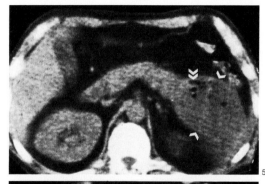

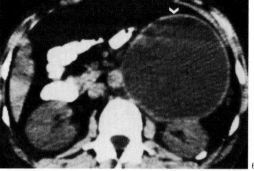

Fig. 73-**5p: Pancreatic abscess.** Enlargement of the tail of the pancreas (>) with demonstration of small air bubbles (≫).

Fig. 73-**6a:** Superinfected, **posttraumatic pseudocyst** of the pancreas (without formation of gas, density: 15 HU).

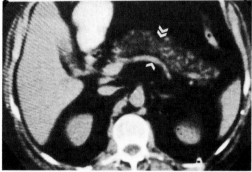

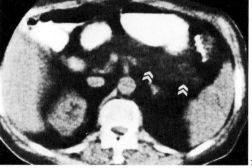

Fig. 73-**7a,b: Lipomatosis.** Duffuse fatty degeneration of the pancreas (b), which differs from lobular pancreatic organs (a) of obese patients (splenic vessels >).

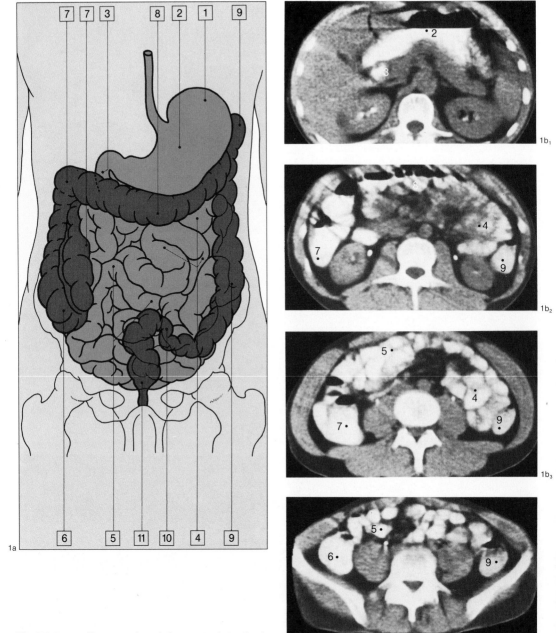

Fig. 74-1 a–c: Topography of the gastrointestinal tract.

Key
1 Fundus of the stomach
2 Body of the stomach, antrum
3 Duodenum
4 Jejunum
5 Ileum
6 Coecum
7 Ascending colon, right flexure
8 Transverse colon
9 Descending colon, left flexure
10 Sigmoid
11 Rectum

1b: Image of the gastrointestinal tract in a patient following total bowel opacification (4-23).

1c: Image of individual sections of the bowel and their positional relationship in different patients.

Gastrointestinal tract (74-00)

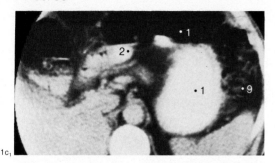

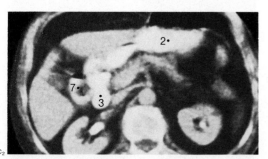

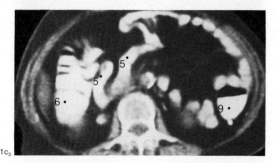

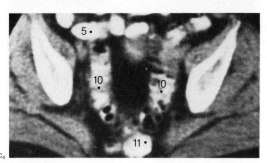

Anatomy and imaging (74-10)
Overall, the gastrointestinal tract with its complicated loops and variable shape represents an unfavourable scanning object for the rigid planar geometry of computerized tomography. Unequivocal differentiation of individual intestinal loops, particularly from cystic masses, is possible only following oral administration of contrast material (4-23). Even, intraluminal distribution of the contrast material leads to the demonstration not only of familiar radiological patterns (Kerckring's folds, haustra), but also of the thickness of the intestinal wall (Fig. 74-1b). In obese patients, individual vessels of the root of the mesentery stand out clearly within the omental fatty tissue. Incomplete fillings of the intestinal lumen and stomach can simulate tumours (494).

Examination technique (74-20)
- **Total bowel opacification** (4-23).
- **Spasmolytics** (scopolamine-N-butyl-bromide 15–30 mg i.v or 1–2 mg glucagon i. v.) in the case of 20-second scanners, as required in the case of shorter scan times.
- **Scanning:** Adjacent slices 10–13 mm thick in the target region (pelvis), 20–30 mm thick in regions of lymph drainage.

Scanning area: dependent on the clinical findings. In postproctectomy status: promontorium to the symphysis.
- **Reduced bolus injection** (4-34) with 5–10 ml Urografin 76% i. v. 10 minutes before the examination to opacify the urinary bladder (in suspected pelvic processes).

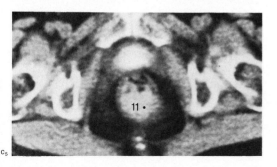

Gastrointestinal tract (74-30)
Anomalies of position, malrotation and fine mucosal changes can be demonstrated much better with the conventional X-ray technique than with computerized tomography. Consequently, **inflammatory** and **early neoplastic** processes are not an indication for computerized tomography.

In special cases (495, 500) and particularly in lymphomatous infiltration, thickening of the

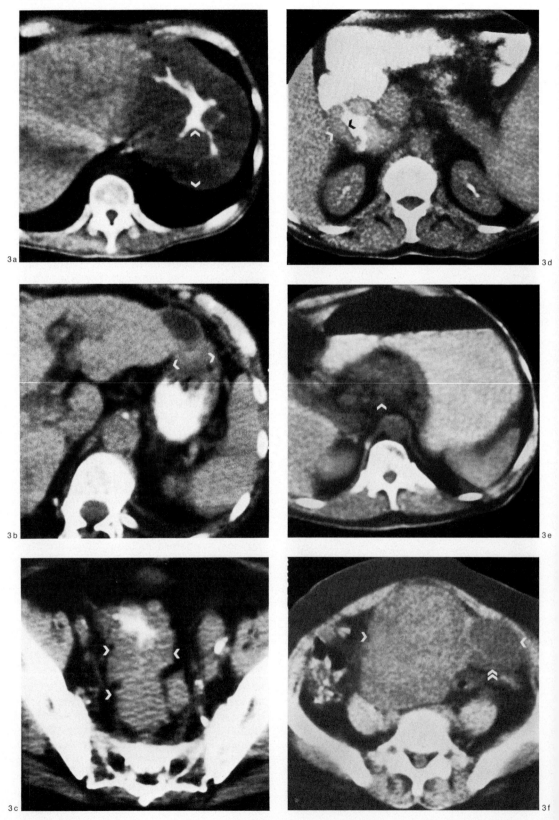

wall can be demonstrated better than with the conventional gastrointestinal examination, the yield of which is based on motility and mucosal surface. In extensive neoplasms which are not restricted to the intestinal lumen, conventional gastrointestinal studies remain dependent on indirect signs. Manifestations in malignant lymphomas in the mesentery, tumor infiltration of the surrounding tissue and regional lymph node metastases can be demonstrated by computerized tomography and are of diagnostic interest.

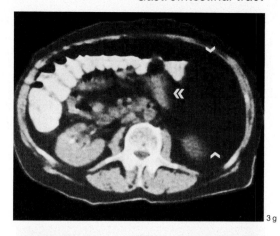

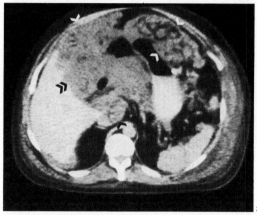

Fig. 74-3 g, h: Fat-containing tumours of the mesenteric space.

3 g: Mesenteric limpoma with displacement of bowel loops to the right (≫).

3 h: Liposarcoma, the tissue density of which is loosened by fatty structures. Infiltration of the right hepatic lobe (≫).

Fig. 74-3 i: Carcinoma of the stomach. Distinct thickening of the wall, particularly of the dorsal wall, with infiltration of the bed of the pancreas (≫).

Fig. 74-3 a–d: **Manifestations of malignant lymphomas** in the region of the gastrointestinal tract.

3 a: Massive thickening of the fundus wall (>).

3 b: Infiltration of the anterior wall of the stomach (<>).

3 c: Involvement of the rectum and sigmoid with ventral displacement of the lumen by the tumour masses (>).

3 d: Isolated involvement of the duodenum with thickening of the duodenal wall (>).

Fig. 74-3 e, f: **Metastases from carcinomas.**

3 e: Regional metastases retrogastric in cardiac carcinoma (>).

3 f: Massive mesenteric lymphomas in recurrence of a carcinoma of the colon with liquefaction of a tumour node (≫).

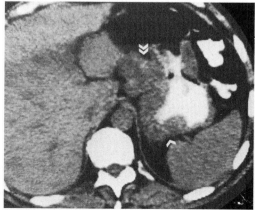

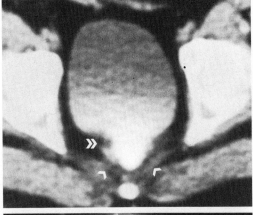

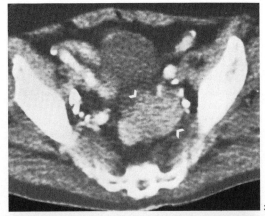

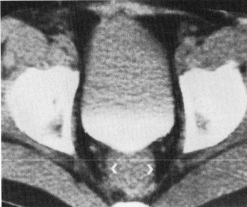

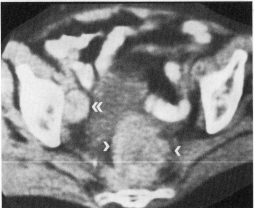

Fig. 74-3 k, l: Status after abdomino-perineal proctectomy.

3 k: In the bed of the rectum only demonstration of fine cord formation (>) and typical stretching of the dorsal wall of the urinary bladder (≫).

3 l: Scar tissue. After secondary healing, demonstration of a fairly large, relatively smooth-bordered soft-tissue structure which was demonstrable only 3 months after surgery and which has not changed for $4^{1}/_{2}$ years.

Fig. 74-3 m: Destruction of the sacrum in carcinoma of the rectum (>).

Fig. 74-3 n, o: Recurrence following abdomino-perineal proctectomy.

3 n: High soft-tissue structure left with polycyclic delimitation and displacement of the pelvic organs. Demonstration of slight but distinct enhancement following administration of contrast medium.

3 o: Soft-tissue zone with polycyclic delimitation in the bed of the rectum without destruction of the sacrum. Demonstration of a regional lymphoma of the obturator group (≫).

Fig. 74-3 p: Recurrence with fistulation in the bed of the rectum. Demonstration of a soft-tissue structure with incorporation of air. Slight presacral fibrosis.

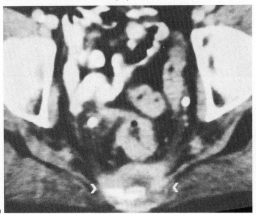

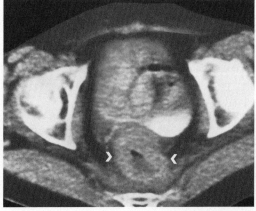

Recurrence following proctectomy (74-31)

The postoperative CT follow-up of proctectomy is of great proven value. No other method of demonstration can provide a better image of the presacral region. Proctectomy is associated with considerable changes in the anatomy. Mobilization of the rectum and sigma and opening of the retroperitoneal space lead to a large presacral wound cavity which, depending on the surgical procedure and the function of the drainage, granulates and heals secondarily. Congestion of secretions and abscess formation lead to retarded healing in up to 60 % of cases (52). Fibrosis of the granulation tissue and organization of abscesses can lead to extensive connective-tissue transformation of the presacral space, a process also known as secondary retroperitoneal fibrosis (86-41). Late abscesses and fistulae are a not infrequent occurence.

● **CT**

If no scar tissue is present – the exception rather than the rule in our patients –, exclusion diagnosis in respect of a recurrence is problem-free and reliable, provided that the bowels and urinary bladder are adequately opacified. The majority of cases, however, display varying amounts of scar tissue which is separated from the sacrum by a narrow layer of fat. The uterus and prostate must be distinguished from this irregular or smoothly delimited soft-tissue zone.

The **suspicion of recurrence** is justified if assymetry of the soft tissue is demonstrated, particularly if this is caused by lymph nodes of the internal iliac group. A compact mass with moderately reduced central density is equivocal: it can signify an incipient (late) abscess or a liquefying tumour. Collections of gas can signal either an abscess or a fistula. The late occurrence of a hydronephrosis is likewise an indication of a recurrence (502).

Unequivocal signs are bone destruction (of the sacrum), infiltration of adjacent organs (bladder, M. piriformis, M. obturatorius internus, M. glutaeus medius) or an increase of soft tissue on follow-up examinations (493). In view of this, computerized tomography should be conducted 2–3 months after surgery to establish the initial finding for later control examinations.

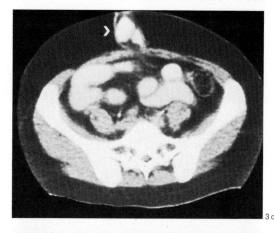

Fig. 74-**3 q: Hernia of the abdominal wall.** Within the subcutaneous layer of fat, demonstration of bowel loops in front of the abdominal wall (>).

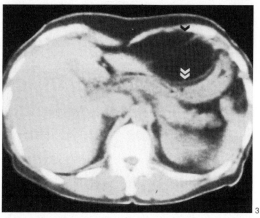

Fig. 74-**3 r: Lipoma of the abdominal wall.** Behind the left M. rectus abdominis, demonstration of a homogeneous soft-tissue structure with fat-equidense density values. Displacement of the transverse fascia in a dorsal direction (≫).

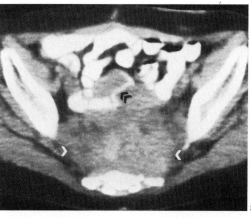

Fig. 74-**3 s: Recurrence following proctectomy.** Large soft-tissue mass with destruction of the sacrum, regional lymphomas and incipient infiltration of the small bowel (≫).

75-00

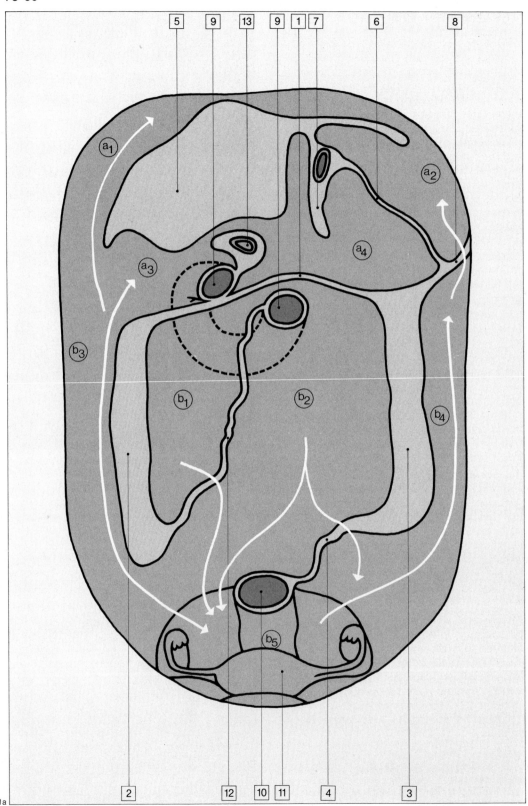

Peritoneal cavity (75-00)

Anatomy and imaging (75-10)

The abdominal cavity is a complicated space which cannot be delineated by computerized tomography in healthy subjects because the peritoneal fold usually follows a crooked course through the computerized tomographic slice. However, the peritoneal cavity can be demonstrated if fluid collections are present.

Supramesocolic spaces

On the right side, the dorsal surface of the liver is attached to the diaphragm by the coronary ligament, giving rise to a **subphrenic** and a **subhepatic space** which communicate ventrally with each other (Fig. 75-1b). Medially, the right subphrenic space is incompletely separated from the left by the falciform ligament. Encapsulated accumulations of fluid are usually found anteriorly and posteriorly below the diaphragm and anteriorly and posteriorly below the liver (Morison's pouch). On the left side, the surface of the liver is divided cranially by a very narrow coronary ligament and inferiorly by the lesser omentum (Fig. 75-1a, c). The lesser omentum covers the **lesser sac,** which is bounded as follows: dorsally by the pancreas, laterally by the gastrolienal and lienorenal ligament, caudally by the mesocolon and gastrocolic ligament, and ventrally by the posterior wall of the stomach and the inferior surface of the liver, including the caudate lobe (Fig. 75-1c,e). In the case of a large left hepatic lobe, the bursa extends dorsally to beneath the diaphragm. It is divided into two sections by a peritoneal fold around the left gastric artery. Depending on their course, the individual boundaries can be identified in the computed tomogram if fluid collections are present.

The **left subphrenic space** embraces the lateral and cranial convexity of the spleen and continues to the surface of the left hepatic lobe, where it is bounded medially by the falciform ligament. Caudally, the fold of the phrenicocolic ligament separates it only partly from the left paracolic gutter.

Fig. 75-**1a**: Topography of the posterior wall of the abdominal cavity.

1 Transverse mesocolon
2 Ascending mesocolon
3 Descending mesocolon
4 Sigmoid mesocolon
5 Coronary ligament
6 Phrenicosplenic ligament
7 Gastropancreatic fold (with oesophagus)
8 Phrenicocolic fold
9 Duodenum
10 Rectum
11 Uterus and adnexa
12 Root of mesentery
13 Hepatoduodenal ligament (with portal vein)

A **Supramesocolic spaces**
a_1 right subphrenic space
a_2 left subphrenic space
a_3 subhepatic space
a_4 lesser sac

B **Inframesocolic spaces**
b_1 right infracolic space
b_2 left infracolic space
b_3 right paracolic gutter
b_4 left paracolic gutter
b_5 Douglas' pouch

The arrows show the movement of fluid between the peritoneal spaces (from Meyers [32]).

75-10

Inframesocolic spaces

Beneath the mesocolon extending laterally up to the border of the colon are the right and left **infracolic spaces** (Fig. 75-1a), which are separated by the root of mesentery. Fluid produced there flows caudally via the mesosigmoid in to the pouch of Douglas. From there it ascends lateral to the ascending and descending colon to the diaphragm, the preferred route being the right paracolic gutter. When the patient is in the horizontal position, non-encapsulated fluids flow early on into the deep-lying recesses (Douglas' pouch and posterior subhepatic space). The ventrolateral circumferences of the liver and spleen and the dorsal angles of the (intraperitoneal) paracolic gutters fill up when the amount of effusion increases (Fig. 75-1h–l).

Fig. 75-**1 b – e: Topography of the upper abdominal spaces.**
1 b: Right paravertebral section
1 c: Median section
1 d: Transverse section (at the level of the porta hepatis)
1 e: Transverse section above the renal hila (5 cm caudalward of d).

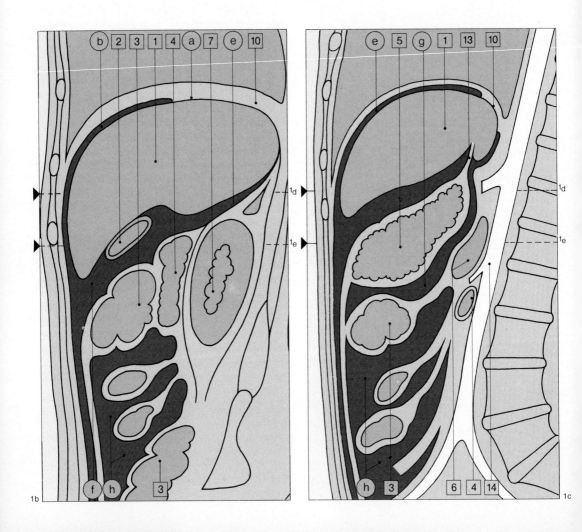

Peritoneal cavity

Key
1. Liver
2. Gallbladder
3. Colon
4. Duodenum
5. Stomach
6. Pancreas
7. Kidney
8. Spleen
9. Falciform ligament
10. Coronary ligament
11. Gastrosplenic ligament
12. Splenorenal (or phrenicosplenic) ligament
13. Lesser omentum
14. Abdominal aorta
15. Portal vein

● Subphrenic spaces
a right dorsal
b right ventral
c left ventral
d left lateral

● Subhepatic spaces
e right dorsal (Morison's pouch)
f right ventral
g lesser sac
h inframesocolic space

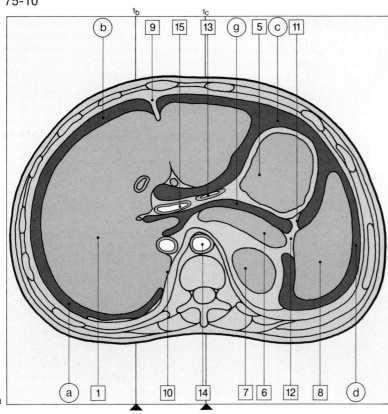

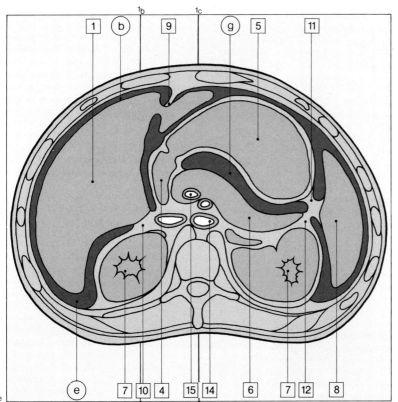

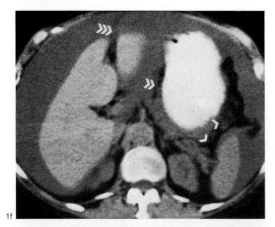

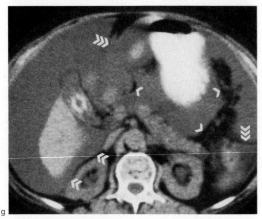

Fig. 75-1 f–h: **Peritoneal spaces in ascites** (cf. Fig. 1 a–e). Subperitoneal fatty tissue facilitates allocation.

1f: Subphrenic spaces (gastrosplenic and splenorenal ligaments >, lesser omentum ≫, falciform ligament ⋙).

1g: Subhepatic spaces (Morison's pouch ≫, lesser sac including the gastrosplenic and splenorenal ligaments and the lesser omentum >, falciform ligament ⋙ and phrenicocolic fold ≫).

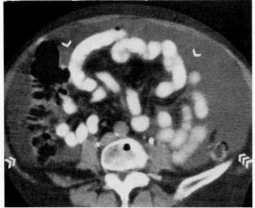

● CT

Fluid collections in the subphrenic spaces and in the dorsal subhepatic recess can be demonstrated sensitively in the computed tomogram from a diameter of 1.5 cm. Small amounts of fluid in the other spaces of the peritoneal cavity can only be clearly demonstrated when the intestinal lumen is unequivocally identifiable as a result of contrast medium administration. This applies in particular to the inframesocolic space, which is difficult to delineate because of the undulating root of mesentery. The intestinal loops and fat-containing mesentery leaves are forced apart by larger amounts of effusion (Fig. 75-1i). The lesser sac usually dilates to a lesser extent in general ascites. If encapsulation occurs, the fluid-filled bursa can protrude like a cyst (73-32). Each of the above-described spaces can adhere if an inflammatory reaction occurs and progress to an abscess on infection. The localization of circumscribed accumulations of fluid is determined by the site of the primary lesion (perforation, inflammation), by the particular intraperitoneal compartment concerned, by gravity and by the position of the body (32).

Examination technique (75-20)
● **Total bowel opacification** (4-23).
● **Spasmolytics** (15-30 mg scopolamine-N-butyl-bromide i. v. or 1–2 mg glucagon i. v.) in the case of 20-second scanners, as required in the case of faster scan times.
● **Scanning:** adjacent slices 10–13 mm thick in the epigastrium and pelvis, 20–30 mm thick in the mesogastrium.
Scanning area: depending on the clinical finding: epigastrium, mesogastrium or pelvis.
● **Reduced bolus injection** (4-34) with 5–10 ml Urografin 76 % i. v. 10 minutes before the examination to opacify the urinary bladder (in suspected pelvic processes).

Ascites (75-30)
A number of diseases (75-3a) can be accompanied by ascites. Low-protein transudations are a consequence of an increase in the venous blood pressure or of reduced colloid-osmotic pressure. Exudations are caused by inflammations of the peritoneum and display a protein content of more than 30 g/l. Neoplastic metastases cause direct irritation of the peritoneum or block the drainage of lymph.

1 h: Inframesocolic spaces (right paracolic gutter ≫, left paracolic gutter ⋙, inframesocolic spaces >). The route of the mesentery is clearly recognizable because of fatty tissue.

Peritoneal cavity

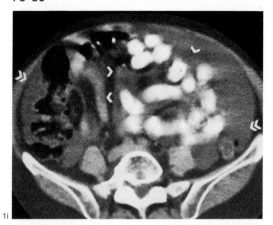

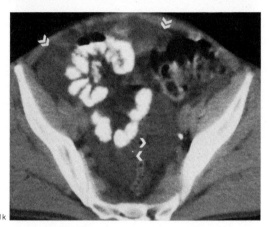

Fig. 75-1 i-l: **Ascites.**
1i: Inframesocolic spaces (right paracolic gutter next to the air-filled coecum ≫, left paracolic gutter next to the small-calibre descending colon ≫), accumulations of ascites between the mesentery (inframesocolic spaces >).
1k: Ascites in the minor pelvis on both sides of the sigmoid colon or mesosigmoid (>) and in front of the ileal loops (≫).
1l: Encapsulated accumulations of ascites. They differ from generalized ascites by virtue of their roundish shape.

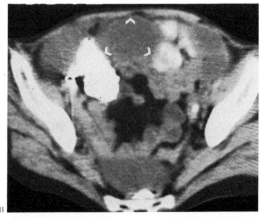

Cardiovascular (incl. hypoproteinaemia)
● Congestive heart failure ● Inferior vena cava obstruction ● Portal vein obstruction ● Budd-Chiari syndrome ● Constrictive pericarditis ● Hypoalbuminaemia ● Liver cirrhosis ● Myxoedema
Inflammatory
● Peritonitis ● Familial paroxysmal peritonitis ● Abdominal vasculitis ● Eosinophilic gastroenteritis ● Tuberculosis ● Pancreatitis ● Intestinal perforation ● Whipple's disease ● Glomerulonephritis
Neoplastic

● Peritoneal carcinosis
  (malignant tumours of stomach, colon, ovary, pancreas)
● Lymphatic obstruction
  (incl. malignant lymphoma)
● Pseudomyxoma peritonaei
● Mesothelioma
● Meigs' syndrome

Fig. 75-3a: Diseases accompanied by **ascites** (modified from [26]).

● **CT**

Ascites appears in the computed tomogram as a hypodense margin around the intraperitoneal organs. The amount of fluid determines the extent to which the physiologically available space is filled. The intestinal loops and the mesentery display harmonic distribution in the abdominal cavity. Increased pressure leads to unilateral and eccentric displacement and compression of the bowels. The mesentery can be identified by its fatty tissue components. In carcinomatous peritonitis, solid components can occasionally be demonstrated within the hypodense zone on the smooth surfaces of the parenchymatous organs, particularly the liver. They are an indication of peritoneal metastases and, under favourable scanning conditions, can be recognized from a diameter of 1.5 cm (355). The radiodensity of the fluid is 5–20 HU, a range determined both by the protein content (3-51) and by the varying measuring sensitivity of the scanners (80).

Not infrequently, the cause of the ascites can be ascertained with the same examination (75-3a). Differentiation of retroperitoneal from intraperitoneal exudations is necessary in acute pancreatitis. However, the relationship of the fascias (86-14) provides unequivocal criteria.

Peritoneal metastases (75-40)

Peritoneal metastases are found in men primarily in advanced stages of tumours of the gastrointestinal tract (stomach, colon, pancreas), and in the woman in tumours of the internal genitals (ovary). The peritoneal implantation follows the flow of the ascites (75-10), although initially only very small and virtually undetectable amounts of fluid serve as the vehicle (32). The predilection sites of peritoneal metastases are the Douglas' pouch, the mesosigmoid, the root of mesentery, the right paracolic gutter and the right subphrenic space.

● CT

Small nodes with a diameter of 0.5 cm cannot be demonstrated by computerized tomography even in easily surveyable regions, e.g. the subphrenic space. Larger secondary soft-tissue tumours from a diameter of about 3 cm can be differentiated from intestinal loops only under optimal oral opacification of the bowels. Intraperitoneal localization cannot normally be confirmed without concomitant ascites, so that differentiation from mesenteric lymph nodes (86-51) is not usually possible.

Intraperitoneal abscesses (75-50)

An intraperitoneal abscess constitutes infected local peritonitis, which develops following perforation of the gastrointestinal wall (ulcer, diverticulum), surgery, or as a result of adjacent inflammations (pancreatitis, adnexitis, pericholecystitis). It develops in the vicinity of the organ concerned, where it first of all becomes encapsulated and can also incorporate the respective peritoneal compartment. Abscesses in the **lesser sac** are usually the consequence of ulcerous perforations of the posterior wall of the stomach or of pancreatitis. They are found in the **left subphrenic space** following ulcerous perforation of the anterior wall of the stomach, anastomotic insufficiency and colonic perforation. **Subphrenic and subhepatic abscesses** can develop in keeping with the intraperitoneal movements of fluid (75-1a) following infra- and supramesocolic affections. They are found 2–3 times more frequently on the right than on the left, the preferred site being the subhepatic (posterior) space (Morison's

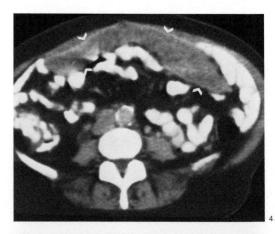

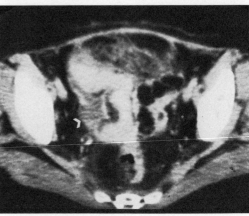

Fig. 75-4a,b: **Peritoneal carcinosis.**
4a: Peritoneal carcinosis in the greater omentum in metastatic carcinoma of the ovary.
4b: Peritoneal carcinosis in the minor pelvis in malignant tumour of the uterus. Encapsulated, irregularly demarcated zones of reduced density with soft-tissue component along the intestinal wall (>). Generally irregular contours of the bowel loops.
Fig. 75-5a: **Subhepatic abscess** in the anterior subhepatic space following cholecystectomy. Discrete accumulation of fluid in Morison's pouch as well (≫); note the thickened wall of the abscess.

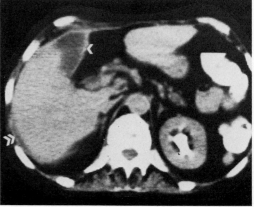

Peritoneal cavity

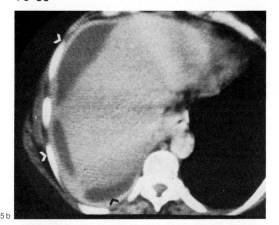

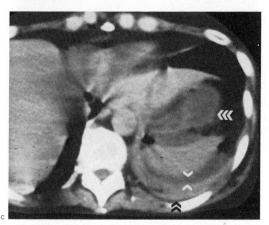

Fig. 75-**5b–d: Intraperitoneal abscesses.**

5b: Subphrenic abscess right. Multiseptate zone of reduced density in the right subphrenic space with compression of the liver surface, which appears flattened. Radiodensity: 35 HU.

5c: Subphrenic abscess left in status after gastric resection. Demonstration of a hypodense zone between the spleen and the limb of the diaphragm (><). (Further effusions [hypodensities] in the lesser sac ≫ and in the angle of the diaphragm ≫).

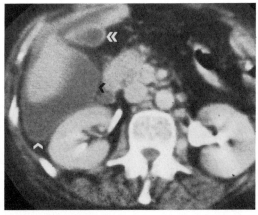

pouch) as the deepest point in the abdominal cavity with the patient lying on his back. The pouch of Douglas abscess develops not only as a result of inflammation of pelvic organs, but also as a consequence of inframesocolic exudations.

● **CT**

Computerized tomography depicts the abscesses as hypodense zones which must be analysed in a similar way to ascites (75-30). While the right subhepatic space is readily identified, in the other sections fluid-filled intestinal loops must be differentiated from possible abscesses; this can only be done reliably following adequate intestinal opacification. In urgent cases, constancy of the position and shape on changing the position of the patient can support the tentative diagnosis of abscess. Collections of gas within an extraluminal hypodense mass are considered to be pathognomonic for an infectious process (3-53). The left subphrenic space can undergo marked cicatricial change as a result of splenectomy, which can be performed by extensive electrocoagulation, and thus escape accurate assessment. Transmigrating pleuritis frequently renders delineation of the diaphragm difficult. Analysis of the image must then be commenced at the medial angle of the diaphragm (Fig. 75-5c). The **radiodensity** of the mass ranges from 20–40 HU (80) and can be considerably lower, particularly under therapy (3-53).

Cystic masses (mesenteric cysts, ovarian cysts) and non-inflammatory peritoneal fluid collection (local peritoneal carcinomatosis) must be considered in the differential diagnosis.

Intraperitoneal haemorrhage (75-60)

Haemorrhage into the abdominal cavity is a consequence of (usually blunt) abdominal trauma (71-60, 76-60) or of intestinal perforation with vascular erosion. The intraperitoneal blood accumulates as described under 75-10 and can be demonstrated particularly sensitively in the subhepatic recess (Morison's). At 40-60 HU, the radiodensity in the fresh stage is distinctly higher than in ascites (690).

5d: Subhepatic abscess (in Morison's pouch). Hypodense zone around the right lower pole of the liver. Moderate thickening of the peritoneum as a sign of a chronic course. Gallbladder (≫).

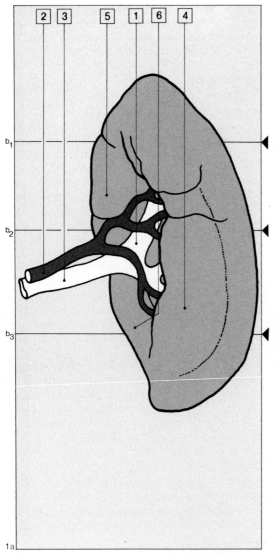
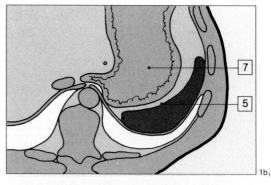
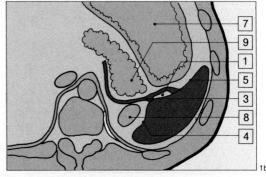
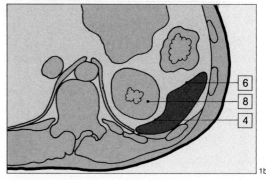
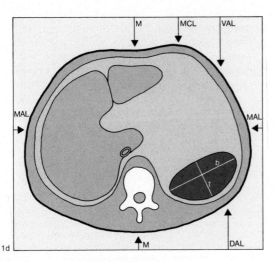

Fig. 76-1 a–c: Normal spleen.

1 a: Dorsal view of the spleen.

1 b: Shape in the transverse section (cf. 1a for level of section).

Key
1 Hilum
2 Splenic artery
3 Splenic vein
4 Facies renalis
5 Facies gastrica
6 Facies colica
7 Stomach
8 Kidney
9 Pancreas

Fig. 76-1 d: Normal dimensions of the spleen.

b = width (longitudinal axis of the ellipsoid cross-section of the spleen)
t = depth (transverse axis of the ellipsoid cross-section of the spleen)
l = longitudinal extent (= scanning area)
b = 7–10 cm, t = 4–6 cm, l = 11–15 cm

Spleen (76-00)

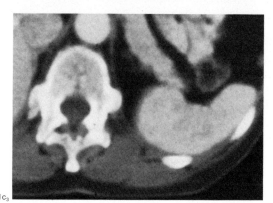

1c: Opacification of the splenic parenchyma after a bolus injection. Transient demonstration of parcelling corresponding to the trabecular and pulpar structure of the parenchyma. (c_1 = 32 sec., c_2 = 52 sec., c_3 = 82 sec. after injection.)

Splenic index
b x t x l ∿ 300 (range 160–440) (686).
M   = Median line
MCL = Medioclavicular line
VAL = Anterior axillary line
MAL = Middle axillary line
DAL = Dorsal axillary line

Anatomy and imaging (76-10)

The **shape** of the spleen, which weighs no more than 200 g in the adult, is influenced by the adjacent organs. The stomach, kidney, diaphragm and the left flexure of the colon lie against the spleen from within their own recesses. The surface of the organ is invested by the peritoneum. The organ vessels reach the spleen via the splenorenal ligament and spread out in the region of the hilum like a longitudinally aligned fan. Vessels pass along the gastrosplenic ligament to the large curvature of the stomach (lesser sac 75-10).

Estimating the size is made difficult by the variable shape. In the horizontal section, the organ figure can be imagined as an ellipse, the longer axis of which should not exceed 10 cm,

Fig. 76-2 a: **Causes of splenomegaly** (from Harrison [55]).

Splenomegaly in inflammations	**(Sub)acute infection** (septicaemia, bacterial endocarditis, abscess, mononucleosis etc.) **Chronic infection** (tuberculosis, syphilis, histoplasmosis, brucellosis, malaria, leishmaniasis etc.) **Others** Lupus erythematodes, rheumatoid arthritis, sarcoidosis, histiocytosis etc.
Splenomegaly in intrasplenic congestion	Cirrhosis of the liver Thrombosis, stenosis of the portal and splenic veins Right heart insufficiency
Splenomegaly in increased storage	Niemann-Pick's disease, Gaucher's disease Amyloidosis, haemosiderosis, haemochromatosis
Splenomegaly in disorders of haematopoiesis and haemolysis	Haemolytic anaemia, thalassaemia Myelofibrosis Polycythaemia vera Thrombocytopenic purpura
Splenomegaly in neoplasia	Cysts (neoplastic pseudocysts) Benign solid tumours (haemangioma etc.) Reticulosarcoma, mal. Lymphoma, leukaemia Myeloma

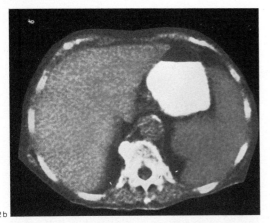

Fig. 76-2b: **Amyloidosis.** Only moderate enlargement of the spleen with homogeneous density. The density values are within the normal range at 36 HU.

Fig. 72-2c: **Thorotrast® spleen.** A rather small spleen with diffuse increase of density (256 HU). Demonstration of opacified lymph nodes along the splenic vessels. Thorotrast® also stored in the right hepatic lobe (>). Compensatory hypertrophy of the caudate lobe (≫).

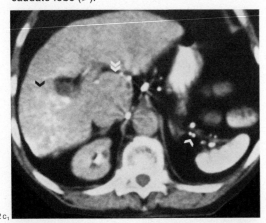

while the shorter axis is regarded as normal up to 6 cm (48). The craniocaudal length in healthy persons is less than 15 cm (26), and can be estimated by the scanning distance required to demonstrate the organ. **Splenomegaly** should be assumed if at least two of the axes described clearly exceed the normal values. A normal-sized spleen does not usually extend beyond the midaxillary line. Only in splenomegaly or hepatomegaly do the surfaces of the two organs come into contact with each other.

The parenchyma displays a homogeneous structure in the plain computed tomogram, the radiodensity being 45 ± 5 HU.

Examination technique (76-20)

- **Spasmolytics** (scopolamine-N-butyl-bromide 30–45 mg i. v. or glucagon 1–2 mg i. v.) immediately before the examination in the case of 20-second scanners, as required in the case of shorter scanning times.

- **Scanning** with slice thicknesses of 8–10 mm in an adjacent slice sequence.

- **Intravenous administration of contrast medium** (facultative)

Normal-dosed infusion with 250 ml Urovison i. v. (4-35) (in unclarified or extensive processes, e. g. trauma etc.).

Guided bolus injection (4-32) to differentiate localized lesions.

- **Total bowel opacification** (facultative, 4-23) within the framework of staging examinations in malignant lymphomas (86-51).

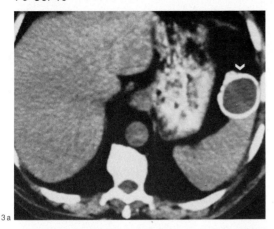

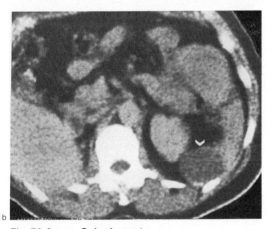

Fig. 76-**3a–c**: Splenic cysts.
3a: Calcified echinococcus cyst.
3b: Histologically unclassifiable epithelialized splenic cyst with thin walls.

3c: Large post-traumatic pseudocyst with irregular delimitation from the splenic parenchyma (≫). The contents of the cysts display density values of 22 HU.

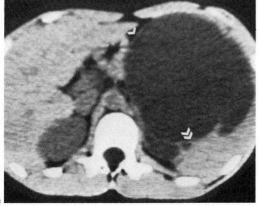

Splenic cysts (76-30)

Splenic cysts are rare and, in the majority of patients, are parasitic in origin (echinococcal cysts). Benign (neoplastic) cysts originate from the lymph or blood vessels (lymphangiomas, haemangiomas). Dermoid cysts have also occasionally been demonstrated (4). Cysts can also develop following trauma (haematoma) or infarction (pseudocysts).

● CT

The cystic masses squash the splenic pulp, giving rise to parenchymal spurs (81-30) (Fig. 76–3a–c). Splenic cysts fulfil the usual CT criteria (3-51). Calcifications are demonstrated mainly in parasitic cysts (echinococcal cysts) (Fig. 76–3a). CT signs of dermoid cysts cf. 61-43 and 85-42. Splenic cysts situated at the hilum are important in the differential diagnosis of pseudocysts of the tail of the pancreas. However, the density value and the soft wall of the cyst, which does not enhance following contrast medium administration, usually permit diagnostic demarcation from pancreatic pseudocysts (73-32).

Solid tumours of the spleen (76-40)

With the exception of **malignant lymphomas** and **plasmocytomas**, which originate from the splenic parenchyma, the spleen is rarely the site of origin of primary tumours. **Haemangiomas** are more frequent than **lymphangiomas**, while **hamartomas, fibromas, myxomas, chondromas, osteomas, malignant haemangioendotheliomas** and **fibrosarcomas** are rarities.

Metastases in the spleen usually occur in the late stage of a malignant disease. They are never an isolated finding. Dissemination is usually haematogenous, but can be lymphatic in individual cases. The lungs, breasts, prostate, ovaries, colon, rectum, stomach and the skin (malignant melanoma) are the sites of the primary tumours. The metastases are of microscopic size in about a third of cases (693) and can enlarge the spleen considerably (4).

● CT

In the majority of cases, circumscribed solitary masses can be identified as hypodense zones within the splenic parenchyma, although contrast enhancement is required in some cases (693). This applies equally to metastases and malignant lymphomas. In diffuse permeation of the splenic pulp with tumour tissue, only splenomegaly indicates splenic involvement, although the latter can also occur in organs of normal or even diminished size (86-51). The CT

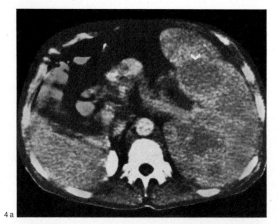

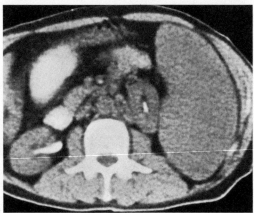

Fig. 76-4 a, b: **Splenomegaly in malignant lymphoma.** Homogeneous tissue density in most cases (b), even after contrast medium administration. In coarse-nodular changes, and particularly in Hodgkin's disease, the neoplastic regions may become visible after a bolus infection (a).

appearance of haemangiomas of the spleen, which has so far not been described in the literature, is probably basically the same as that of hepatic haemangiomas (71-43).

Inflammatory diseases of the spleen
(76-50)

In acute and chronic infections, reactive hyperplasia of various cell elements leads to varying degrees of splenomegaly (Fig. 76-2a). Granulomatous inflammations cause only moderate enlargement of the spleen. Disseminated calcifications can frequently be demonstrated in the healing stage, mainly in tuberculosis, histoplasmosis and brucellosis.

In the majority of cases and particularly in patients with reduced immune defence, a **splenic abscess** develops as part of a generalized infection (septicaemia). An abscess rarely develops on the basis of necrotic splenic tissue (region of infarction, pseudocysts, haematomas).

● CT

Computerized tomography reveals a circumscribed hypodense zone which does not enhance. The density values of the lesion lie within the range of 30 HU (3-53). Differentiation from an older haematoma or a pseudocyst can present difficulties if no gas bubbles – which are regarded as pathognomonic – are demonstrated, in which case the clinical finding is the decisive factor (Fig. 76-5a).

Fig. 76-5a: **Splenic abscess.** Demonstration of a liquefaction cavity with fluid level (≫) in splenomegaly consequent on myeloid leukaemia.

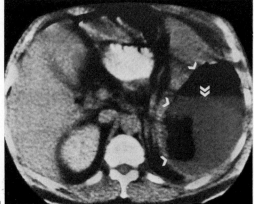

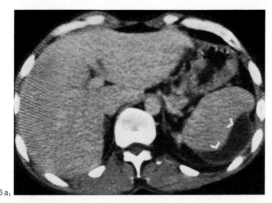

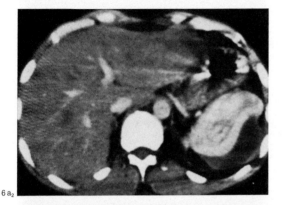

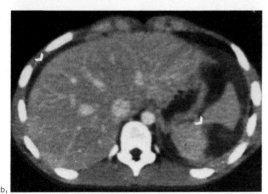

Trauma (76-60)

Splenic injury occurs most frequently following blunt abdominal trauma – particularly after car accidents. A spleen which is enlarged by inflammation, e.g. in mononucleosis, can rupture even as a result of minor trauma. Injuries to the vascular stem can lead to detachment or thrombosis of the major vessels. Depending on its extent, the thrombosis can lead to infarction (76-70) or to the formation of a venous collateral circulation. Intraparenchymal or subcapsular haematomas are demonstrated most frequently. A feared complication is rupture of the capsule (immediate or late), which can result in life-threatening haemorrhage into the abdominal cavity.

Splenic haematoma (76-61)

● CT

In its fresh stage, the haematoma can appear hyperdense in comparison to the splenic tissue (100, 164). Frequently, however, it is isodense, necessitating the administration of contrast medium (e.g. as an infusion) to demarcate the enhanced splenic tissue with its blood supply from the accumulation of blood. Older haematomas are hypodense and readily identifiable in the plain computed tomogram (Fig. 76-6b).

Impression and deformation of the splenic parenchyma are usually found in the case of a subcapsular haematoma; the capsule is usually recognizable and stands out as a circle (Fig. 76-6a). Intraparenchymal haemorrhages appear as irregularly demarcated, partly wedge-shaped zones. If a parenchymal rupture remains undetected and no rupture of the capsule takes place, the haematoma can progress into a (pseudo)cyst. In a reported case (164), subsequent – as opposed to immediate – splenic rupture was recognized by the fact that the intraperitoneal accumulation of blood displayed higher density values than the intra- or perisplenic haematoma (3-52).

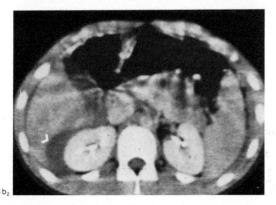

Fig. 76-6a, b: **Haematoma of the spleen.**

6a: Subcapsular haematoma of the spleen. Demonstration of a hypodense subcapsular zone (a_1) which becomes clearly demarcated from the opacified, compressed splenic parenchyma following contrast medium administration (a_2).

6b: Complete splenic rupture with haemorrhagic effusion into the abdomen. Extensive subphrenic zone of reduced density on laceration of the spleen (b_1>). Demonstration of hypodense zones at the upper edge of and below the liver (b_2>). The density values of the intraperitoneal accumulation of fluid are 38 HU.

Vascular lesions (76-70)

Splenic infarction (76-71)
Splenic infarctions are the consequence of thromboembolic occlusions of the splenic artery or its branches. Embolisms usually originate from the chambers of the heart (mitral valve defect, myocardial infarction) or from an aortic aneurysm. Thromboses can be caused by arteriosclerosis, subendothelial infiltration in myeloid leukaemias, inflammatory and neoplastic lesions of the pancreas, trauma (76-60) and haemagglutination in sickle cell anaemia. Infarction regions can liquefy and develop into pseudocysts (76-30). The formation of abscesses occurs in infections (e.g. infected embolisms) (76-50).

● **CT**
Apart from equivocal parenchymal retraction, older splenic infarctions cannot be seen in the plain computed tomogram. A segmental hypodense area can sometimes be demonstrated following administration of contrast medium (Fig. 76-7a).

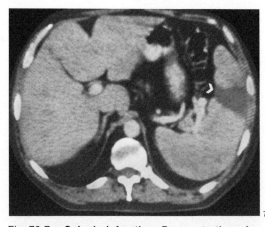

Fig. 76-**7a**: **Splenic infarction.** Demonstration of a segmental zone of reduced density which contrasts distinctly with the splenic parenchyma following contrast medium administration.

Thrombosis of the splenic vein (76-72)
Splenic vein thrombosis occurs as a result of the spread of an inflammatory or neoplastic pancreatic process to the spleen, peritonitis or trauma. A venous collateral circulation (including oesophageal varices) and considerable splenomegaly develop.

● **CT**
The splenomegaly and, frequently, the extensive collateral circulation can be demonstrated by computerized tomography. The collateral network can be enhanced and the patency of the splenic vein checked by a guided bolus injection.

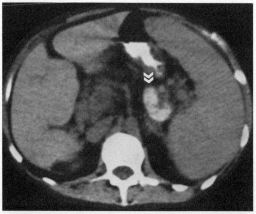

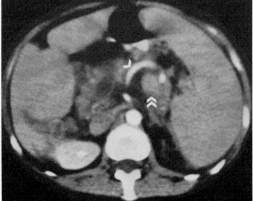

Fig. 76-**7b**: **Splenic vein thrombosis.** Marked splenomegaly and signs of chronic pancreatitis. Plain scan demonstration of a distinctly dilated, hyperdense splenic vein (≫) which does not enhance further following a bolus injection (b_2). Hypervascularity at the splenic hilus extending in part to the thickened gastric wall (collaterals). The hyperdensity of the splenic wall is an indication of a fresh thombosis (cf. 3–52).

Splenic anomalies (76-80)

In the majority of cases, the very rare condition of **asplenia** is accompanied by anomalies of the heart and abdominal cavity. In **polysplenia**, the spleen is divided into 2 to 10 separate parenchymal lobes which can develop on both sides of the dorsal mesogastrium. Accessory spleens are found with comparative frequency (10–30% of anomalies) at autopsy. They consist of functional splenic parenchyma and are encountered in or near the splenic hilum in 75% of cases and in the tail of the pancreas in 20% of cases. They usually display a diameter of 1 cm, although they can achieve a size of up to 10 cm.

● **CT**

An accessory spleen appears in the computed tomogram as a homogeneous, smoothly bordered soft-tissue structure displaying the same radiodensity as the splenic parenchyma (Fig. 76-8a). It is of differential-diagnostic importance and must be differentiated from masses of the pancreas, kidney and adrenal. Differentiation from renal processes is possible following administration of contrast medium as a result of renal accumulation of the material. Frequently, however, there is no definite differentiation possible between an accessory spleen and tumours of the adrenals or the pancreas. In practice, demarcation can often be achieved by scintigraphy. (Oily contrast media which accumulate in the spleen have also been proposed for further computerized tomographic clarification [160].)

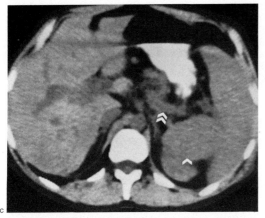

Fig. 76-**7 c**: **Splenic vein thrombosis.** Splenomegaly with accessory spleen (>). The dilated splenic vein exhibits faint central linear hypodensity as a sign of thrombosis (≫).

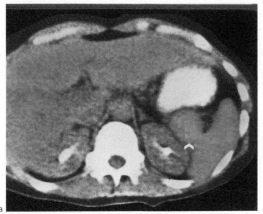

Fig. 76-**8 a**: **Accessory spleen.** Spherical, smoothly bordered soft-tissue structure isodense with the spleen and compressing the fundus of the stomach from dorsal.

Fig. 76-**9 a**: Diseases which can lead to **calcification of the spleen** (from [27,47], modified).

Infections
Echinococcus cysticus
Abscess
Granulomas (multiple) in
– tuberculosis
– brucellosis
– histoplasmosis
Tumours
Lymphangioma
Haemangioma
Non-parasitic cysts
Vascular diseases
Arteriosclerosis
Aneurysm (splenic artery)
Haematoma
Pseudocyst
Infarct
Phleboliths
Other diseases
Sickle-cell anaemia
Haemosiderosis
Capsular calcifications

**Urogenital tract,
retroperitoneal space** (80-00)

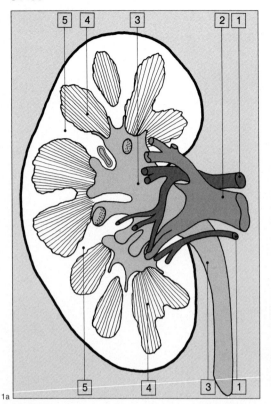
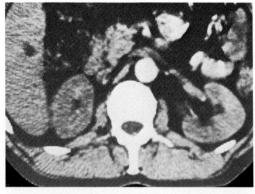
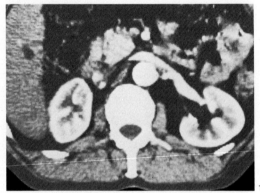
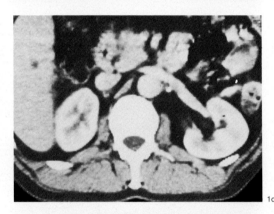
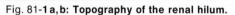
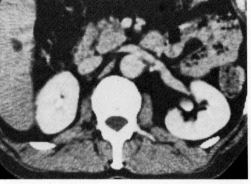

Fig. 81-1 a, b: **Topography of the renal hilum.**
1 a: Longitudinal section
1 b: Transverse section

Key
1 Renal artery
2 Renal vein
3 Renal pelvis and ureter
4 Medullary pyramids
5 Renal cortex

Fig. 81-1 c: **Opacification of the renal parenchyma** following a bolus injection. The well-supplied renal cortex becomes demarcated from the renal medulla for 60–80 seconds (c_1 = plain scan, c_2 = 22 seconds p. i., c_3 = 52 seconds p. i., c_4 = 182 seconds p. i.).

Kidney (81-00)

Anatomy and imaging (81-10)

The kidneys, each of which weighs about 150 g in the adult, are marked by regular architecture. The renal parenchyma surrounds the **renal sinus** like a mantle. It consists of up to 18 **medullary pyramids**, which contain the collecting tubules and fuse to 6–12 papillae in the renal sinus, and the highly vascularized renal cortex, which envelops the medullary cone and accomodates the vascular system, the glomerulae and tubular structures. The calyceal system, which unites – for the greater part intrarenally – to form the renal pelvis, runs through the renal sinus. The **main renal arteries**, which pass behind the renal veins to the kidney, ramify close to the hilum like the veins into a ventral and dorsal branch which surrounds the renal collecting system bilaterally. They enter the parenchyma between the papillae as interlobar vessels (Fig. 81-1 a, b).

● **CT**
In the computed tomogram, the kidneys appear to be transverse-oval at the poles and sickle-shaped in the hilum region. The parenchyma, which displays **radiodensity** of 30 ± 10 HU depending on the state of hydration, exhibits homogeneous density in the plain scan. Following contrast medium administration opacification of the cortical regions, which leaves out the medullary pyramids as hypodense zones, takes place in the early arterial phase – in analogy to arteriography (Fig. 81-1 c_2). The opacification of the cortex decreases in the later phases due to accumulation of the contrast medium in the tubular system, which leads to an increase of density of the renal medulla. The medullary pyramids, the tips of which are orientated concentrically towards the renal sinus, can be demonstrated in their full length from the base to the tip only at the level of the renal hilum. They are intersected in various planes to their long axis in the vicinity of the renal poles. Consequently, the surrounding enhanced renal cortex appears in different oval or annular shapes. The fibrous capsule cannot be demarcated by computerized tomography. The outer renal boundary appears to be smooth when scanned tangentially.

At the level of the renal hilum, the normal transverse diameter measures 5–6 cm frontally and 4 cm sagittally (anteroposteriorly). A value of 1.5 cm is regarded as normal for the width of the parenchyma. The craniocaudal axis, which measures 10–12 cm in healthy persons, can be determined by the scanning distance required to demonstrate the whole organ.

Perirenal and pararenal space see 86-14.

Examination technique (81-20)

● **Reduction of intestinal gas** by means of a low residue diet 48 hours before the examination, particularly with 20-second scanners.

● **Intravenous contrast medium administration** (obligatory).
Normal dose infusion (4-36) with 250 ml Urovison i. v. (in uncircumscribed processes).
Guided bolus injection (4-32) in localized processes for further differentiation.
Exception: no contrast medium needed to demonstrate concrements.

● **Spasmolytics:** Scopolamine-N-butyl-bromide 30–45 mg i. v. or glucagon 1–2 mg i. v. immediately before the examination in the case of 20-second scanners, as required in the case of shorter scanning times.

● **Scanning** with slice thicknesses of 8–10 mm in an adjacent slice sequence
Scanning area: the entire renal bed.

● **Partial bowel opacification** (4-23) in special cases (e. g. post-nephrectomy status).

Cystic diseases of the kidney (81-30)

Benign renal cysts fulfil the following criteria in the computed tomogram:

1. Smooth border in the region of tangential demonstration in comparision to the surrounding tissue and the parenchyma (formation of cortical spurs).

2. Thin walls which are just or not recognizable.

3. Density of the cystic contents approximately that of water (5 ± 5 HU), but less than 15 HU independent of enhancement.

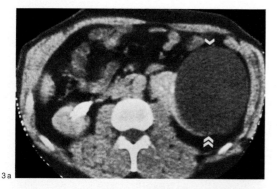

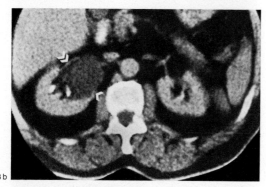

Fig. 81-3a–d: Renal cysts.
3a: Solitary renal cyst with cortical spurs (≫).
3b: Central peripelvic renal cyst right with displacement of the cavity system and the vessels (≫).

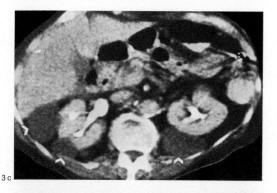

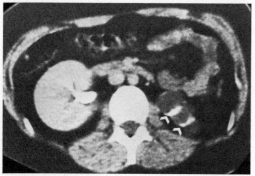

Solitary cysts (81-31) (Fig. 81-3a–c)

Solitary parenchymal cysts must be regarded as acquired disease in which the incidence increases with age. They are frequently found by chance. Infection must be considered if the density values are above 20 HU, particulary if wall thickening is present. The latter is also demonstrable in necrotic hypernephromas (81-41). Fibrolipomatosis must be included in the differential diagnosis of cysts adjacent to the collecting system (81-56).

Polycystic diseases of the kidney (81-32)

The infantile (congenital) form is always bilateral and leads to symmetrical enlargement of the kidneys. The kidneys are permeated by minute cysts with a maximum size of 1–2 mm, which places them below the limit of resolution of computerized tomography.

The adult form causes clinical symptoms and exhibits cystic spaces of varying size and distinct enlargement of both kidneys in the computed tomogram (Fig. 81-3d–f). Unilateral forms have been reported in 4–14% of cases (29). Calcification of individual cysts is a common finding, while malignant degeneration is rare. Nephrolithiasis and infection of cysts are not infrequent complications.

Other cystic masses (81-33)

The **multicystic kidney** (blastemic cyst) occurs unilaterally and is urographically and arteriographically silent. The cysts, which are arranged like a bunch of grapes, tend towards calcification, causing typical annular figures in the plain film. The urinary ducts are atretic or end blindly. In contrast to the polycystic renal diseases of infancy and adulthood, the cause is not held to be genetic.

Multilocular renal cysts are rarely demonstrated. The affected kidney displays local cystic transformation with multiseptate spaces of varying size filled with thick myxomatous material. The septa and the capsule of the mass are hypervascularized and therefore frequently create the angiographic impression of tumour vessels. Because of this appearance the disease is also known as benign multilocular cystic nephroma.

3c: Subcapsular renal cysts, bilateral.
3d: Multicystic kidney with calcified renal cysts (>).

• CT

Only few computerized tomographic observations have so far been made (521), and differentiation from a neoplasia has proved impossible where the cystic spaces were very small.

Calyceal cysts and **medullary sponge kidneys** can be diagnosed unequivocally by urography and are not an indication for CT.

Solid parenchymal tumours (81-40)

The overwhelming majority of solid tumours of the renal parenchyma are malignant. Hypernephromas also form the largest group of renal malignomas, accounting for 80 % of cases. Renal adenomas classified as benign tumours are considered to be potentially malignant once they exceed a diameter of 3 cm. Angiomyolipomas, on the other hand, are benign and degenerate only in extremely exceptional cases (29).

Hypernephroid carcinomas (81-41)

• CT

Hypernephromas appear in the computed tomogram as space-occupying masses which deform the renal parenchyma. They are usually irregularly demarcated or lobulated and, unless they have liquefied, are virtually isodense with the renal parenchyma in the plain scan. As a result of the accumulation of contrast material following infusion the functioning renal parenchyma becomes demarcated from the mass, which then appears (relatively) hypodense. The density gradient depends on the dosage of contrast medium and the degree of vascularity of the tumour. The majority of hypernephromas ($\sim$ 60 % of cases) display marked vascularity and consequently appear temporarily hyperdense in the early phase of a guided bolus injection (509). An adequate and even infusion or bolus injection of contrast material is absolutely essential if anomalies of shape are to be reliably distinguished from tumours which cause only moderate bulging of the renal cortex (4-36).

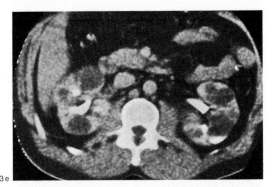
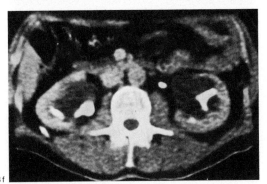

Fig. 81-3 e–h: **Polycystic disease.**
3 e: Moderately enlarged kidneys with intraparenchymal renal cysts of varying size.
3 f: Central arrangement of the renal cysts bilateral.

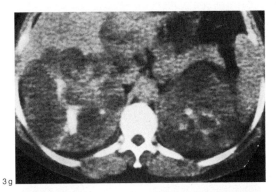
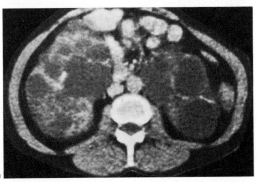

3 g, h: Cystic degeneration with marked enlargement of the kidney and expansion of the renal cavity system.

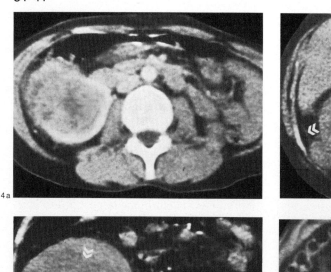
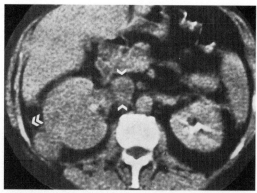
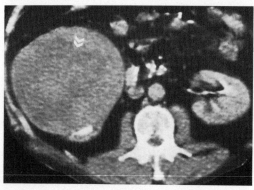
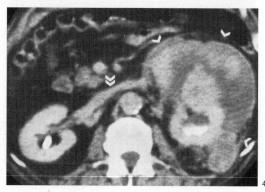

Fig. 81-4 a–f: Hypernephroid carcinoma.

4 a: Hypervascularized tumour with hyperdense peripheral areas and moderate (central) necroses. No demonstration of regional lymph node metastases.

4 b: Large hypernephroma with smooth borders and irregular, hypodense necrotic zones (≫).

4 d: Infiltration of the hypernephroma through Gerota's fascia (≫). Hypodense, dilated inferior vena cava indicative of a partial thrombosis (>).

4 e: Extensive tumour with central necroses and hypervascularized peripheral areas. Gerota's fascia has not been penetrated in this slice (>), the patent renal vein opacifies after administration of contrast material (≫).

4 c: Cystic hypernephroma with thickened wall (><) and homogeneous, reduced density values. Demonstration of multiple paraaortic lymph node metastases (≫).

4 f: Cystic hypernephroma with smooth but thickened walls and occasional septa. No regional lymph node enlargement. At 23 HU, the radiodensity of the tumour is clearly above that of water.

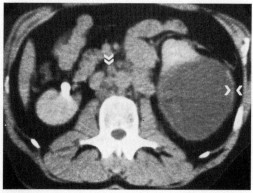
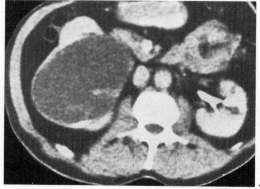

The CT image of the perirenal space is so good that tumour-staging can be performed, e. g. according to the classification proposed by Robsen et al. (545) and developed for the prognosis of the patient:

I: Tumour limited to the renal parenchyma (tunica fibrosa renalis intact).
II: Tumour expansion into the perirenal space (Gerota's fascia intact).
III: Invasion of the renal vein or metastasis into regional lymph nodes.
IV: Expansion or metastases into adjacent organs.

Regional lymph nodes mask the contours of the large **vessels**. The inferior vena cava can be distinctly opacified and its patency checked following rapid contrast medium infusion via a leg vein (155), although a more reliable method is to give a bolus injection and to employ a sequential slice technique above the junction of the renal vein with the inferior vena cava. With large tumours, Gerota's fascia is often moderately thickened — probably due to concomitant inflammation — and can consequently be readily identified in most cases. The perirenal fatty tissue is consumed by the expanding tumour and not displaced (haematomas 81-61).

Unenhanced **hypodense areas** are frequently found within extensive hypernephromas and correspond to zones of necrosis (Fig. 81-4a, b) (530). Tumour disintegration can be so complete that the existence of a neoplasm is signalled only by generally moderate thickening of the wall or by a solid cone (Fig. 81-4c, f). Until evidence to the contrary is forthcoming, the thickened wall of a cystic space must be diagnosed tentatively as a malignant growth. A specific search must therefore be made for secondary criteria of malignancy, e. g. enlargement of regional lymph nodes and involvement of adjacent organs.

Calcifications of whatever shape (shell-like, amorphous) situated within and not at the periphery of a solid renal mass must be taken as a further indication of malignancy (Fig. 81-4h).

In **postnephrectomy patients,** a local recurrence can be seen in the computed tomogram as a mass of soft-tissue density following adequate opacification of the bowel, which usually fills the empty renal bed. If the postoperative course is complicated, however, an organized haematoma or fatty tissue necrosis (530) can appear as a mass of soft-tissue density which is indistinguishable from a recurrence. Unless signs of malignancy are present (regional lymphomas, metastases, muscle infiltrations, bone destruction) (Fig. 81-4g), only guided puncture, angiography or CT follow-up studies can provide further information.

Fig. 81-**4g: Recurrence of a hypernephroma** right (≫) with liver metastases (>).

Fig. 81-**4h: Hypernephroid carcinoma with tumour calcifications** (≫).

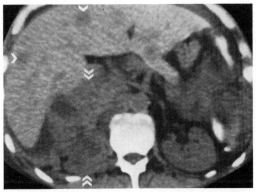

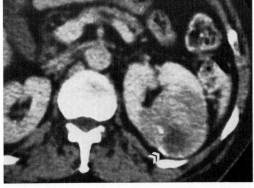

The following masses must be considered in the **differential diagnosis:**
Solid tumours: organized abscess, organized haematoma, renal metastases, renal adenoma, xanthomatous pyelonephritis, malignant lymphoma, (fibroma, leiomyoma).
Cystic hypernephroma: infected cysts, abscess, tuberculosis.

Adenoma and cystadenoma (81-42)
These benign tumours are not rare (7 % of autopsies) and are frequently encountered together with benign nephrosclerosis or pyelonephritis. The majority are microscopic in size, but they can achieve a diameter of several cm. They are regarded as potentially malignant from a diameter of 3 cm. Cystic forms, which can calcify (530), are a minority finding. Larger adenomas – which are still a rare clinical observation – are usually poorly vascularized and difficult to distinguish from malignant tumours even with angiography.
● **CT**
With contrast medium enhancement, computerized tomography can demonstrate adenomas and cystadenomas from a diameter of 1–2 cm. No differential-diagnostic criteria have so far been established in respect of a malignant tumour (solid or cystic hypernephroma) (530, 535).

Angiomyolipoma (81-43)
Angiomyolipomas are regarded as a type of hamartoma and occur in 50–80 % of cases of tuberous sclerosis (Bourneville-Pringle's disease). Bilateral or multifocal development is a frequent finding. In addition to fatty tissue, mixed tumours also contain arteries with maldeveloped walls (aneurysmatic degeneration).
● **CT**
The fatty tissue component of the tumour can be clearly demonstrated by computerized tomography, and this greatly facilitates diagnosis of the type (505). Enhancement varies following administration of contrast medium depending on the degree of vascularization and aneurysmatic degeneration (60) (Fig. 81-4 i, k).

Fig. 81-4 i, k: **Angiomyolipomas.** Demonstration of extensive, smoothly bordered fatty tissue components with some thin septa within the enlarged organs (>).

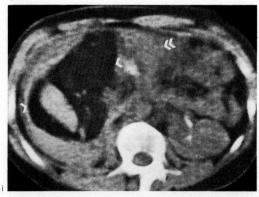

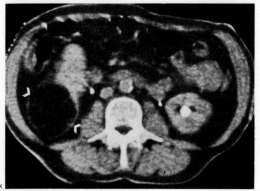

Mesenchymal tumours (81-44)
Fibromas, lipomas, leiomyomas and haemangiomas are usually benign masses with a diameter not exceeding 1 cm which occur very rarely and represent a chance postmortem finding. Only the lipoma can be identified by computerized tomography, and an angiomyolipoma must be considered in the differential diagnosis.

Wilms' tumour (nephroblastoma) (81-45)
Wilms' tumour is the renal tumour of infancy and occurs with about the same frequency as the neuroblastoma. These two kinds of tumour account for 16–20 % of infantile malignant growths. Wilm's tumour occurs bilaterally in 5–10 % of cases and gives rise to early haematogenous metastasis into the lung and liver, the subsequent clinical picture being

dominated by local tumour growth and metastases to regional lymph nodes (33). The tumour consists of embryonal renal cells, stands out relatively smoothly from the renal parenchyma in the initial stage and frequently displays necrotic and haemorrhagic regions. Punctiform and annular calcifications are found in 10–20% of cases (33).

● **CT**

The computed tomogram reveals a solid mass originating from the kidney which appears hypodense in comparison to the enhanced renal parenchyma (Fig. 81-4 l). Zones of reduced density represent necrosis. Partial and complete hydronephrosis is frequently demonstrated, and this can also involve the contralateral kidney as the tumour expands beyond the mid-line. Tumour-staging is possible since the computed tomogram can also reveal infiltration into the adjacent tissue through the renal fascia, regional or paraaortic lymph node metastases and liver metastases.

Tumours of the renal pelvis (81-46)

Like those of the urinary bladder, papillomas of the renal pelvis tend to degenerate. Carcinomas of the renal pelvis constitute the smaller group of malignant growths of the kidney, accounting for 8–10% of cases. Transitional epithelium is the site of origin in 80–85% of cases. Carcinomas originating from squamous epithelium, which are a less frequent finding, tend to infiltrate the renal parenchyma at an early stage. Regional (paraaortic) lymph node involvement is found even in the case of very small tumours.

● **CT**

As in the urogram, tumours of the renal pelvis are seen in the computed tomogram as filling defects of the enhanced cavity system (Fig. 81-4 n). The resolution of the image matrix prevents recognition of fine structures of the tumour surface. The renal cavity system is not an ideal object for computerized tomography because of its ramified margins which mainly run obliquely in the scanning plane. Consequently, tapetum-like growing carcinoma in particular can escape computerized tomographic detection. A positive urogram of the renal pelvis is not invalidated by a normal computed tomogram. Computerized tomography can, however, demonstrate infiltration of a tumour of the renal pelvis into the adjacent parenchyma, although differentiation from a hypernephroma which has invaded the renal pelvis can be difficult or even impossible in

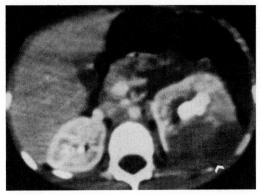

Fig. 81-4 l: **Wilms' tumour:** Hypodense zone, relatively sharply demarcated from the renal parenchyma. Moderate, uneven enhancement of 30 HU.

Fig. 81-4 m, n: **Carcinoma of the renal pelvis.**

4 m: Area of soft-tissue density in the region of the upper group of calyces left (>). No enhancement. Demonstration of perirenal, inflammatory changes and regional lymph node enlargement (≫).

4 n: Papillary carcinoma recognizable as a filling defect within the renal pelvis (>), with general pyelonephritic changes of the kidney.

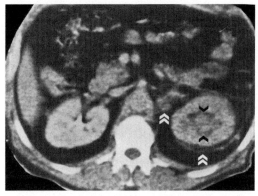

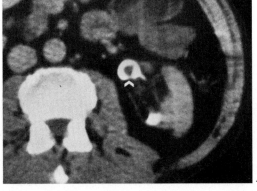

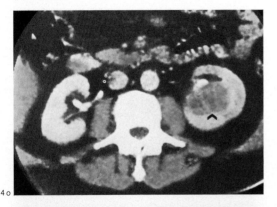

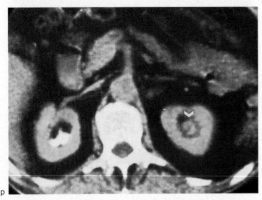

Fig. 81-4 o–q: Carcinoma of the renal pelvis.
4 o: Relatively dense, smoothly bordered mass with displacement of the cavity system left. At 46 HU, the density values are distinctly higher than those of cysts.
4 p: Unenhanced, soft-tissue structure within the upper calyceal group without demonstration of invasion of the renal parenchyma.

4 q: Smoothly bordered filling defect in the region of the right calyceal group with density values of 48 HU – well above those of a central renal cyst. Incidental finding: lobar dysmorphism (≫).

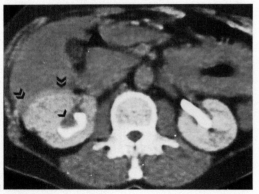

such cases. Of importance for the differential diagnosis is the fact that tumours of the renal pelvis display only slight enhancement following bolus injection because of their poor vascularity, and frequently cause partial obstruction of the collecting system. The density values must be carefully analysed because of the partial volume effect since these tumours are usually small. Small slice thicknesses of 4–5 mm should be chosen in critical cases, and the hilum of the kidney must be inspected for lymph node enlargement (metastases).

Secondary tumours of the kidney (81-47)

Metastases to the kidneys occur most frequently from bronchial carcinoma, followed by mammary and gastric carcinoma.

Renal metastases, which are seen at autopsy twice as frequently as primary tumours, usually occur within generalized carcinomatosis. Bilateral involvement is observed in more than 50% of cases. At autopsy, renal involvement is found in a third of malignant lymphoma cases.

● **CT**

Hypovascularized metastases appear as hypodense masses (Fig. 81-4 r) and cannot be differentiated from hypovascularized hypernephromas (even after a bolus injection). The diagnosis is facilitated by bilateral involvement, the demonstration of other metastases and awareness of the primary tumour. Differential diagnosis from renal manifestation of a malignant lymphoma is likewise simple in most cases due to the retroperitoneal pattern of involvement. Malignant lymphomas can break through fascial boundaries and penetrate directly into the renal parenchyma.

Inflammations (81-50)

A number of acute inflammations – particulary glomerulonephritis, abacterial interstitial nephritis and pyelonephritis – cause nothing more than enlargement of the organ, and are not an indication for computerized tomography. The final state of chronic inflammatory processes with atrophy of the organ is, however, easily recognizable and assessable in the computed tomogram.

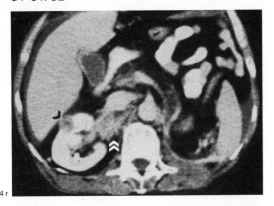

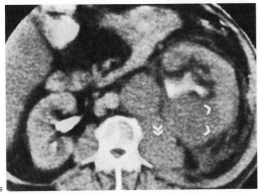

Fig. 81-4 r, s: **Secondary renal tumours.**

4 r: Renal metastasis in contralateral metastatic disease from an excised hypernephroma. Its appearance cannot be distinguished from that of a primary hypernephroma. Hilar lymphomas (≫).

4 s: Invasion of the left kidney by a malignant lymphoma (>). Demonstration of extensive retroperitoneal lymphomas and infiltration of the psoas muscle (≫).

Fig. 81-5 a: **Chronic pyelonephritis.** Renal atrophy right with parenchymal contraction above the calyces (>) and compensatory regeneration nodes (≫).

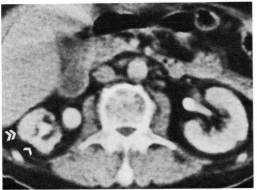

Local bacterial nephritis, abscesses, carbuncles (81-51)

Non-specific pyogenic abscesses — usually unilateral — develop haematogenously in the majority of cases and via the ascending route in some. A local increase of renal volume is found in the acute stage. On progression of the disease, reversible interstitial infiltration gives way to irregular liquefaction which finally forms a cavity with an abscess membrane. As the course of the disease progresses, the abscesses can become organized with connective tissue, invade the renal cavity system or erupt into the perirenal space. Renal carbuncles are marked by dry necrosis and an abundance of granulation tissue.

● CT

The different phases give rise to different CT aspects. Irregularly demarcated, partly linear unenhanced regions of parenchyma are found in the acute stage of infiltration or incipient liquefaction (533) (Fig. 81-5b). The healing process under antibiotic therapy can be supervised. The chronic course with the formation of an abscess membrane offers the picture of a thick-walled cyst with higher density values ($\sim$ 30 HU) which cannot be distinguished from an infected cyst (Fig. 81-5f). Spontaneous healing can occur on eruption into the cavity system. If, however, drainage is obstructed by necrotic material and pus, the condition deteriorates into pyonephrosis.

Xanthogranulomatous pyelonephritis (81-52)

Multiple abscesses usually of one kidney and stained yellow macroscopically by lipid-containing xanthoma cells are typical of xanthogranulomatous pyelonephritis, an etiologically unclarified disease. Organ enlargement, urinary stasis with concrements, impaired excretory function, intrarenal calcifications and perirenal inflammation are further features (29), all of which can be demonstrated by computerized tomography. No density values have yet been reported for the (lipid-containing) abscesses.

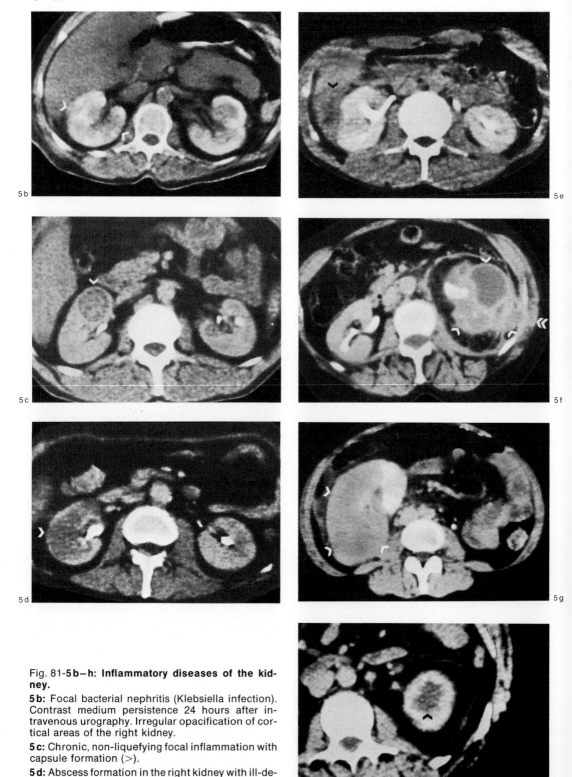

Fig. 81-5b–h: **Inflammatory diseases of the kidney.**

5b: Focal bacterial nephritis (Klebsiella infection). Contrast medium persistence 24 hours after intravenous urography. Irregular opacification of cortical areas of the right kidney.

5c: Chronic, non-liquefying focal inflammation with capsule formation (>).

5d: Abscess formation in the right kidney with ill-defined delimitation from the opacified renal parenchyma. Completely reversible under antibiotic therapy.

Kidney

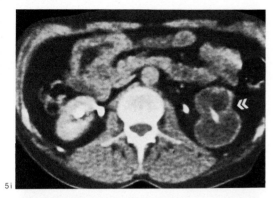

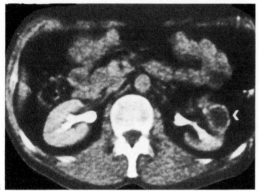

Fig. 81-5 i, k: **Ulcero-cavernous tuberculosis of the kidney.** Demonstration of hypodense, smoothly bordered, septated spaces at the lower renal pole left (≫). The walls display signs of calcification. The density values of the necrotic material are 12 HU. Demonstration of only slight enlargement of hilar lymph nodes.

5 e: Subcapsular abscess of the right kidney with concomitant inflammation of the right lower hepatic lobe (>).

5 f: Multiple abscesses of the left kidney with perirenal infiltration and simultaneous inflammatory involvement of the thoracic wall (≫). The abscessed areas display ring-shaped enhancement as a sign of granulation tissue.

5 g: Carbuncle of the right kidney. The inflamed zone (>) is poorly demarcated from the opacified renal parenchyma, but its borders to the fibrous capsule are smooth.

5 h: Abscess at the lower renal pole left with poor demarcation from the renal parenchyma (>).

Chronic pyelonephritis (81-53)

The diagnosis of chronic pyelonephritis is made clinically and by urography. Computerized tomographic diagnosis is based on the current radiological criteria (Fig. 81-5a).

1. Loss of parenchyma (narrowing of the parenchymal cortex extending to shrinkage of the organ).
2. Cicatricial contractions over deformed calyces which can extend as far as the fibrous capsule.
3. Regeneration nodes (acquired pseudotumours).
4. Impaired excretory function.

Slight calyceal deformations escape computerized tomographic detection because of the limited spatial resolution.

Renal tuberculosis (81-54)

Postprimary tuberculosis does not become manifest in the kidneys for 5–20 years following haematogenous dissemination. In the productive course the usually miliary tubercles permeate the renal parenchyma diffusely, while the liquefying, caseogenous course is marked by a loss of parenchyma. Calyceal destruction visible in the urogram usually signifies extensive parenchymal changes of the renal segment concerned. Concomitant productive processes or strictures which can lead to encapsulation of groups of calyces are typical of tuberculosis. Progression of the disease culminates in tuberculous pyonephrosis (caseous pyonephrosis with thickening of the necrotic material).

● CT

Only the ulcerocavernous forms are visible in the computed tomogram. The cross-sections of the kidney present a mulberry- or clover-leaf appearance on loss of several segments (Fig. 81-5 i, k). The marked tendency of the caseogenous necrotic material to calcify can be employed to narrow down the differential diagnosis. Fine calcification of the walls of the cavities is also frequently demonstrable. Differentiation from non-specific abscesses and pyonephroses may be impossible in the individual case, particularly in the case of focal liquefaction.

Transplanted kidney (81-55)

Computerized tomography can supply certain diagnostic information when the excretory function of the transplanted kidney is reduced. Acute enlargement together with the clinical findings is an indication of acute rejection, while a gradual decrease in size is indicative of chronic rejection (556). Haematomas (Fig. 81-5 m), abscesses and lymphoceles can be demonstrated just as in a normal renal bed and can also be differentiated to the usual extent (81-51, 81-61). If there are no contraindications from a clinical point of view, contrast medium administration is recommended to achieve better demarcation of the renal parenchyma (524, 539).

Fibrolipomatosis (81-56)

Fibrolipomatosis constitutes proliferation of the fatty and connective tissue in the renal sinus. As regards its pathogenesis, some authors (32a) ascribe it the function of a filling tissue (filling fat) following atrophy of the renal parenchyma, e. g. as a result of pyelonephritis. The high coincidence of fibrolipomatosis in prostatic adenoma, chronic pyelonephritis and nephrolithiasis makes reflux into the renal sinus the principal factor in the pathogenesis (49a): repeated extravasation of urine into the peripelvic and pericalyceal space due to urinary congestion leads to a chronic inflammatory reaction and proliferation of the normally sparse fatty tissue in the renal sinus.

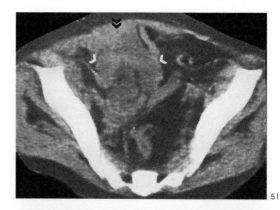
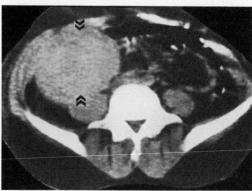

Fig. 81-5 l, m: **Transplanted kidneys.** Renal sinus oriented in a dorsal direction. Normal density values and size of the kidney (>). Demonstration of an accompanying haematoma on the renal capsule (≫) which can be diagnosed by increased density values (5 m).

● CT

Computerized tomography reveals distinct dilation of the renal sinus, through which the (enhanced) and usually stretched renal cavity system runs. The changes are generally present to a similar degree in both kidneys. In contrast to peripelvic cysts, there are no unequivocal signs of displacement. The fibrolipomatous tissue surrounds the calyces and the renal pelvis in the same way, giving the appearance of a cuff (Fig. 81-5 n).

To avoid the partial volume effect, the density values must be measured exactly next to the structures of the collecting system and in the case of thin slices. They can be the same as those of the surrounding perirenal fatty tissue. Frequently, however, they are considerably higher – sometimes above those of water. The renal sinus can then be demarcated septally from the perirenal fatty tissue in a medial direction and creates the impression of an expansive growth because of its protrusion (Fig. 81-5 o, p). The relatively high density values in

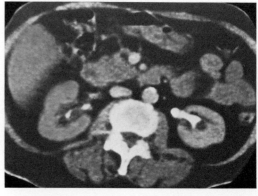

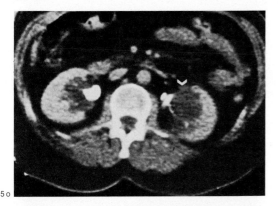

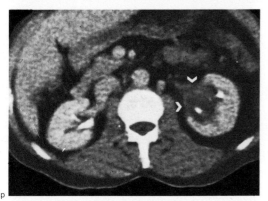

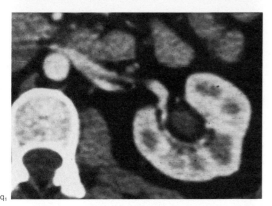

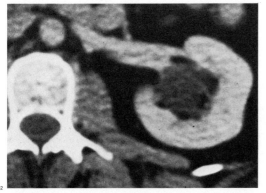

comparison to fat may result from a fibrous component. If one accepts Voegeli's suggestion (49a), the increased density of the fibrolipomatous structures to above the values of the fatty tissue represents the extent of the chronic inflammatory changes, which can therefore be demarcated from the pure filling fat engendered by atrophy of the parenchyma. The differential diagnosis must discriminate between fibrolipomatous tissue – which can display the density of water – and peripelvic cysts. The diagnosis can usually be made on the basis of the distribution of the fat-containing tissue around the renal collecting system, the absence of signs of displacement and the fact that the condition is usually bilateral. From personal experience, the administration of contrast medium even as a specific bolus injection makes no contribution to the differential diagnosis, since it does not lead to unequivocal enhancement of the fibrolipomatous tissue (Fig. 81-5q).

Renal trauma (81-60)

Trauma – usually blunt – can lead to contusion or rupture of the renal parenchyma and, less frequently, to detachment of the arterial or venous stem. Isolated lacerations of the renal collecting system or detachment of the ureter are found only in certain constellations. Vascular injuries are usually accompanied by haematomas of varying size and may cause local thrombosis. Lacerations of the renal cavity system cause urinary extravasation, particularly in the simultaneous presence of obstructed flow (86-32).

Fig. 81-5n–q: **Fibrolipomatosis**.

5n: The fat-containing tissue in the renal sinus is distinctly denser than that surrounding the renal fatty tissue (here + 8 HU). Symmetrical involvement of the kidneys and elongation of the necks of the calyces.

5o, p: Tumour-like protrusion of the fibrolipomatous fatty tissue (8/10 HU).

5q: No noticeable enhancement of the fibrolipomatous tissue following a bolus injection (q_2).

Renal haematoma (81-61)

Haematomas develop either as a result of trauma or spontaneously. According to a study by Polky and Vynallek (32), 80% of non-traumatic haematomas are situated peri- or pararenally, while 20% are found beneath the capsule. Etiological factors reported by the authors are nephritis, neoplasms, aneurysms of the renal artery, arteriosclerosis, hydronephrosis, panarteriitis nodosa, tuberculosis, renal cysts and coagulopathies. Traumatic causes of haematomas are stab wounds, iatrogenic puncture and particularly blunt abdominal trauma. The renal capsule (fibrous capsule) may remain intact in parenchymal rupture, giving rise to a subcapsular haematoma. However, rupture of the parenchymal capsule leading to a perirenal haematoma is frequently demonstrable. A subcapsular haematoma may invade the perirenal space secondarily. Frequently, the only clinical indication of a subcapsular or perirenal haematoma is hypertension resulting from compression effects (page kidney) – particularly in spontaneous haemorrhages.

● CT

Damage to the renal parenchyma due to trauma can be identified by inhomogeneities of opacification. Irregular contours are indicative of a rupture (Fig. 81-6a). Fine parenchymatous lacerations, detached vessels and thromboses are only accessible to angiography, while the extent of a subcapsular or perirenal haematoma can be readily demonstrated by computerized tomography. Its expansion into the adjacent area and displacement of retroperitoneal organs can be assessed particularly well. A subcapsular haematoma is identifiable by impression of the renal parenchyma, the outer capsule and the parenchyma forming – in contrast to the renal cyst – an acute angle (Fig. 81-6b). Perirenal haematomas can develop locally or diffusely in the adipose capsule (511).

The **radiodensity** is dependent on the age and type of the haematoma (clot, suggillation). Fresh compact haematomas can remain hyperdense for 1–2 days in comparison to unenhanced muscle or renal tissue. Because they are avascular lesions, their density does not change following enhancement and they usually appear hypodense in comparison to enhanced renal parenchyma. In the further course they can liquefy (reduction of density, formation of capsules), calcify (Fig. 81-6c) and be absorbed or become organized.

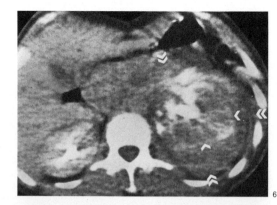

6a

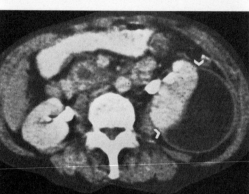

6b

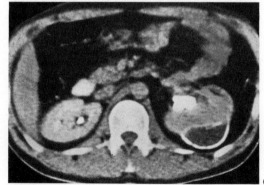

6c

Fig. 81-**6a–c: Renal haematoma.**
6a: Rupture of the renal parenchyma with perirenal haematoma (≫). Because of its horizontal course, the parenchymal rupture can be demonstrated better in the angiogram.
6b: Subcapsular haematoma with acute-angled bending of the fibrous capsule of the kidney. The density values are distinctly above those of water at 17 HU. Flattening of the renal parenchyma.
6c: Subcapsular haematoma with calcification.

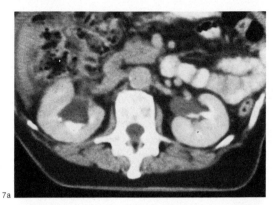

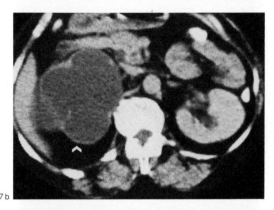

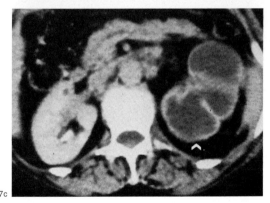

Fig. 81-7 a–c: **Obstructive uropathy.**

7 a: Congested kidney bilateral with dilated, protruding renal pelvis. Substratification phenomenon caused by delayed elimination of the contrast medium.

7 b: Hydronephrotic sacciform kidney right with non-functioning renal parenchyma. The density values of the liquid contents are 14 HU.

7 c: Pyonephrosis with septum-like parenchymal remnants. The density values of the purulent contents are 18 HU.

Obstructive uropathy (81-70)

Hydronephrosis (congestion kidney) (81-71)

By far the most frequent cause of urinary congestion is a mechanical obstruction to flow, e. g. occlusion of the lumen (lithiasis, tumour, trauma), intramural processes (strictures – congenital, inflammatory, radiogenic –, atresias) and compression of the ureters (retroperitoneal tumours, lymphomas, retroperitoneal fibrosis, pelvic tumours, trauma, atypical course of the ureter). Purely functional causes (neurogenic, vesicoureteral reflux) are very rare and are encountered mainly in younger patients. Individual calyces, the renal pelvis, ureters and urinary bladder are affected depending on the site of the obstruction. The increase of intraluminal pressure leads first of all to atrophy of the papillae, which become hollowed out, and then to rolling-out of the medullary pyramids, leaving only the renal columns intact as parenchymatous bridges. The kidneys may be enlarged to varying degrees in chronic urinary congestion, but are smaller than usual in the majority of cases – not infrequently with compensatory hypertrophy of the opposite side. It is disputable whether the renal shrinkage in urinary congestion is due to inflammatory processes alone. The onset and duration of the obstruction in relation to the age of the patient appear to be of pathogenetic importance (12, 43).

● CT

The computed tomogram reveals the dilated collecting system as a central, hypodense (about the density of water) zone orientated on the calyceal system. The duration and extent of the (chronic) congestion determine the deformation of the collecting system, which finally merges to form a mulberry-like figure, the excavations corresponding to the atrophic medullary pyramids. The final stage is a destructured, liquid-filled sac consisting of connective tissue (Fig. 81-7 b).

Slight dilations of the collecting system are not reliably recognizable in the computed tomogram because of the unfavourable scanning geometry (81-46). The renal pelvis protrudes extrarenally in a medial direction at a relatively early stage – a sign which therefore merits attention despite the fact that it is not specific. Substratification of the contrast medium occurs following its administration in urinary stasis (Fig. 81-7 a) because the specific gravity is higher than that of urine. It may be very minimal and in this situation indicates the residual function of the kidney. In the case of a low-lying obstruction, a dilated ureter can be followed in the caudal direction if it takes an axial course and the lumen displays a calibre of 0.5–1 cm (Fig. 81-7f).

Differential diagnosis from central (parapelvic) cysts presents no difficulties when the collecting system is opacified, since the signs of displacement of the enhanced collecting system are plain to see. The points to watch for as regards polycystic kidneys with excretory insufficiency are that hydronephroses represent a communicating cavity system with centrally open and aligned septa, while cystic septa are always closed but cannot be completely delimited in the computed tomogram because of the partial volume effect.

The density value, which lies within the range of that of water, makes no contribution to the differential diagnosis.

Pyonephrosis (81-72)

Pyonephrosis arises as a result of the simultaneous occurrence of obstruction and inflammation, e. g. in inflammatory changes of the renal parenchyma (pyelonephritis, tuberculosis, abscess and carbuncle) following secondary obstruction by necrotic material, in strictures or in secondary infection of hydronephrosis. Pyonephrosis is marked by a pus-filled collecting system which, depending on the degree of congestion and parenchymatous destruction, assumes a sac-like configuration. Not infrequently, the inflammatory changes spread to the perirenal and pararenal space. Progression to an atrophic kidney is possible in chronic forms, a condition which can be recognized even in the general X-ray film by amorphous and shell-like calcareous infiltrations.

● CT

In analogy to hydronephrosis, the computed tomogram reveals varying degrees of dilation of the renal collecting system. Reduction or inflammatory destruction of the renal parenchyma can be assessed. While the **density values** in hydronephrosis are similar to those of water, those in pyonephrosis are higher (Fig. 81-7c), ranging from 20–70 HU depending on the viscosity of the necrotic material. Computerized tomography cannot usually discriminate between specific and nonspecific pyonephrosis (calcifications 81-54). In contrast, its spread to the perirenal and pararenal space can be demonstrated at an early stage (86-31). Hypertrophy of the perirenal fatty tissue has been described in pyonephrosis (532).

Urolithiasis (81-73)

90–95% of all renal stones consist of calcium-containing carbonates, phosphates, oxalates and magnesium ammonium phosphate. Phosphate stones devoid of calcium display distinctly reduced density and are, like cystine stone, just recognizable in urograms free from overshadowing. Only xanthine and urate concrements escape diagnosis by plain urography.

● CT

Due to the higher density resolution, computerized tomography is able to demonstrate calcium-containing structures more sensitively than conventional radiological techniques (72-42) – provided that the concrement is detected in the slice as a whole. The same goes for cystine and magnesium ammonium phosphate calculi. The demonstration of larger xanthine and urate concrements, which display density values between 60 and 80 HU, in the plain scan appears to be at least partly possible, whereas their differentiation from blood clots is unsuccessful (560).

Shadows in the renal sinus must be differentiated from vascular calcifications (renal artery), which frequently display a linear arrangement in keeping with the course of the vessel. Coarser and shell-like (extrapelvic) shadows are an indication of an aneurysm of the renal artery (530).

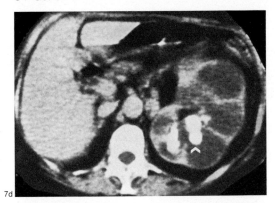

Vascular processes (81-80)

Although renal artery stenosis is not usually recognizable in the computed tomogram, the haemodynamic effects can be assessed. If **sequential computerized tomography** is used (in analogy to sequence scintigraphy), the intravascular arrival of the contrast medium can be demonstrated and analysed quantitatively together with other kinetic parameters (143, 531). This method is in the initial stages of clinical investigation.

Renal infarct (81-81)

Thromboembolic occlusions of the renal artery or its branches result in a renal infarct. The emboli usually originate from the heart (defect of the mitral valve, myocardial infarct etc.) or from an aortic aneurysm.

● CT

The principle signs in the computed tomogram are the absence of enhancement of an area of parenchyma in the fresh stage (528) and contraction in the cicatricial stage. The infarct may escape computerized tomographic detection if only one renal segment is affected — particularly when it is situated at the poles.

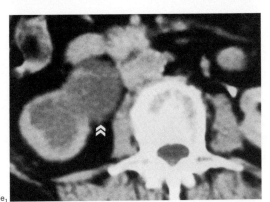

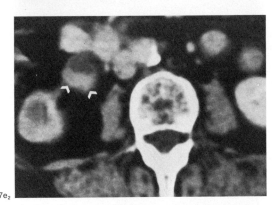

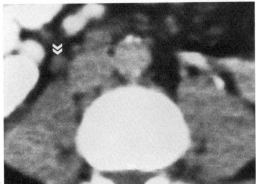

Fig. 81-**7 d: Hydronephrotic sacciform kidney with calculi** (>).

Fig. 81-**7 e: Carcinoma of the ureter** close to its point of departure. Demonstration of a sickle-shaped soft-tissue structure surrounding the congested ureter like a cuff (>). Chronic congested kidney right (e_1) with the renal pelvis outside the kidney right.

Fig. 81-**7 f: Dilated ureter** caused by distal obstruction (here: metastatic carcinoma of the prostate).

Variants, anomalies (81-90)

Renal **agenesis** means the absence of a kidney, **aplasia** the lack of development of the rudiment of a kidney. **Hypoplasia** means an underdeveloped but perfectly formed kidney, while **lobar dysmorphism** is defined as hypertrophy or duplication of a renal segment (medullary pyramid with surrounding cortex).

Anomalies of position (**ectopias**) can be congenital or acquired (ptosis). If a kidney is malpositioned on the opposite side the term crossed dystopia is used, a condition which can also display anomalies of rotation and shape. **Horseshoe kidneys** – in which the lower poles are joined together – display collecting systems aligned ventrally in a typical manner. Their vascular supply is highly variable.

● CT

In the case of unilateral silent kidney, computerized tomography can normally discriminate between a kidney which is present but not functioning and **agenesis or aplasia,** since the renal bed can be surveyed precisely. The demonstration of a small structure of soft-tissue density with aortic vascular supply opposite the point of departure of the renal artery of the functioning kidney is an indication of aplasia. In the case of agenesis the renal bed appears empty. In both anomalies the adrenal is present bilaterally in more than 90% of cases.

Overall, **hypoplasia** appears in the computed tomogram as a diminutive version of a normally shaped kidney. Parenchymal changes (81-53) can assist in the differential diagnosis from a pyelonephritic atrophic kidney.

A **horseshoe kidney** can be diagnosed even in the plain scan on the basis of the bridge formation and the rotatory anomaly. Differentiation from parenchymatous and fibrous connections is possible following rapid contrast medium infusion, particularly after a guided bolus injection. However, angiography remains indispensable prior to surgery, since the highly variable vascular supply cannot be reliably demonstrated by computerized tomography.

Lobar dysmorphism, which can lead to tumour-like distention of the renal parenchyma, behaves like normal renal tissue. Synchronous enhancement of the renal parenchyma is found following contrast medium administration. The nature of the anomaly becomes more distinct after a guided bolus injection, which also permits differentiation of medullary and cortical structures (509). Persistent foetal lobulation can be confirmed in a similar way.

Fig. 81-9a: **Pelvic kidney.** Slightly enlarged kidney with the renal sinus extending in a ventral direction.

Fig. 81-9b: **Agenesis of the right kidney.** Empty right renal bed into which the right flexure of the colon (≫) has moved. No demonstration of (rudimentary) vessels opposite the point of departure of the renal vein left.

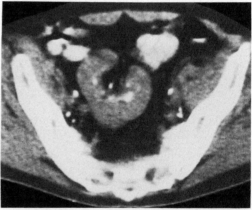

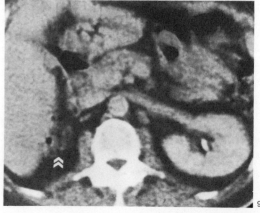

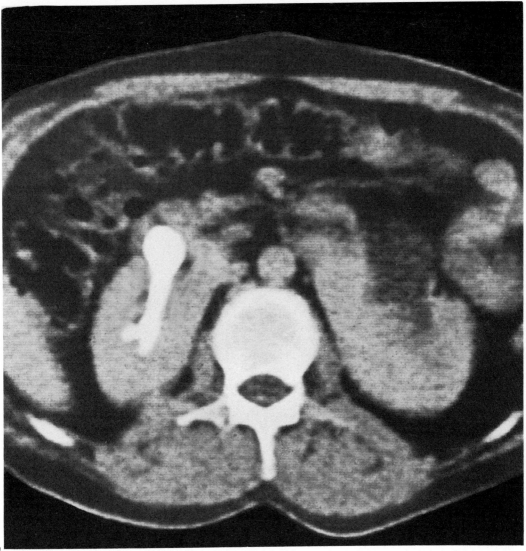

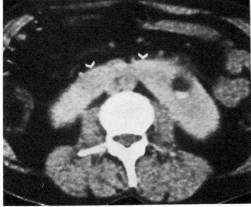

Fig. 81-9c: **Horseshoe kidney.** Renal sinus extending in a ventral direction. Also demonstration of congestion in the cavity system with substratification of contrast material on the left side. On deeper slices, demonstration of a parenchymal bridge (c_2) which has enhanced and therefore contains functional parenchyma.

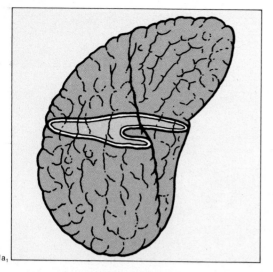

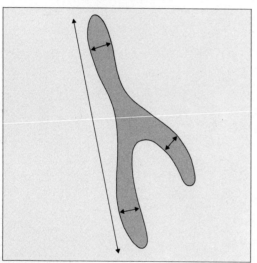

Width (of limb)	left (mm) ± SD	right (mm) ± SD
Karstaedt (585)	21.5 ± 4.6	22.8 ± 6.3
Montagne (589)	21.5 ± 3.2	22.1 ± 4.6
Heuck (583)	24.3 ± 7.9	26.8 ± 6.4

Thickness (of limb)	left (mm) ± SD	right (mm) ± SD
Karstaedt (585)	6.7 ± 1.7	5.1 ± 1.1
Montagne (589)	~ 10	< 10
Heuck (583)	5.7 ± 1.2	5.5 ± 1.0

Fig. 82-1a: **Normal adrenal.**
1a₁: Ventral view of the left adrenal.
1a₂: Measurement of the length and thickness of the limb in the transverse section.
1a₃: Dimensions of adrenal of normal size based on the data of various authors.

Right side:

triangular (3 %)

linear (9 %)

linear (36–87 %)

v-shaped (9–52 %)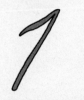

Left side:

v-shaped (50–60 %)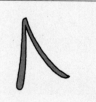

delta-shaped (32 %)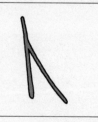

triangular (9–40 %)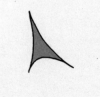

Adrenals (82-00)

Anatomy and imaging (82-10)

The adrenals weigh 12–16 g in an adult (4). They can almost always (95–100 %) be identified in the computed tomogram if a narrow slice technique is chosen. Their identification may be difficult only in cachectic patients with greatly reduced retroperitoneal fatty tissue or in cases in which artifacts overshadow the organs. The adrenals have a variable shape, the basic forms being linear, V, delta and triangular configurations (Fig. 82-1b). The complicated turned-in surface gives rise to varying sectional structures in different sectional planes of the same organ (Fig. 82-1c). The thickness and length of the limb of the organ can be increased in hyperplasia (Fig. 82-1a for normal values). The left adrenal extends deeper in front of the ipsilateral kidney, from which it is separated by a gap of about 0.5 cm (575). The adjacent splenic vessels can simulate an enlarged adrenal (administer contrast medium if necessary). The right adrenal is situated directly behind the inferior vena cava and is recognizable as a linear structure between the crura of the diaphragm and the hepatic capsule (Fig. 82-1c). The craniocaudal extension is 20–40 mm long (584, 585, 589).

Examination technique (82-20)

- **Spasmolytics** (scopolamine-N-butylbromide 15–45 mg i.v. or glucagon 1–3 mg i.v.) immediately before the examination in the case of 20-second scanners, as required in the case of shorter scan times.

- **Scanning** of adjacent, thin slices (i.e. 4 [to 8] mm). If only greater slice thicknesses are available, overlapping slices (table advance 5–8 mm).

- **Contrast medium** optional (guided bolus technique (4-32) or infusion (4-36)).

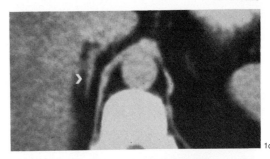
1c₁

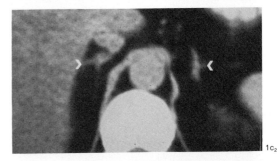
1c₂

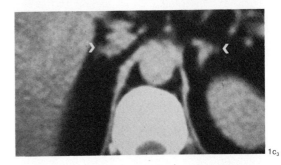
1c₃

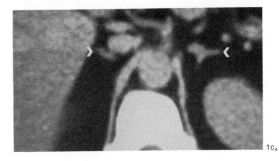
1c₄

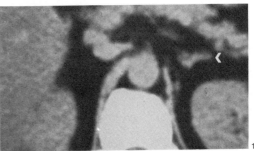
1c₅

Fig. 82-1c: **Normal adrenal.** Relationship of the shape of the adrenal to the level of the slice.

Fig. 82-1b: **Shapes of normal adrenals** in the transverse section after Montagne (589) and Karstaedt (585).

Hyperplasia and adrenocortical tumours (82-30)

Hyperplasia is usually the result of increased hormone production. All the different kinds of primary cortical tumours can be both active and inactive from an endocrine point of view. The histological section cannot reveal whether a neoplasm is hormone-producing or not, so that indirect signs, e.g. concomitant hypoplasia or atrophy of the rest of the adrenal tissue, must be used to clarify the situation. Differentiation between nodular hyperplasia and multiple adrenocortical adenomas is usually made on the basis of clinical aspects (suppression tests). With the exception of haematogenous metastases, the histological differentiation of malignant from benign adrenocortical tumours is frequently just as difficult.

Cushing's syndrome develops on the basis of an ACTH-producing pituitary tumour in 70–75% of cases, and results in diffuse or nodular hyperplasia. Other causes of the elevated glucocorticoid levels are adenomas in about 20% and carcinomas of the adrenals in 5–10% of cases. Primary hyperaldosteronism is based on an adenoma (classical Conn's syndrome) or on micro- to macronodular hyperplasia, while carcinomas are extremely rare. The reported relative incidence of adenoma to hyperplasia varies (1:1 – 4:1). This uncertainty is probably attributable to the fact that mild hyperaldosteronism in adrenocortical hyperplasia cannot be sharply demarcated from essential "hypertension" with low plasma renin levels.

The **adrenogenital syndrome (AGS)** is caused either by congenital or later developing hyperplasia (enzyme defects) or by cortical tumours. An AGS with its onset in childhood is usually caused by a tumour (carcinoma more frequently than adenoma). Adrenal feminization is usually due to a carcinoma of the adrenal cortex.

Adrenocortical hyperplasia (82-31)

Occurrence: Cushing's syndrome, AGS, primary hyperaldosteronism (less frequently in thyreotoxicosis, acromegaly, diabetes mellitus).

● CT

A general increase in the size of the adrenal can be detected only by measuring the horizontal and vertical dimensions. The length and width of the limb of the organ provide an indication (Fig. 82-1a). However, the overwhelming majority of cases of clinically con-

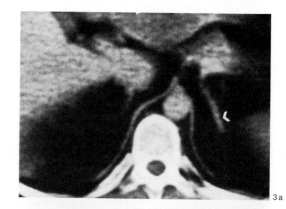

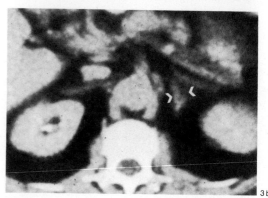

Fig. 82-3 a–c: **Adrenocortical hyperplasia.**
3 a: Hyperplasia of the adrenals with broad and long limbs.
3 b: Nodular hyperplasia in the Conn's syndrome.

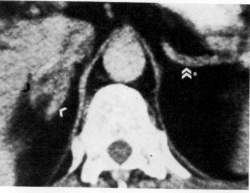

3 c: Nodular hyperplasia in Conn's syndrome. Histologically, the hyperplasia is of varying nodularity. The computed tomogram reveals broadening of the limbs. (Splenic artery ≫.)

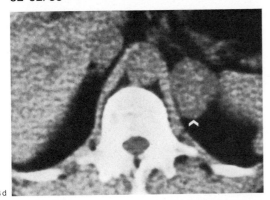

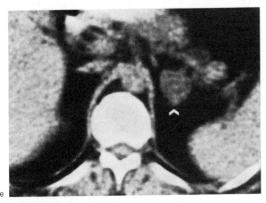

Fig. 82-3 d–f: **Adenomas.**

3 d: Conn's adenoma. Smoothly bordered mass (>) with density values in the muscle range (49 HU).

3 e: Spongiocytic adrenocortical adenoma. Silent in laboratory tests. Histologically, demonstration of spongiocytic cells. Density values generally reduced compared to muscle tissue (24 HU).

3 f: Cushing's adenoma. Distinct enhancement on administration of contrast material. The plain scan likewise reveals slightly reduced density values compared to muscle tissue (26 HU).

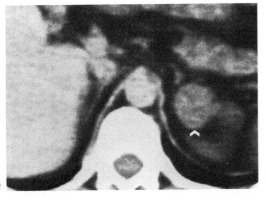

firmed bilateral adrenocortical hyperplasia does not display unequivocal signs of enlargement in the computed tomogram (586).

Because of the variability of the shape of the adrenals (Fig. 82-1b) only definite and bilateral enlargement should be interpreted as hyperplasia (Fig. 82-3a–c).

Adrenocortical adenomas (82-32)

Clinical picture in hyperfunction: Cushing's syndrome, Conn's syndrome, AGS.

Benign neoplasms of the adrenal cortex are usually discovered at a size of 2–5 cm, although they can assume considerable proportions. Necrosis and cystic degeneration can then be demonstrated frequently, calcifications less frequently. Adenomas are occasionally encountered bilaterally (1–2% of cases).

● **CT**

They can be clearly identified in the computed tomogram from a size of 10 mm under favourable imaging conditions (adequate periglandular fatty tissue, peripheral location) and from 15 mm in the majority of cases (Fig. 82-3 d–f).

Adrenocortical adenomas, especially in Conn's syndrome, are particularly rich in lipoids and consequently display reduced tissue density which is dependent on the lipid content. This ranges from the vascularized soft tissue (60 HU) to the negative density range (– 15 HU). Radiodensities in the range of water therefore necessitate the administration of contrast material to differentiate fatty tissue-containing tumours from cysts. Marked enhancement can be achieved in Cushing's adenoma (582) because vascularization is usually high. As angiographic practice shows, Conn's adenomas are usually hypovascularized.

Adrenocortical carcinomas (82-33)

Clinical picture in hyperfunction: Cushing's syndrome, AGS, frequently mixed pictures.

More highly differentiated, hormone-producing carcinomas predominate in childhood, while the absence of clinical symptoms in the case of older, hormone-inactive malignant tumours means that they are frequently not discovered until they have reached an inoperable stage. Extensive necrosis, haemorrhage and calcifications are encountered more frequently in carcinoma than in adenoma. The prognosis of adrenocortical carcinoma is unfavourable because of the massive and early spread.

CT

Computerized tomography cannot always distinguish between carcinoma and adenoma. Bulbous, polycyclic and poorly defined delineation is an initial sign of malignancy, while invasion of adjacent organs and the paraaortic space and regional metastases are unequivocal signs. Depending on the degree of differentiation, accumulation of lipids is also possible in a carcinoma, which means that the tissue density may be reduced. However, no definite correlation can be established between the lipid content and the density value (varying degrees of vascularization?) (591). In contrast to fat-containing tumours, hypodense regions corresponding to necrotic zones (Fig. 82-3g) do not enhance.

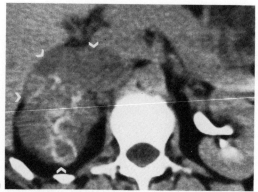

Fig. 82-3 g, h: Adrenocortical carcinomas.

3 g: Carcinoma (highly differentiated) with calcifications, distinct necrotic zones after contrast medium administration and displacement of upper abdominal organs (liver, vena cava). No demonstration of lymph node metastases.

3 h: Carcinoma with smooth borders and uncharacteristic density values. Encirclement of the renal vessels (≫) is the only striking feature.

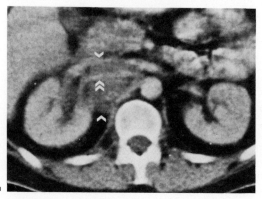

Adrenomedullary tumours (82-40)

Myelolipomas (82-41)

The myelolipoma, which is regarded as mesenchymal metaplasia, is a very rare, benign tumour and is usually found by chance at autopsy. Only when it achieves a substantial size does it cause clinical symptoms. Endocrine disturbances have been described (573). Haemorrhage and calcifications can infiltrate the predominantly lipid component.

CT

The computed tomogram shows a lipid mass surrounded by a smooth capsule. The tissue density of the fatty tissue component is the same as or slightly above that of the retroperitoneal space (−50 to −80 HU). The rare calcifications are usually shell-like. Marked haemorrhagic infiltration stands out well from the fatty tissue component and can be organized or calcify (577).

The renal angiomyolipoma (81-43), the retroperitoneal lipoma (86-71) and the liposarcoma (86-71) must be considered in the differential diagnosis.

Phaeochromocytoma (82-42)

This chromaffin tumour occurs intraadrenally in 90 % and extraadrenally in 10 % of cases and develops bilaterally in 10 %.

The main age at manifestation is the 5th decade of life. The phaeochromocytoma is usually highly vascularized and has an early tendency to necrosis or cystic degeneration even when the diameter is small. Fibrosing, haemorrhagic infiltration and peripheral, sometimes shell-like calcifications have likewise been described (6).

CT

The computed tomogram reveals a smooth-bordered lesion which usually enhances significantly (Fig. 82-4b). Necrotic zones within the tumour are clearly demarcated. Fine punctiform and coarser shell-like calcifications are visible in a third of the cases (30, 577). On average, phaeochromocytomas are considerably bigger than adrenal adenomas.

The clinical features (hypertensive crises), the age of the patient and the enhancement narrow the field down as regards the differential diagnosis, in which above all the adrenal adenoma must be considered.

Adrenals

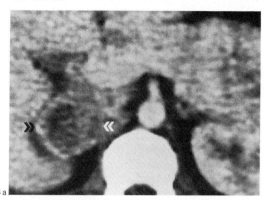

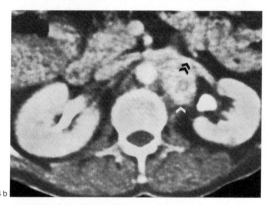

Fig. 82-4 a, b: **Phaeochromocytoma.**
4 a: Demonstration of a hypodense central zone (necrosis) following contrast medium administration. Only slight enhancement in the periphery of the tumour (atypical).
4 b: Recurrence of a phaeochromocytoma with distinct enhancement of the tumour and ventral displacement of the renal vein left (≫).

Fig. 82-4 c: **Bilateral metastases from a squamous-cell carcinoma** of the lung. The density values are distinctly reduced due to the necrosis.

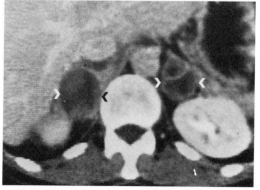

Phaeochromoblastoma (82-43)
The phaeochromoblastoma can be regarded as the malignant variant of the phaeochromocytoma. Metastases from this hormone-inactive tumour occur early. Its appearance in the computed tomogram is similar to that of the phaeochromocytoma – apart from the malignancy criteria (584).

Neuroblastoma (82-44)
Histologically, the neuroblastoma sympathicum differs only slightly from the sympathicoblastoma. It is one of the most important highly malignant tumours of infancy and is usually fatal. The tumours tend to necrosis, haemorrhagic infiltration, pseudocysts and, in more than half the cases, to distinct calcifications (30). Early lymphatic (regional, mediastinal) and haematogenous dissemination to the liver and bones is usual.

● **CT**
Calcifications and necrotic zones can be seen in the majority of computed tomograms. Other metastatic diseases of infancy are the main differential diagnostic consideration.

Metastases (82-45)
Metastases are a not infrequent cause of adrenal space-occupying lesions. They originate (in order of frequency) from tumours of the bronchial system (30–50 %), mammary glands and adjacent organs (stomach, pancreas, kidney) and from lymphomas and melanomas. The metastases are usually disseminated through the blood stream, and both sides are involved in more than 50 % of cases.

● **CT**
The striking feature in the computed tomogram is frequently the great extent (Fig. 82-4 e) of metastases, which makes it difficult to determine the organ of origin. Necrotic zones are usual, and the poor vascularity of the metastatic tissue means that only moderate enhancement can be expected. Bilateral involvement, the demonstration of other metastases and a knowledge of the primary tumour usually facilitate the diagnosis.

Adrenal cysts (82-50)
Cystic masses of the adrenals are very rare in comparison to those of the kidneys. They usually measure 3–4 cm, but can attain considerable proportions. Shell-like calcifications are demonstrable in 15 % of cases – considerably more frequently than in renal cysts –, the

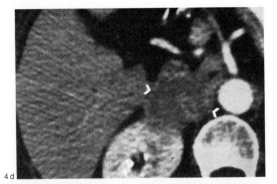

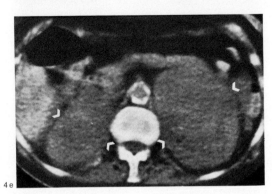

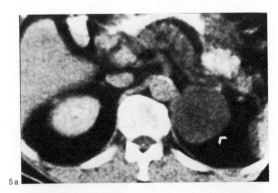

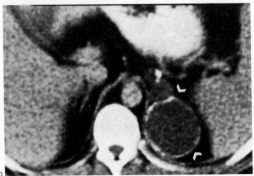

reason for this being that only few of them are of epithelial origin. The other adrenal cysts are subdivided into parasitic cysts (echinococciasis), endothelial cysts (lymphangiomatous, angiomatous), pseudocysts following haemorrhage caused by trauma and pseudocysts caused by necrosis or haemorrhage within a tumour.

● CT

The computed tomogram shows the usual signs of a cyst (Fig. 82-5a). Differentiation is not usually possible if the walls are thin. Thick walls are indicative of pseudocysts (Fig. 82-5b). Contrast material must then be administered to establish whether vascularized tumour tissue is present as in the phaeochromocytoma, which can calcify in a similar way (82-42). Concentric septation (71-33) and calcifications indicate parasitic origin.

Haemorrhage (82-60)

Birth trauma, coagulation defects, anticoagulant therapy, malignant hypertension, septic abortion and toxaemia are the main causes of adrenal haemorrhage. In the Waterhouse-Friderichsen syndrome – which occurs classically in meningococcal septicaemia but also with other gram-negative pathogens –, massive bilateral haemorrhage finally leads to complete destruction of the adrenals.

● CT

In their fresh stage, haemorrhages appear in the computed tomogram as hyperdense swellings of the adrenal. Demarcation of the contours of the gland from the surrounding fatty tissue may be blurred. In the later course, the attenuation values are of no assistance in the differential diagnosis from other adrenal masses, and resort must then be made to the case history and the tendency of the lesions to regress (Fig. 82-6a). Since adrenal haematomas can display attenuation values in the water range (3-52), the administration of contrast

Fig. 82-4d, e: **Adrenal metastases.**
4d: Metastasis from a hypernephroma with irregular enlargement of the adrenal and only slight peripheral enhancement (compare Fig. 86-7h, however).
4e: Bilateral metastasis with considerable enlargement of the smoothly bordered adrenals.

Fig. 82-5a, b: **Adrenal cysts.**
5a: Thin-walled cyst with density values of 15 HU.
5b: Calcified adrenal cyst with plaque-like mural calcifications.

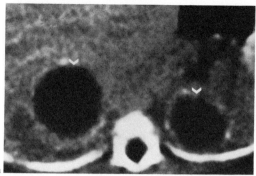

Fig. 82-6a: **Haemorrhagic cysts** following birth trauma. Demonstration of fine plaque-like mural calcifications (>). Spontaneous regression of the hypodense zones after 4 weeks.

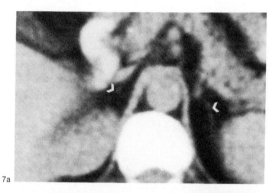

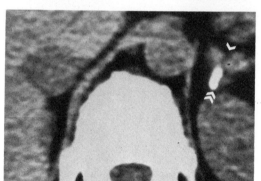

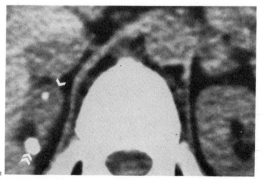

medium may become necessary to differentiate them from cystic or fat-containing masses.

Inflammation, atrophy (82-70)

Inflammation (82-71)

Exudative inflammation of the adrenals fails to occur because of the increased content of corticosteroid. Granulomatous inflammations run a protracted course and tend to produce focal necrosis. Initially, infantile toxoplasmosis, leprosy, histoplasmosis and coccidioid mycosis as well as tuberculosis lead to enlargement of the gland. In the course of the healing process, the gland is subject to fibrosis, partial calcification and, depending on the loss of parenchyma, to atrophy. Idiopathic atrophy is the most common, and is regarded as a sequel to lymphocytic adrenitis due to an autoimmune disease.

● CT

The adrenals are enlarged in the stage of florid inflammation and can be delineated accordingly in the computed tomogram (Fig. 82-7a). Calcifications are an indication of a past granulomatous inflammation. The reduction in the size of the glands can be demonstrated in the computed tomogram (584) (82-72).

Hypoplasia, atrophy (82-72)

Hypoplasias occur either congenitally or during childhood (idiopathic Addison's disease of childhood). Atrophy is usually the sequel of chronic inflammation (82-71) and haemorrhage (82-60), and the weight of the glands in the adult can fall to 1.2–2.5 g. Anterior pituitary insufficiency leads to secondary atrophy of the adrenals (Sheehan's syndrome).

● CT

Even small or shrunken adrenals can be demonstrated if a low slice thickness and reduced sector scan are chosen. However, there are no generally accepted data as regards the size which can be regarded as a definite indication of atrophy.

Fig. 82-7a: **Atrophy.** Only discrete, barely demonstrable adrenals in clearly visible adrenal beds. Status after autoimmune adrenalitis.

Fig. 82-7b: **Adrenal tuberculosis.** Demonstration of enlarged adrenals bilaterally with plaque-like calcifications (≫). The granulomatous inflammation has not yet led to atrophy of the organ.

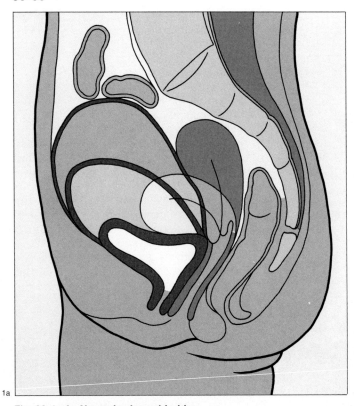

Fig. 83-**1a, b: Normal urinary bladder.**

1a: When the bladder is filled to absolute capacity, larger sections of the bladder wall become aligned almost axially and can then be depicted better in the computed tomogram. Similarly, the vesicouterine space and the circumference of the upright uterus can also be evaluated more accurately.

1b: Tangential projection with a well-filled bladder usually allows for evaluation of the wall of the bladder in the direction of the lumen as well (b_1). After intravenous administration, the contrast medium with its high specific gravity leads to the substratification phenomenon in the resting patient (b_2).

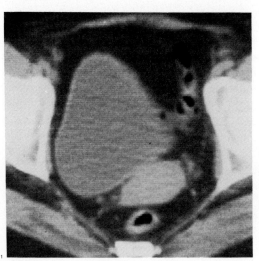

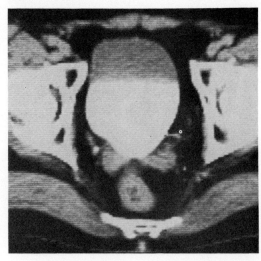

Urinary bladder (83-00)

Anatomy and imaging (83-10)
The configuration of the urinary bladder depends on its state of filling (Fig. 83-1a). After micturition, the roof of the bladder collapses and runs almost horizontally (transversally), so that only a small part of the bladder wall is seen tangentially in the computed tomogram. The imaging conditions for the bladder are considerably better when it is completely full, since the greatest part of the bladder wall runs more or less axially through the computerized tomographic slice. Small areas of the floor and roof of the bladder are then the only regions difficult to demonstrate due to partial volume effects. The wall is 1–3 mm thick when the bladder is completely full. Outwardly it is demarcated by perivesical fatty tissue. Assessment is rendered difficult by impression effects of intestinal loops, particularly when the bladder is not completely full. The inner contours of the bladder wall can be clearly demarcated following opacification of the lumen to 150–200 HU (4-21, 4-35).

Examination technique (83-20)
- **Retrograde opacification of the bladder lumen** (4-21)
- **Spasmolytics:** Scopolamine-N-butyl-bromide 30–45 mg i. v. or glucagon 1–2 mg i. v. immediately before the examination in the case of 20-second scanners, as required in the case of shorter scan times.
- **Scanning:** with slice thicknesses of 5–8 mm.

Scanning area: the entire bladder area (including the floor of the pelvis).

To demonstrate lymph node metastases: Slice intervals of 20–25 mm above the cavity of the bladder up to the pelvic inlet.

Changes of position (83-30)
Positional changes of the bladder are established by urography. They are caused by masses of the adjacent organs, e. g. by tumours of the female genitals (85-30/40), prostatic lesions (84-30), tumours and abnormal extension of the bowel – mainly of the sigmoid and rectum –, aneurysms of the pelvic vessels (86-71), primary and secondary tumours of the osseous pelvis (93-62), pelvic lipomatosis (86-42) and neurofibromatosis.

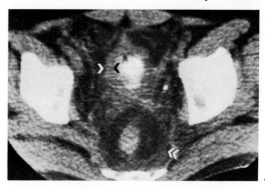

Fig. 83-**4a: Radiogenic contracted bladder.** Distinct thickening of the wall (><) in status after irradiation for carcinoma of the bladder. Also, demonstration of typical perifocal fibrosis (≫). Reduced bladder lumen.

Inflammations of the urinary bladder (83-40)
Inflammations can usually be unequivocally diagnosed on the basis of dysuric complaints and are **not an indication** for computerized tomography. They are caused usually by bacteria and less frequently by parasites, chemical substances and irradiation. The various acute forms (necrotic, haemorrhagic and purulent) can progress into a chronic (proliferative) stage and lead to a contracted bladder with thickening of the wall. Schistosomiasis causes polypous filling defects of the bladder lumen in addition to cicatricial changes. Thin-walled, water-filled cysts with a diameter of 1 to a maximum of 10 mm are usually found in cystic cystitis. Calcifications of the wall of the bladder can be demonstrated in ulcerative forms, particularly in schistosomiasis, tuberculosis and, but less frequently, following irradiation.

- **CT**

The thickness of the urinary bladder wall depends on the state of filling (Fig. 83-1a). Consequently, only retrograde cystography can provide a comparable standard. The wall is normally several millimeters thick when the bladder is full to capacity. Thicknesses in excess of 0.5 cm on capacity filling must be regarded as pathological. Frequently, fibrosis of adjacent tissues (e. g. perirectal fibrosis) is also observed following irradiation. Of interest as regards the differential diagnosis is schistosomiasis, which can assume a tumour-like appearance. Complete thickening of the bladder wall must be demarcated from hypertrophy (trabeculated bladder) resulting from obstruction.

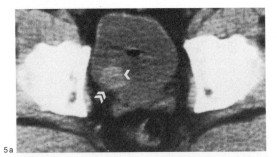

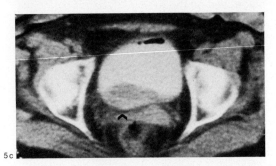

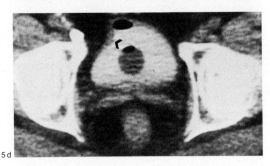

Tumours of the urinary bladder (83-50)

Papillomas, carcinomas (83-51)

Over 90 % of the tumours originate from the mucosa. Most of them – 80 % – are papillary urothelial carcinomas which occur mainly in advanced age groups and, overall, increase in frequency. The lateral wall of the bladder is affected in 40–50 % of cases, the trigonum vesicae and the neck in about 25 % and the roof of the bladder in 5–10 %. Initially, metastases occur via the lymphatic route and affect the parametric, iliac and paraaortic chains. The size of the tumour and its metastatic potential do not correlate. In addition to histological criteria of malignancy (grading G_0–G_3), staging is important for the surgical procedure.

TNM staging	
TiS	superficial carcinoma
T_1	tumour infiltration subepithelial
T_2	tumour infiltration of the inner muscle layer
T_3	tumour infiltration as far as the outer muscle layer
T_4	tumour infiltration of the perivesicular fatty tissue and adjacent organs
N	tumour metastases to regional lymph nodes
M	remote metastases

● CT

The tumour, which is usually confirmed by cystoscopy, is depicted as a filling defect in the bladder lumen and as a protrusion towards the perivesicular fatty tissue. Expansion beyond the wall of the bladder (T_4) is present when the external contours of the unaffected adjacent wall are surmounted. Asymmetry of the contours of the bladder, local retraction or a plateau phenomenon demonstrated on capacity (retrograde) filling of the lumen is an indication of deep tumour invasion of the muscles (T_2, T_3). The regional (iliac and presacral) lymph nodes must always be evaluated at the same time. Comparison of the contralateral chains and control of the course plays an im-

Fig. 83-5a: **Papilloma of the bladder.** Within the unenhanced bladder, demonstration of the tumour shadow. Smooth contours of the outer wall of the bladder (≫).

Fig. 83-5b–d: **Carcinoma of the bladder.**
5b: Smoothly bordered filling defects of 2 cm with smooth outer contours of the bladder (histology P_2).
5c: Broad filling defect of the dorsal wall of the bladder with smooth outer contours. Bladder surroundings normal (histology P_2).
5d: Contraction of the bladder wall with local thickening in status after transurethral tumour resection (histology P_3, but perivesical carcinomatous lymphangiosis).

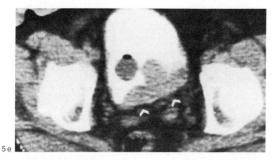

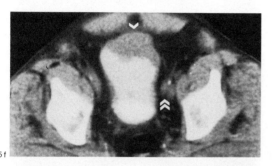

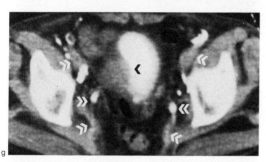

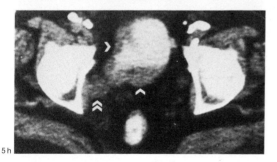

Fig. 83-5 e–h: **Carcinoma of the bladder.**

5 e: Polypous tumour of the bladder with smooth outer contours (histology P₃).

5 f: Broad tumour of the anterior wall of the bladder about 2.5 cm thick extending beyond the contours of the bladder (>). Possible lymph node enlargement left. External iliac (≫). Otherwise no demonstration of metastases.

5 g: Tumour extending beyond the wall of the bladder right. No demonstration of regional lymph node enlargement in ectatic vessels (≫). Ureters (≫).

5 h: Tumour extending beyond the wall of the bladder right with involvement of the lateral and dorsal wall and regional lymphoma of the obturator group right (≫).

portant role in the case of border-line findings (nodular structures of 1–2 cm). Staging presents no difficulty if invasion of the adjacent organs, osseous destruction or unequivocal lymph node enlargement (> 2 cm in diameter) is present.

Tumours of the adjacent organs (uterus, prostate), which can infiltrate the wall of the bladder, create differential-diagnostic difficulties. Determination of the primary tumour can be highly problematical or even impossible in individual cases. Since carcinomas of the bladder can also appear as flat lesions, diagnostic demarcation from inflammatory oedema (e.g. due to irritation by an indwelling catheter) becomes impossible in individual cases, making it essential to resort to the cystoscopic and histological findings. Impression effects and protrusions of the bladder wall require thorough analysis (84-10) and, perhaps, lateral positioning of the patient as well.

Mesenchymal tumours (83-52)

The rare mesenchymal tumours originate from muscle tissue. The benign **leiomyomas** and **rhabdomyomas** are smoothly demarcated, sometimes pedunculated masses and are of clinical relevance only when they cause symptoms of obstruction. Malignant variants, e.g. **leiomyosarcomas** and **rhabdomyosarcomas**, display rapid, bulbous, sometimes ulcerative growth and have, in general, a poor prognosis. These neoplasias, which usually occur in the fourth decade of life, have an infantile counterpart, the embryonal rhabdomyosarcoma, which is marked by particularly aggressive infiltration of the adjacent organs. Phaeochromocytomas and primary malignant lymphomas of the urinary bladder are rarities. Fibromas, neurofibromas, lipomas and haemangiomas are occasional chance findings.

● **CT**

Apart from the (extremely) rare lipoma, the nature of the tumour cannot be diagnosed by computerized tomography, the main role of which is to determine the size, extent and metastases of the tumour.

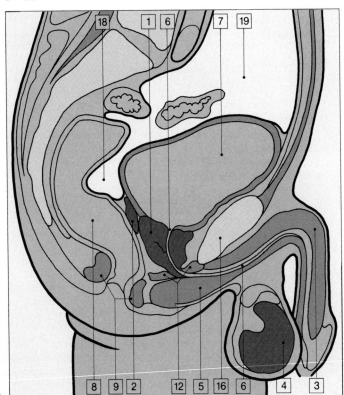

Fig. 84-**1a–c: Topography of the male pelvis.**

1a: Lateral view.

1b: Frontal section.
b_1 lies 3 cm in front of b_2.

1c: In the tranverse computed tomogram.

Key
1. Prostate
2. Seminal vesicle
3. Cavernous body of the penis
4. Testes
5. Cavernous body of the urethra
6. Urethra
7. Urinary bladder
8. Rectum
9. M. sphincter ani
10. M. obturatorius internus
11. M. levator ani
12. M. transv. perinei prof. (Diaphragma urogenitale)
13. M. ischiocavernosus
14. A. V. pudenda
15. Fossa ischiorectalis
16. Os pubis
17. Plexus prostaticus
18. Spatium rectovesicale
19. Abdominal cavity
20. Ductus deferens
21. Os coxae
22. A. V. obturatoria
23. A. dorsalis penis
24. Tuber ossis ischii

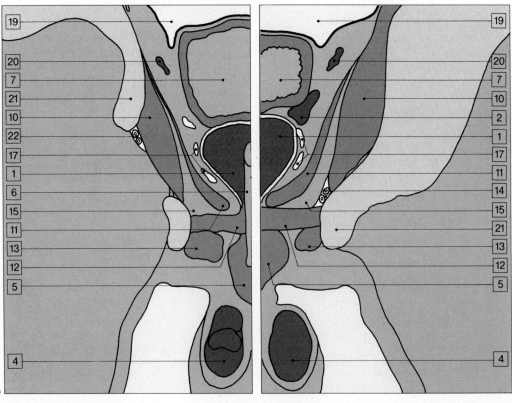

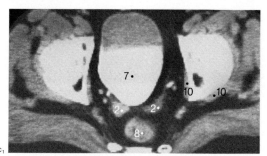
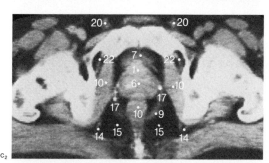
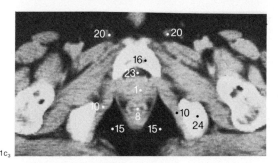
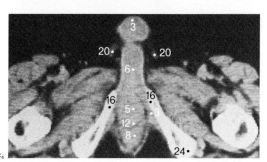
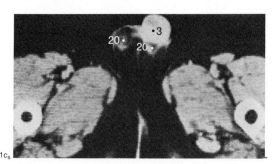

Prostate (84-00)

Anatomy and imaging (84-10)

The **prostate** appears infravesically as a smoothly bordered structure which is approximately transverse-oval in shape and has a soft-tissue density. Its lateral diameter is about 4 cm and can increase to 5 cm in advanced age (519). The boundary surface to the bladder runs almost horizontally or ascends dorsalward in a slight cranial direction. Optimal demonstration of the prostate in the computed tomogram is impossible because of partial volume effects: Slight irregularities of the bladder wall due to expansion of a prostatic tumour can escape CT demonstration. Lateral delimitation is frequently made difficult by the close contact with the fascia of the M. levator ani, whereas unequivocal bilateral demarcation from the internal obturator muscle is always possible. Peripheral calcifications lying against the capsule of the prostate correspond to phleboliths within the periprostatic venous plexus.

The **seminal vesicles** lie above the prostate and, with the patient in the supine position, can be demarcated from the wall of the bladder due to the interposition of fatty tissue. The angle of the seminal vesicles to each other changes when the patient is repositioned (561). The size of the vesicles is subject to considerable variation. The vas deferens cannot usually be clearly identified.

Examination technique (84-20)

● **Retrograde opacification** of the urinary bladder lumen (4-21), possibly (4-34).

● **Spasmolytics:** Scopolamine-N-butyl-bromide 30–45 mg i.v. or glucagon 1–2 mg i.v. directly before the examination in the case of 20-second scanners, as required in the case of shorter scan times.

● **Scanning:** with slice thicknesses of 5 – (max.) 8 mm.

Scanning area: The entire bed of the prostate (including the floor of the urinary bladder and pelvis).

Demonstration of lymph node metastases: Slice intervals of 20–25 mm above the bed of the prostate up to the pelvic brim.

Adenoma and carcinoma of the prostate (84-30)

Adenoma of the prostate is a benign neoplasm of the central sections of the prostate which can cause a bulbous impression in the floor of the bladder. It is the main cause of infravesicular obstruction to flow. Following enucleation, the compressed prostatic tissue remains conserved as a surgical capsule. **Carcinoma of the prostate,** which is the fourth most frequent malignant neoplasm of man, develops in the majority of cases from the peripheral regions of the prostatic parenchyma. It expands incessantly into the vicinity and invades the seminal vesicles at an early stage. Lymphography fails to demonstrate the first and second regional chains of lymph nodes, and in particular the presacral chain. **Sarcomas** are very rare and more likely to be encountered in infancy (embryonal rhabdomyosarcomas). The histology and aggressiveness of these tumours are the same as the bladder neoplasms of the same name.

● CT

Adenoma of the prostate appears in the computed tomogram as a smoothly bordered, infravesical mass. Not infrequently, polycyclic protrusions into the floor of the bladder can be seen.

Carcinoma of the prostate tends rather to protrude asymmetrically into the periprostatic space. Polycyclic demarcation of the external contours, leading eventually to obliteration of the contours at the internal obturator muscle, can occur. The seminal vesicles must be checked for symmetry, and any differences between the sides as regards demarcation and definition must be interpreted as infiltration. Symmetrical and normal-sized seminal vesicles do not rule out tumour infiltration (Fig. 84-3 b_2). The boundary surface to the urinary bladder can be adequately assessed and any infiltration of the bladder recognized only in the case of distinct cranial expansion. The pararectal and presacral soft tissue structures may be increased in healthy persons. Any asymmetry must be interpreted as suspect and, if the diameter of a soft tissue mass exceeds 2 cm, as lymph node metastases. However, no large-scale comparative case studies with surgical lymph node staging are yet available. The criteria described under 86-15 apply to the higher lymph node chains (internal and common iliac groups), the assessment of which should be included in the diagnosis.

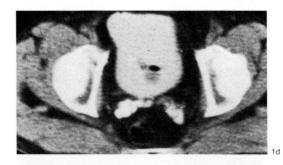
1d

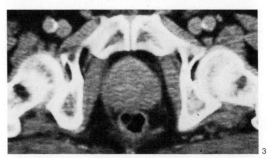
3a

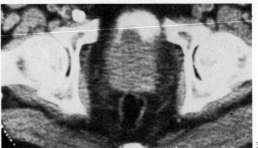
3b₁

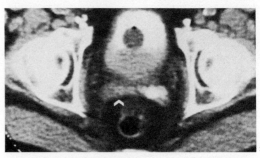
3b₂

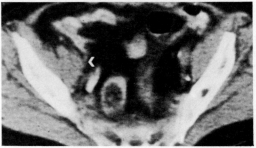
3c

Inflammations of the prostate (84-40)

Urethrovesical, haematogenous and lymphatic spread of infections lead to diffuse **catarrhal** inflammation of the prostate which, depending on the pathogen, can progress into a **phlegmon** or an **abscess**. In the chronic stage, connective-tissue transformation and the formation of scar tissue eventually lead to contraction of the prostate. Concomitant specific prostatitis develops in the course of genital tuberculosis. Calcifications of inflammatory, particularly tuberculous necroses (secondary prostatic concrements) are found especially in ulcerous-cavernous prostatitis, which can lead to fistula formation with the urethra, rectum and perineum. In the majority of cases, secondary prostatic stones can be demarcated from primary stones (prostatic secretion concrements) by their amorphous character, extent and configuration (50).

● **CT**

In the acute stage, computerized tomography reveals congruous enlargement of the prostate which does not displace the urethra. The density values do not permit differentiation from adenoma of the prostate. The surgical capsule does not contrast with the inflamed prostatic tissue as regards its density (564). Hypodense zones and localized protrusions are demonstrated in inflammatory liquefaction (Fig. 84–4a).

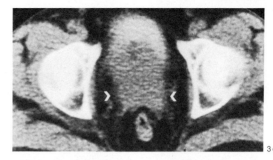

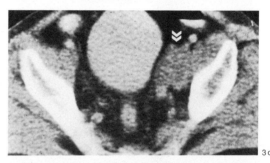

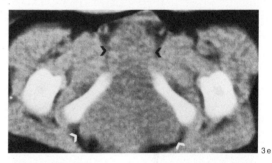

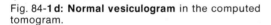

Fig. 84-1 d: **Normal vesiculogram** in the computed tomogram.

Fig. 84-3 a: **Prostatic adenoma.** Smooth borders and homogeneous radiodensity of the moderately enlarged prostate.

Fig. 84-3 b–e: **Malignant tumours of the prostate.**
3 b: Carcinoma of the prostate extending beyond the capsule. Enlarged prostate with irregular shape. Demonstration of infiltration of the right seminal vesicle which is not enlarged and does not enhance after vesiculography (b_2).

3 c: Lymph node metastases (>) with enlargement of the lymph nodes in the region of the internal iliac and obturator right.

3 d: Metastatic carcinoma of the prostate which is clearly enlarging and deforming the gland (>) with external iliac metastases (≫).

3 e: Rhabdomyosarcoma. Homogeneous soft-tissue mass invading the floor of the pelvis and displacing the pelvic organs in a cranial direction.

Fig. 84-4 a: **Prostatic abscess.** Demonstration of an enlarged prostate with hypodense areas extending to the seminal vesicle (a_2>). Deformation and enlargement of the seminal vesicles as well.

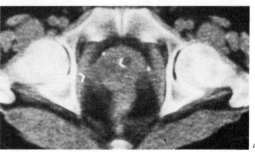

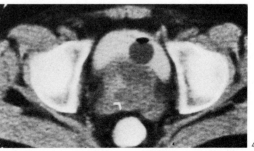

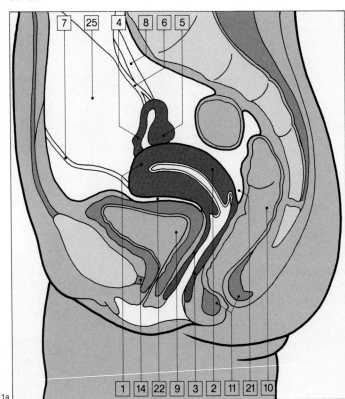

Fig. 85-1a–d: **Topography of the female pelvis.**
1a: Median section
1b: Frontal section
1c: Frontal section 5 cm behind 1b
1d: Transverse CT sections

Key
1 Corpus uteri
2 Cervix uteri
3 Vagina
4 Tuba uterina
5 Ovarium (mesosalpinx)
6 Lig. suspensorium ovarii
7 Lig. teres uteri
8 Ureter
9 Urinary bladder
10 Rectum
11 M. sphincter ani
12 M. obturatorius internus
13 M. levator ani
14 M. trans. perinei prof. (Diaphragma urogenitale)
15 M. ischiocavernosus
16 M. bulbocavernosus
17 A. V. pudenda
18 Fossa ischiorectalis
19 Os pubis
20 Plexus uterovaginalis
21 Excavatio rectouterina
22 Excavatio vesicouterina
23 Os coxae
24 A. V. obturatoria
25 Abdominal cavity
26 Lig. sacrouterinum

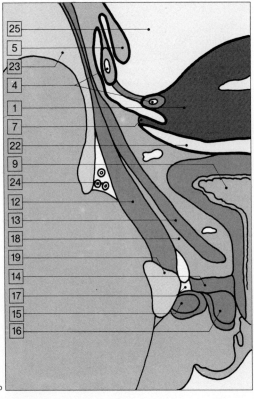

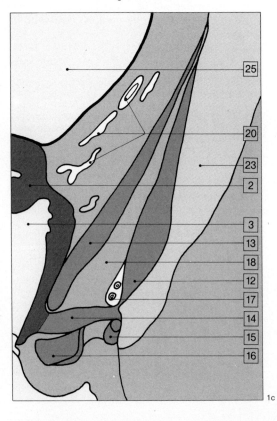

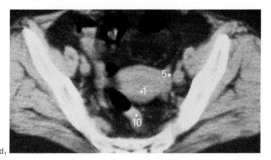
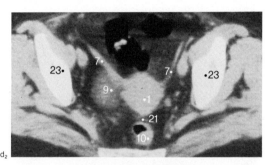
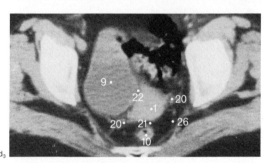
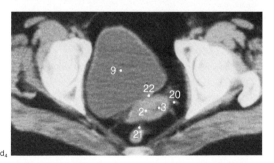
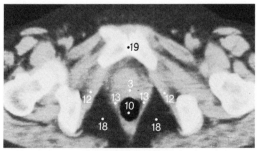

Female genital organs (85-00)

Anatomy and imaging (85-10)

Together with the urethra and rectum, the **vaginal canal** is bounded laterally by the crura of the M. levator ani. Due to poor interposition of fat, it is demarcated to varying degrees from these adjacent structures as a transverse-oval soft-tissue structure. The lumen can be marked by a tampon which contains air. The junction with the uterine cervix is ill-defined and, without marking, cannot be clearly identified in the computed tomogram. Demonstration of the **uterus** depends to a great extent on the state of filling of the urinary bladder (Fig. 83-1a). The uterine axis turns upright when the bladder is completely full, so that the circumference of the uterine body is met tangentially. When the bladder is empty, the uterine axis may run in the scanning plane. The boundary surfaces to the bladder (vesico-uterine space) and rectum can then no longer be assessed due to partial volume effects. For the same reasons, caution must be exercised when estimating the size of the uterus, since various sectional areas are demonstrated depending on its position. A sagittal image reconstruction[1] (secondary slice) can facilitate matters in critical cases. The muscles of the uterus are depicted as a homogeneous soft-tissue mass of about 50 HU.

Parts of the normal **adnexae** can be identified only in exceptional cases because of the intraperitoneal position with intestinal superimposition. The ligamentum latum cannot be identified because of its curved course, but the ligamentum teres uteri can be seen in individual cases (adipose patients). Similarly, the ovarian tubes cannot be recognized unequivocally. A normal-sized **ovary**, which lies against the pelvic wall below the iliopsoas muscle in the ovarian fossa, cannot be demonstrated. Its approximate position can be determined by means of infusion urography to opacify the ureter, which passes directly behind the ovary along the pelvic wall to the urinary bladder (512) (Fig. 85-1a).

---

[1] cf. CT terminology (97-00)

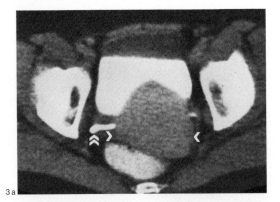

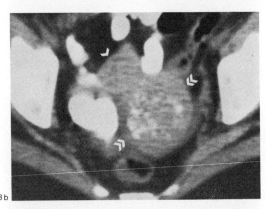

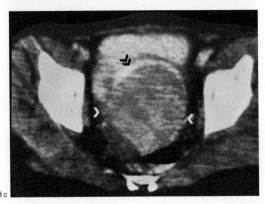

Opacification of the small and large bowel is an important condition for unequivocal demarcation of uterine and ovarian lesions. This can be dispensed with in cervical lesions only in the subperitoneal space, which is clearly structured by muscles and fatty tissue (ischiorectal fossa). Complete filling and adequate opacification of the lumen is important in suspected involvement of the urinary bladder (83-20).

Examination technique (85-20)
● **Reduction of intestinal gas** by means of a low residue diet, if possible from 48 hours before the examination (particularly with 20-second scanners).

●**Total bowel opacification**
Oral administration of about 1,000 ml of a dilute Gastrografin solution 40–60 minutes before the examination (4-23).

● **Marking of the vagina** by a tampon which contains air.

● **Spasmolytics** (scopolamine-N-butyl-bromide 30–45 mg i. v. or glucagon 1–2 mg i. v.) immediately before the examination in the case of 20-second scanners, as required in the case of shorter scan times.

● **Scanning**
At slice intervals of 8–10 mm in an adjacent slice sequence.
Scanning area: the entire area of the uterus from the pelvic floor to at least the level of the piriform muscle (departure of the internal iliac vessels).

To demonstrate lymph node metastases cranialward, slice intervals of 20 mm up to the level of the renal hila.

● **Intravenous contrast medium administration** (facultative)

Infusion (4-36) for opacification of the ureters (see below).

Guided bolus injection (4-32) for differentiation of the degree of vascularization in mass lesions.

Fig. 85-3 a–c: **Uterine myoma.**
3 a: Swelling of the cervix and uterine body displaying isodensity with the uterine muscles. Ureter (≫).
3 b: Swelling (≫) displaying isodensity with the uterine muscles (>) at the level of the uterine fundus with plaque-like calcifications.
3 c: Following contrast medium administration, inhomogeneous enhancement of a uterine mass with peripheral hyperdensity (≫) (hypervascularized myoma).

Fig. 85-3d: **Recognizability of tumour stages** (UICC) **of cervical carcinoma** in the computed tomogram. ∅ = unrecognizable, ○ = rarely or not clearly recognizable, ◐ = recognizable in some cases, ● = recognizable in the majority of cases.

Tumours of the uterus (85-30)

Myoma (uterine leiomyoma) (85-31)

Uterine myomas can be found in 20 % of women over 30 years of age, the location being subserous or intramural in 95 % of cases. The size of the tumours varies from a few millimeters to more than 20 cm. Pedunculate forms are found where the location is submucous and subserous. Myomas are seldom found in the broad ligament or in the cervix.

In 30 % of cases the myoma is subject to benign changes, e.g. myxomatous and fatty degeneration, necrosis, haemangiomatous transformation and oedematous saturation mainly of the central parts. Infection with abscessing or putrefaction of the regressive parts of the myoma is a clinically serious condition. Calcifications can be demonstrated only exceptionally in submucous myomas, but frequently in intramural and subserous forms. With increasing degeneration, the initially punctate and irregularly disseminated pattern gives way to larger, plaque-like calcifications which conglomerate and occasionally assume a peripheral shell-like configuration. The myomas may be hypervascular or hypovascular in comparison with the uterine tissue (42). Sarcomatous degeneration is rare, occurring in less than 0.5 % of cases.

● CT

Myomas deform and displace the uterus depending on their size. Bulbous protrusions of the same density as uterine tissue are indicative of a myoma only if calcifications are also demonstrated, since the latter rarely occur in solid malignant tumours. The absence of regional lymphadenopathy and symptoms supports the tentative diagnosis.

Regressive changes (myxomatous or necrotic transformation) or oedema lead to hypodense zones. Since this picture is equivocal, the differential diagnosis in the individual case can only be made with careful reference to the clinical data.

Rapid expansive growth suggests a uterine sarcoma (85-33), although it is also possible in the case of a myoma. Regional lymphadenopathy can be used as a criterion of malignancy, but not ascites, which also occurs (rarely) in myomas.

Cervical carcinoma (85-32)

The uterus is involved in 75 % of cases of genital cancer in the woman.

Initially, **cervical carcinoma** expands locally in the lateral wall of the cervix before invading the parametrial and paravaginal tissue. As long as the growth of the carcinoma remains restricted to the uterus, lymph node metastases in the minor pelvis can be expected in 8.5–26 % of cases (23). The hypogastric and obturator lymph nodes are affected first of all, followed later by the iliac and paraaortic lymph nodes. Not infrequently, the parauterine lymph nodes remain unaffected by regional metastases. Remote metastases, particularly in the liver, lung, brain and bones, are found only in the late, advanced stages.

UICC-category		Tumour growth		Recognizability in the computed tomogram
T_1		Restricted to the cervix	∅	
T_2	a	Infiltration of the upper two-thirds of the vagina	○	Uncertain even when a vaginal tampon is used
	b	Infiltration of the parametria	◐	Incipient infiltration uncertain
T_3	a	Expansion to the lower third of the vagina	◐	When a vaginal tampon is used
	b	Infiltration of the parametria up to the pelvic wall	●	
T_4		Expansion to the urinary bladder/rectum/beyond the pelvis	●	Incipient infiltration of the hollow organs not usually recognizable
N_1		Regional lymph node metastases	●	Cf. 86–15
N_2		Juxtaregional lymphomas (including paraaortic lymph nodes)	●	Cf. 86–15
M_1		Distant metastases	●	Within parenchymatous organs (cf. relevant section)

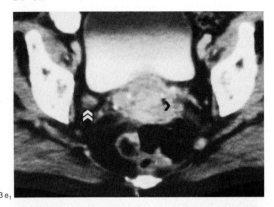

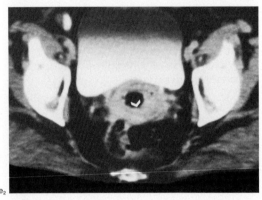

Fig. 85-3 e: **Cervical carcinoma Stage II b***. Demonstration of a thickened vaginal wall in the upper third (e_2 >), incipient infiltration of the parametria (e_1 >) and regional lymph node enlargement (≫). Invasion of the adjacent hollow organs is not yet clearly recognizable. ($T_{2b}N_1M_0$).

Fig. 85-3 f: **Uterine carcinoma Stage III***. Considerable enlargement of the fundus and body of the uterus. Like the uterine cavity, the tumour is recognizable as a hypodense, excentric zone (>). Invasion of the tube right (≫). Bowel, rectum (≫). ($T_3N_0M_0$).

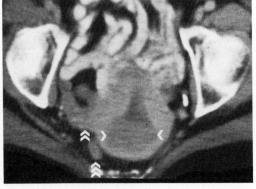

● **CT**

The tumour, which is usually confirmed gynaecologically, cannot be detected by computerized tomography until it has caused distinct dilation of the uterine cervix, which measures normally about 4 cm. Poorly defined and asymmetrical protrusions into the parametrial or paravaginal fatty tissue is an indication that the tumour has invaded the surrounding tissue. The advance of the tumour tissue towards the pelvic wall can be demonstrated by computerized tomography, making it possible to classify the tumour as Stage II b, III a or III b. Computerized tomography can also reveal enlargement of the internal iliac, obturator, presacral, external iliac and paraaortic lymph nodes, but cannot detect lymph nodes of normal size with micrometastases. The claim that computerized tomography is superior to lymphography (529) has not gone undisputed (627).

Uterine carcinoma (85-33)

Uterine carcinoma, which occurs 3 times less frequently than cervical carcinoma, remains restricted to the uterine cavity for a relatively long time before spreading to the cervix. Break-through into the free abdominal cavity is an occasional finding. Lymph node metastases do not usually occur until the outer third of the uterine wall is infiltrated. As in ovarian carcinoma, they can then be found in the paraaortic and lumbar groups and, occasionally, in the regional external iliac group. Tubal or ovarian carcinomas are simultaneously present in about 13% of cases. A complication of the condition is pyometra (infection of necrotic tumour tissue).

● **CT**

The tumour, which is usually confirmed gynaecologically, cannot be detected by computerized tomography until it is in an advanced stage, since it remains restricted to the uterus for a relatively long time and does not metastasize until later. Slight enlargement of the uterus cannot be reliably demonstrated (85-10). Diagnosis is aided by round deformation and distention of the uterus.

A central reduction of density corresponding to necrotic tumour tissue or congested secretion (blood) is not infrequent (85-51). However, invasion of neighbouring tissue (parametria, pararectal fatty tissue, bladder, rectum) can be adequately identified. Regional and paraaortic

*) FIGO

UICC-category	Tumour growth		Recognizability in the computed tomogram	
T_1 a b	Restricted to the uterus Uterine cavity < 8 cm in diameter Uterine cavity > 8 cm in diameter		○ ●	As an uncharacteristic mass from a diameter of 5 cm
T_2	Expansion to the cervix		○	
T_3	Expansion beyond the uterus to the vagina to parametria to the adnexae		○ ● ◐	Uncertain even when a vaginal tampon is used Incipient infiltration uncertain As a mass from a diameter of 3 cm
T_4	Expansion to the urinary bladder/rectum/beyond the pelvis		●	Incipient infiltration of the hollow organs not usually recognizable
N_1	Regional lymph node metastases		●	Cf. 86–15
M_1	Involvement of more distant organs		●	Within parenchymatous organs (cf. relevant section)

Fig. 85-3g: **Recognizability of tumour stages (UICC) of uterine carcinoma** in the computed tomogram. ∅ = unrecognizable, ○ = rarely or not clearly recognizable, ◐ = recognizable in some cases, ● = recognizable in the majority of cases.

lymph nodes are demonstrated more frequently by computerized tomography than by lymphography (529).

As regards the differential diagnosis, computerized tomography cannot distinguish between other malignant tumours of the uterus, e. g.:

1. **Chorioepithelioma,** which penetrates the uterine wall in an early stage, causes moderate enlargement of the organ and metastasizes early to the lung (case history: abortion, delivery, hydatidiform mole).

2. **Uterine sarcoma** (2 % of uterine malignant tumours) as a mucosal sarcoma which leads to considerable enlargement of the uterus and undergoes early necrotic adhesion, and uterine myosarcoma, which is indistinguishable from a myoma in the early stage. The tumour's tendency for rapid growth is an important clinical sign.

Uterine adenomyomatosis can have a similar appearance to that of uterine carcinoma. The central (hypodense) parts which can be observed are due to mucosal hyperplasia of the endometriosis. Enlargement of regional lymph nodes is unlikely because of the benign nature of the tumour.

Recurrence of malignant uterine tumours (85-34)

2–3 months after (total) hysterectomy, the computed tomogram usually reveals only a thin layer of connective tissue representing the stump of the vagina. The uterine bed, which is best assessed with a completely full urinary bladder, is largely filled with fatty tissue and, rarely, with compacted cicatricial cords. Recurrent tumours appear as roundish masses of soft-tissue density situated within the uterine space or against the wall of the pelvis. Optimal bowel opacification is essential for unequivocal identification. Depending on the extent of pelvic fatty tissue, recurrent tumours can be seen in the computed tomogram above a diameter of 2–4 cm. Post-operative scars and particularly extensive radiogenic fibrosis are difficult to differentiate from a recurrent tumour. Consequently, the reliability of the diagnosis can be considerably improved by basal findings after surgery or prior to radiation therapy. The presence of enlarged regional lymph nodes in addition to a mass of soft-tissue density must be regarded as a sign of malignancy.

The differential diagnosis must include haematoma and abscesses. These are hypodense in the majority of cases and resemble other accumulations of fluid in the retroperitoneal space (86-30) as regards their morphology and density.

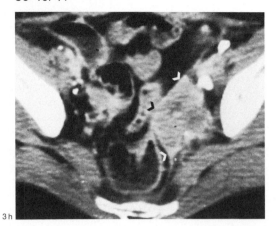

Ovarian tumours (85-40)

Cysts (85-41)
Retention cysts

Retention cysts are the most frequent cause of ovarian masses. **Follicular, lutein** and **corpus luteum cysts** are thin-walled and contain a serous secretion. They usually measure a few cms, rarely exceeding a diameter of 6–7 cm. **Chocolate cysts** can, however, be larger (up to 12 cm) and are usually present bilaterally. Their values correspond to those of components of coagulated blood which have failed to be absorbed following periodic bleeding of the ectopic endometrium (endometriosis). In general, enlargement of bilateral **polycystic ovaries** (Stein-Leventhal syndrome) due to cystic transformation is only moderate (up to a maximum of twice the normal diameter) and symmetrical. The very small retention cysts found in the ovaries rarely exceed a diameter of 0.5 cm.

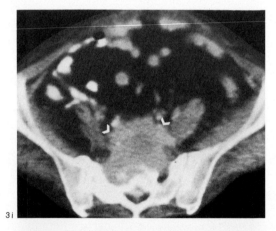

Neoplastic cysts

The **cystoma serosum simplex** is the most frequent neoplasm of the ovary, occurring in 20–25% of cases. Less frequent (5–12% of cases) is the **cystoma serosum glandulare ciliatum**, which displays a high rate of malignant degeneration of 20–30% of cases. Minute calcifications (psammoma bodies), which – depending on their extent – can accumulate to form a fine haze in the X-ray film and which are encountered in 12% of serous cystadenomas, are frequently found within the fine papillae in the wall of the cyst. Serous cystadenomas can assume considerable proportions, are unilocular or multilocular and present bilaterally in 20–50% of cases. The **cystoma pseudomucinosum glandulare**, which is usually multilocular and marked by glassy and gelatinous contents, occurs less frequently than serous cystadenomas, accounting for 10–18% of cases. It is rarely

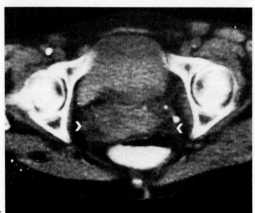

Fig. 85-3 h–k: Tumour recurrence.

3 h: Recurrence in the pelvic wall following total hysterectomy. Soft-tissue zone in the region of the internal iliac vessels, displaying inhomogeneous enhancement following administration of contrast medium.

3 i: Presacral recurrence following hysterectomy. Enhancement after contrast medium administration and demonstration of oseous destruction.

3 k: Recurrence of an ovarian carcinoma with regional, polycyclically delimited soft-tissue masses in the region of the uterine cervix.

found bilaterally (12%) and malignant degeneration is found in 5 (– 15)% of cases. **Pseudomyxoma peritonaei** is a serious complication which occurs in 7% of pseudomucinous cystomas. Calcifications are very rare and, where they do occur, are of the amorphous type (calcified mucin).

● **CT**

Small **retention cysts** can be detected from a diameter of 2–3 cm if they are looked for specifically and optimal enhancement of the bowel is present. The slice level selected must include the uterine fundus. The usual criteria of a cyst (with the exception of the chocolate cyst, see below) apply.

The size of the usually extensive **cystadenomas** can be determined in the computed tomogram. The walls are usually just recognizable, and often moderately thickened in mucinous cystadenoma. Calcifications and bilateral and unilocular development are important signs of a serous cystadenoma.

In vivo, the **density values** do not usually permit unequivocal differentiation between serous and mucinous contents, although the higher glycoproteid content of mucin would lead one to expect an increase of the density values (serous secretion 0–15 HU, mucin 10–20 HU). Because their density values lie within the soft tissue range, chocolate cysts are usually seen in the computed tomogram as solid masses.

Differential diagnosis: Mucinous and serous cystadenocarcinoma (85-43)

Parovarian and **paroophoric cysts** are remnant cysts originating from the Wolffian ducts. They display density values within the water range.

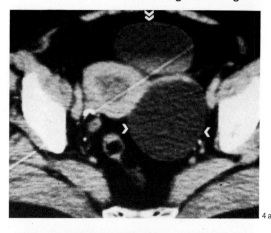

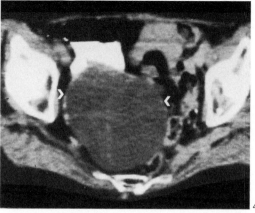

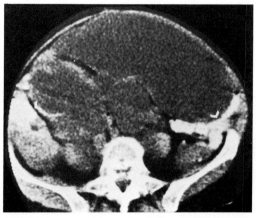

Fig. 85-4a–c: **Cystic masses of the ovary.**

4a: Simple cyst of the ovary. Smoothly bordered, thin-walled cyst lying dorsally against the tube (>). The uterine lumen is dilated and recognizable as a hypodense zone. Density of the cystic contents: 7 HU. Bladder (≫).

4b: Pseudomucinous cystoma. Smoothly bordered, thin-walled mass with multiple septa and density values of 23 HU.

4c: Peritoneal pseudomyxoma. Demonstration of extensive hypodense zones displacing and compressing the bowel (>). Density of the mucin: 32 HU.

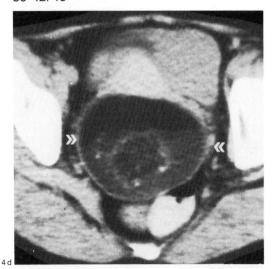

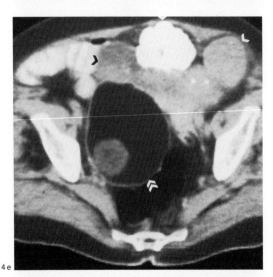

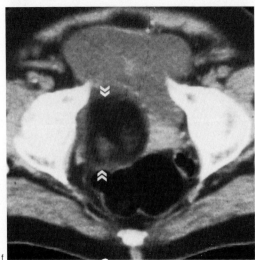

Dermoid cysts (85-42)

Dermoid cysts are not rare, accounting for 5–10 % of ovarian neoplasias. They are encountered bilaterally in 25 % of cases and usually have a diameter of between 12 and 15 cm. The contents consist of epidermal organ tissue of various kinds and varying differentiation. 36–70 % of the cases examined histologically exhibited lipoid- and sebum-containing matter which can increase the radiolucency of the cysts even on the general film. The dermoid cysts are calcified in 50 % of cases, either as shell-like or (in about 30 % of cases) as organoid formations (teeth, bones). No CT correlation has yet been found to the so-called capsule sign of the X-ray film, in which the wall of the cyst is marked inwards and outwards (in 10 % of cases according to Sloan[42]).

● CT

The demonstration of fat-containing matter by measuring the densities in the computed tomogram with values in the negative range is more reliable than on the general X-ray film. If eggshell calcifications of the wall of the cyst are also found, the diagnosis is virtually infallible. The demonstration of ectodermal relicts (bones, teeth) is likewise pathognomonic.

Malignant and hormone-producing tumours of the ovary (85-43)

Malignant tumours

55 % of all **ovarian carcinomas** arise primarily in ovarian tissue – 20 % as a result of malignant degeneration of cystadenomas and 25 % from metastases (Krukenberg tumours with primary location in the gastrointestinal tract in up to 75 % of cases). Overall, they account for 25–35 % of all genuine blastomas of the ovary, are frequently present bilaterally and sometimes extremely difficult to distinguish from benign ovarian tumours. They usually achieve a diameter of 5–7 cm, and are rarely more than 10 cm in diameter. The tumours are usually nodular, mainly of solid consistency, and permeated to varying degrees by cystic formations. Granular (psammoma bodies) or plaque-like calcifications are a not infrequent finding. Advanced stages are usually accom-

Fig. 85-4 d–f: **Dermoid cysts.** Demonstration of smoothly bordered tissue zones of varying density. Fatty tissue components (»), calcareous structures and other mixed tissues are typical.

panied by ascites resulting from peritoneal carcinosis. Lymphogenous metastasis takes place primarily via the ovarian lymph vessels, i.e. initially paraaortically and only secondarily into the pelvic lymph nodes.

Dysgerminoma (seminoma) is found primarily in young women in their twenties and thirties who not infrequently display signs of intersexuality.

The **malignant teratoma** is a solid tumour which consists of all three blastodermic layers and tends towards marked invasive growth into the surrounding tissue and to early metastasis.

Hormone-producing tumours

The most frequent hormone-producing tumour is the **granulosa cell** and **theca cell tumour**, with accounts for 10% of solid ovarian neoplasias, can attain a diameter of up to 15 cm and undergoes malignant degeneration in 25% of cases. The tumour can recur even after a protracted remission. Particularly when it has achieved a substantial diameter, the mainly solid, usually unilateral tumour displays cystic areas resulting from necrosis. The clinical picture is marked by elevated estrogen levels.

The rare **arrhenoblastoma** produces androgens and causes virilization mainly in 20–40-year old women. It usually occurs unilaterally, can contain cystic spaces and normally attains a diameter of only a few cms.

Gonadoblastomas are also rare. They likewise cause virilization and can be recognized radiologically in an early stage by their tendency to calcify (psammoma bodies). They are encountered bilaterally in 30% of cases and are generally benign.

Virilizing **hypernephroid tumours** tend towards necrosis and – like **struma ovarii**, which causes hyperthyroidism – are usually marked by malignant growth.

● CT

Unilateral or bilateral, solid or cystic-solid masses situated 2–3 cm from the tubal angle are signs of an ovarian tumour. On enlargement, the uterus is displaced from the median plane and is sometimes difficult to spot in the region of extensive masses. Paraaortic and regional lymphadenopathy are signs of malignancy. Ascites is found in advanced stages due to peritoneal carcinomatosis and can be recognized as such when – rarely – isolated solid elements of soft tissue density are observed on the smooth serosa-covered surfaces of the intraabdominal organs (529). The density values of ascites are of no assistance as regards the differential diagnosis (75-30).

Bilateral ovarian malignant tumours, most of which display cystic components, are found in more than 25% of cases.

The value of computerized tomography in the **differential diagnosis** is limited: Krukenberg tumours occur bilaterally in 80% of cases, are

Fig. 85–4g: Recognizability of tumour stages (UICC) **of ovarian malignant tumours** in the computed tomogram. ∅ = unrecognizable, ○ = rarely or not clearly recognizable, ◐ = recognizable in some cases, ● = recognizable in the majority of cases.

UICC-category		Tumour growth		Recognizability in the computed tomogram
T_1	a b c	Restricted to the ovaries Restricted to one ovary Restricted to both ovaries Accompanied by ascites	∅ ∅ ●	If at all, then as a mass more than 3–5 cm diameter
T_2	a b c	With expansion to the pelvis to the uterus and/or tubes other pelvic tissues accompanied by ascites	○ ◐ ●	Differentiation between T_1 and T_{2a} is usually impossible
T_3		With expansion to the small bowel and omentum	◐	Frequently recognizable as a conglomerate tumour, but not tumour invasion of the bowel
		Intraperitoneal metastases	○	Rarely within ascites
N_1		Regional lymph node metastases	●	Cf. 86–15
M_1		Distant metastases	●	Within parenchymatous organs (cf. relevant section)

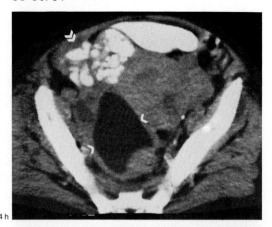

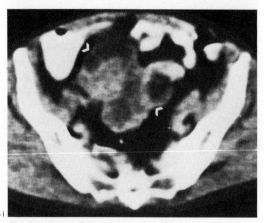

Fig. 85-4 h–k: Ovarian carcinoma.

4 h: Extensive cystadenocarcinomas with mainly solid component. Smoothly bordered zone of reduced density (cystic component >). The calcifications (≫) correspond to a uterine myoma. Demonstration of paraaortic lymph node enlargement on higher slices.

4 i: Demonstration of cystic and solid components (>). No indication of regional lymph node metastases. Computerized tomography was unable to demonstrate the invasion of the large bowel.

usually solid and frequently accompanied by ascites. Serous and mucinous cystadenocarcinomas are similar in appearance to their benign counterparts. However, their solid components are usually more pronounced. Without histological confirmation, a definitive diagnosis is impossible in the majority of cases in the absence of secondary signs of malignancy (metastatic lymph nodes). Marked calcification (psammomas) is an indication of malignancy (exception: gonadoblastoma).

Since the nature of hormone-producing tumours can usually be assumed, computerized tomography merely has the role of locating them.

Inflammations (85-50)

Inflammations of the uterus (85-51)

When the flow of secretion from endometritis or from the infected necrotic material of a uterine carcinoma is blocked, the pus accumulates in the uterine cavity. This results in pyometra, an acute condition which can cause considerable enlargement of the uterus.

● **CT**

Computerized tomography demonstrates not only the space occupation, but also a hypodense zone corresponding to the exudate-filled uterine cavity. Irregular and asymmetrical delineation of the zone of reduced density is indicative of a necrotic tumour.

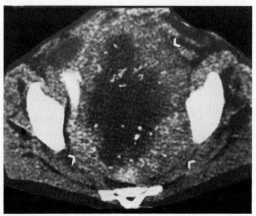

4 k: Serous cystadenocarcinoma. Massive lesion in the small pelvis with cystic and solid components. Demonstration of typical fine, disseminated granular calcifications. Demonstration of regional lymph node enlargement on higher slices.

Inflammations of the adnexa (85-52)

Ascending and haematogenous infections give rise to exudative thickening of the salpinx, which can close on progression of the disease and cause an intraluminal collection of pus **(pyosalpinx)**. Where surgery is not performed, successful medicinal therapy converts the pus to a serous liquid, usually with simultaneous thinning of the wall **(hydrosalpinx)**. The region of the focus of inflammation can adhere in the acute stage (perisalpingitis, perioophoritis) or the liquefactive process can be conducted **(tuboovarian abscess, Douglas's abscess)**. Inflammatory conglomerate tumours which also include sections of bowel are an expression of inflammatory involvement of a larger area of surrounding tissue (pelviperitonitis). Spontaneous rupture into the vaginal vault or the rectum is the natural way of abscess drainage.

● CT

Hydrosalpinx and pyosalpinx can only be seen in the computed tomogram from a size of 2–3 cm and when looked for specifically. In most cases they cannot be distinguished from other cystic masses of the ovary (85-41, 85-42). The density values lie within the range of those of water (0–15 HU) when the contents are serous, higher in pyosalpinx (15–40 HU). Inflammatory conglomerate tumours can assume the appearance of an ovarian tumour in the computed tomogram, so that adequate enhancement of the bowel and reference to the clinical finding are essential for the correct diagnosis.

Inflammations of the parametrium (85-53)

The pathogens gain entry via wounds and lacerations of the cervix and vagina following delivery or surgery. Inflammation of the parametria via bowel and bladder is rare. The exudation can spread in various directions: into the lateral parts of the parametrium **(lateral parametritis)**, into the dorsal parts **(posterior parametritis)**, into the fatty tissue around the neck of the bladder **(anterior parametritis)** and into the perirectal fatty tissue **(paraproctitis)**. After some time and following expansive growth the inflammation finally spreads to the psoas muscle (86-37) or the exudate ascends in the retroperitoneal space (opposite direction to the gravitation abscess) into the pararenal, perirenal and properitoneal spaces (cf. 86-14). The abscess can drain spontaneously following colliquation and encapsulation, i.e. erupt into the hollow organs (rectum, bladder, uterus) or rupture the abdominal or dorsal wall.

● CT

Computerized tomography usually differentiates well between the various subperitoneal spaces, making it possible to determine the extent of the exudation. Since it is difficult to distinguish between inflammatory and tumourous infiltration in the early stages, clinical parameters must also be used for the diagnosis. In extensive processes an inflammatory origin is highly probable if spread is shown to be restricted to various retroperitoneal spaces and the fascial boundaries are not perforated.

Fig. 85-5 a, b: **Inflammation of the adnexae.**
5a: Multiseptate hypodense zones corresponding to a tuboovarian abscess. Uterus (≫), urinary bladder (≫).
5b: Pyo-ovarium right. Smooth mass extending beyond the terminal line of the pelvis, with central hypodensity of 36 HU.

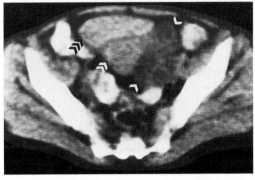

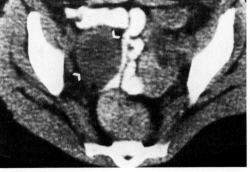

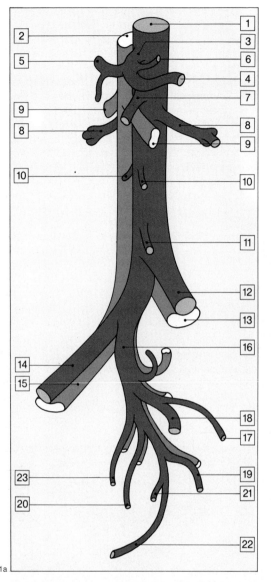
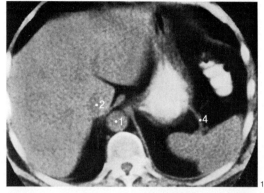
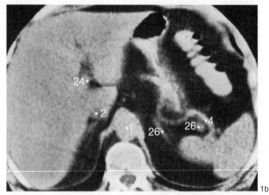
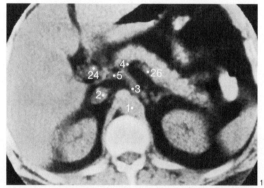
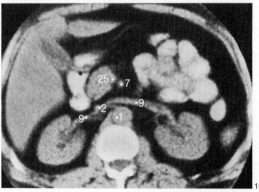

Fig. 86-1a, b: Retroperitoneal vessels.

1a: Location

1b: The vessels in the computed tomogram

Key

1. Aorta abdominalis
2. V. cava inferior
3. Truncus coeliacus
4. A. lienalis
5. A. hepatica communis
6. A. gastrica sinistra
7. A. mesenterica superior
8. A. renalis
9. V. renalis
10. A. testicularis
11. A. mesenterica inferior
12. A. iliaca communis
13. V. iliaca communis
14. A. iliaca externa
15. V. iliaca externa
16. A. iliaca interna
17. A. sacralis lateralis
18. A. glutaea superior
19. A. glutaea inferior
20. A. obturatoria
21. A. rectalis media
22. A. pudenda interna
23. A. vesicalis superior
24. V. portae
25. V. mesenterica superior
26. V. lienalis

Retroperitoneal cavity (86-00)

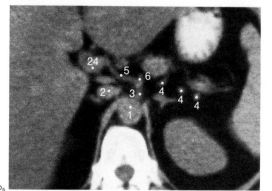

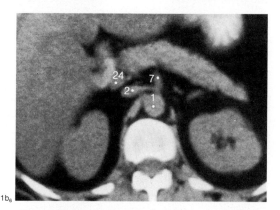

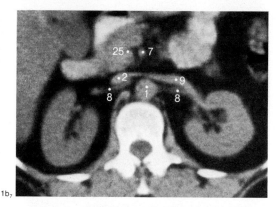

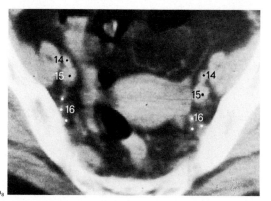

Anatomy and imaging (86-10)

Retroperitoneal vessels (86-11)

The **abdominal aorta** lies left paramedian directly in front of the lumbar vertebrae. Its diameter measures 2–3 cm depending on age and decreases caudalward. The axial course of the vessel offers optimal scanning conditions with sharp demarcation. The **inferior vena cava** runs on the right next to the aorta. Its lumen usually displays a transverse oval shape but is variable depending on the intraabdominal pressure, becoming slit-shaped on inspiration and round on expiration and in Valsalva's manoeuvre. The abdominal aorta branches at the level of the 4th lumbar vertebra. The left common iliac vein crosses under the right common iliac artery and then lies dorsally against the left pelvic artery. In fact, all **pelvic veins** lie dorsal to their arterial namesakes. The departure of the internal iliac vessels at the level of the terminal line is seldom directly recognizable. The vessels can, however, be localized as a convolution on the piriform muscle (Fig. 86–1b).

The **coeliac trunk**, which arises at the level of the phrenic aortic hiatus ventral to the abdominal aorta and at a varying angle to the body axis, is visible together with its branches – depending on their course – in the computed tomogram. As long as its alignment is virtually horizontal, the left gastric artery can frequently be traced in one CT slice up to the dorsal wall of the stomach. The **common hepatic artery** can often be demarcated up to the point of departure of the gastroduodenal artery – before it branches off cranialward together with the portal vein into the hepatoduodenal ligament, when it can only be intersected obliquely. The **splenic artery** is marked by its greatly tortuous course. Consequently, only certain stretches of it can be identified. It runs along the upper (and ventral) boundary of the pancreas and branches out in the splenic hilum like a fan. The **splenic vein** is enveloped by pancreatic tissue or lies dorsally against the pancreas. The splenic vein can be identified in the plain scan to a degree dependent on the

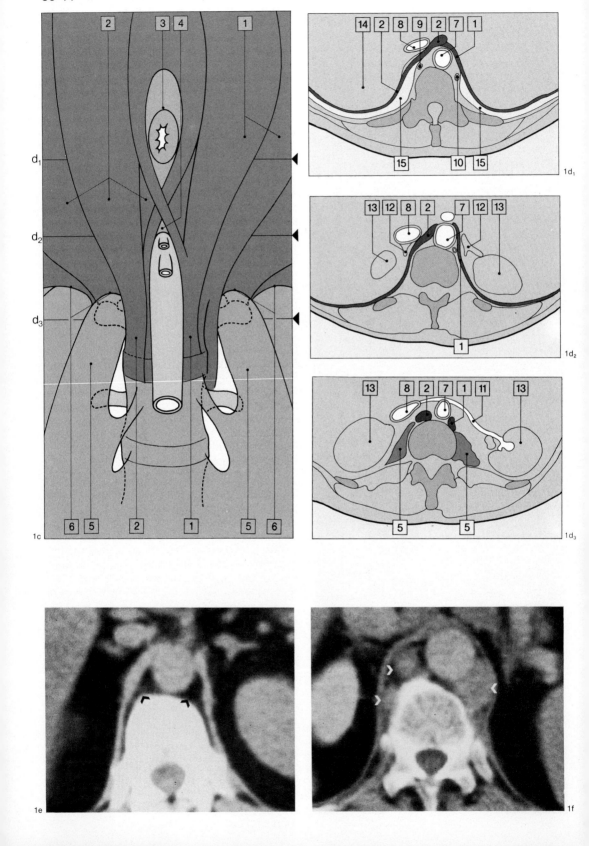

amount of retroperitoneal and intrapancreatic fat (Fig. 73-7a, b). Because it is always enveloped in fat, the **superior mesenteric artery** is usually recognizable even in cachectic patients, while the **superior mesenteric vein** is less distinct. If the amount of fatty tissue is insufficient for demarcation, all the vessels so far mentioned can be unequivocally identified by a **guided bolus injection**. On the other hand, the inferior mesenteric artery cannot always be demonstrated even after the administration of contrast medium (721).

The **renal arteries** can be clearly identified in the plain scan. The **renal veins** run in front of them. The left renal vein crosses over the abdominal aorta at the level of the pars inferior duodeni. The main renal vessels and anomalies (717) can be depicted in their entirety in just a few adjacent slices. The **lumbar vessels**, which depart latero-dorsally from the inferior vena cava and the abdominal aorta, can occasionally be identified following administration of contrast medium (721). The longitudinal structures of the **azygos and hemiazygos veins** are recognizable at the level of the phrenic angle depending on their calibre.

The retrocrural space (86-12)
The retrocrural space (Fig. 86–1d) lies between the phrenic angles and the ventral circumference of the 11th and 12th thoracic vertebra. It represents the lowest recess of the mediastinum. After passing through the aortic hiatus, the abdominal aorta is accompanied on the right by the **azygos vein** and on the left by the **hemiazygos vein**. These veins run directly prevertebrally and display a varying calibre which, in the majority of cases, is below

---

Fig. 86-1c, d: **Anatomy of the diaphragm** (lumbar section).

1c: Location
1d: The diaphragm in the transverse section (cf. 1c for level of section)
Key
1 Crus sinistrum
2 Crus dextrum (medium, intermedium, laterale)
3 Hiatus oesophageus
4 Hiatus aorticus
5 M. psoas
6 Ligamentum arcuatum
7 Aorta
8 V. cava inferior
9 V. azygos
10 V. hemiazygos
11 V. renalis
12 Adrenal
13 Kidney
14 Liver
15 Lung

Fig. 86-1e: **Normal retrocrural space** in the computed tomogram.

Fig. 86-1f: **Retrocrural lymphomas** (>).

the limit of resolution of the scanners. Unless collateral circulation via the azygos vein system can be demonstrated, lymphadenopathy must be assumed above a diameter of 6 mm. The question of whether longitudinal vascular structures are present can be answered by analysing the adjacent slices or by means of guided administration of contrast medium. The **thoracic duct**, which runs on the right dorsal to the aorta and displays a diameter of about 2 mm, is sometimes demonstrable following lymphography, but not usually in the plain scan.

The diaphragm (86-13)
The diaphragm is attached in the lumbar region to the anterior surface of the 1st to 4th lumbar vertebrae and to the transverse processes of the 1st lumbar vertebral body. The left medial column is not so pronounced as the contralateral one, which reaches more deeply – down to the level of the 3rd and 4th lumbar vertebrae. The aorta passes through the diaphragm between the medial columns. These muscular structures can usually be clearly identified by virtue of their course (Fig. 86-1c, d). On cursory analysis of the image, however, they can also be misinterpreted as lymph nodes.

Fascial spaces of the retroperitoneum (86-14)
The subperitoneal fascia (situated laterally between the transverse fascia and the peritoneal cavity) divides into an anterior and a posterior leaf **(anterior and posterior renal fasciae)** (Fig. 86-1g). The posterior leaf inserts into the fascia of the psoas muscle, the anterior into the prevertebral, perivascular connective tissue, thus encircling the **perirenal space**. The peritoneum, which extends over the colon and pancreas and envelops the abdominal organs, creates another, **anterior pararenal space** (Fig. 86-1g). The **posterior pararenal space** lies behind the posterior renal fascia and continues without interruption into the properitoneal fatty tissue. The lateral section (Fig. 86-1h) clearly shows that the perirenal space tapers caudalward like a cone, while the posterior pararenal space increases in width. Although the fascial cone, which is attached to the diaphragm, is not tightly closed caudally, the two fascial membranes quickly fuse on inflammatory irritation. The anterior and posterior (and properitoneal) spaces are connected to each other at about the level of the

86-14

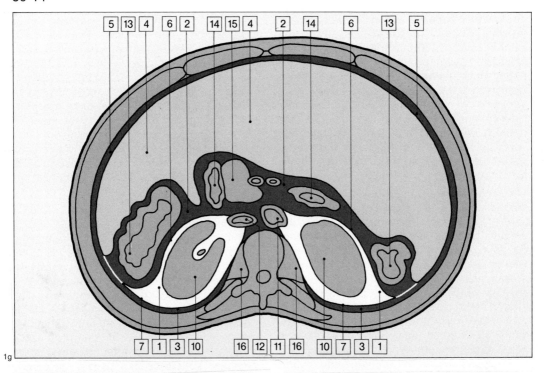
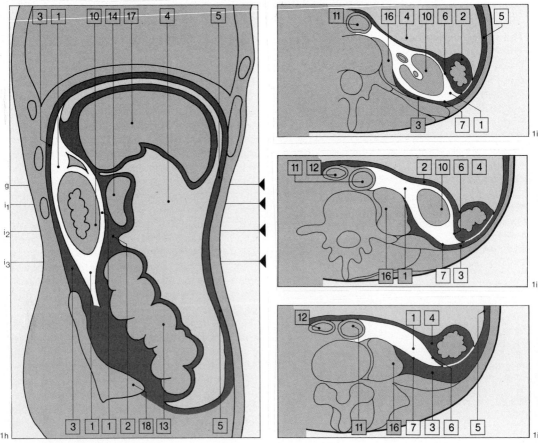

iliac crest (Fig. 86–1h). Communication between the right and left perirenal spaces has occasionally been described (623). The possibility of a connection between the retrocrural and the posterior pararenal space has been discussed (597).

In normal cases, the individual fasciae are no thicker than 1 mm and can then only be depicted by computerized tomography when they run vertically through the CT slice. As Fig. 86–1h demonstrates, however, this applies only to short sections of the curved and oblique renal fasciae. Adequate fatty tissue in the individual retroperitoneal spaces is a further pre-requisite for demonstration of the fasciae (Fig. 86-1k). For the reasons just mentioned, the complicated course of the peritoneal surface cannot usually be depicted. When thickened by exudative and haemorrhagic processes (e.g. in irradiation, infection etc.), the fasciae themselves as well as the spaces which they surround are usually clearly identifiable.

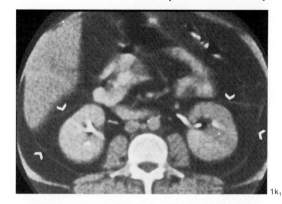

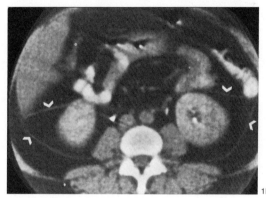

Fig. 86-1k: **Fasciae of the retroperitoneum.** The fascial membranes (><) are often easy to follow in obese patients.

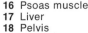

Fig. 86-1g–i: **Fascial spaces of the retroperitoneum.**

1 g, i: Transverse sections (cf. 1h for level of the sections).

1 h: Right paravertebral longitudinal section.

Key
- 1 Perirenal space
- 2 Anterior pararenal space
- 3 Posterior pararenal space
- 4 Abdominal cavity
- 5 Properitoneal fatty tissue
- 6 Anterior renal fascia
- 7 Posterior renal fascia
- 8 Subperitoneal fascia
- 9 Peritoneum
- 10 Kidney
- 11 Aorta
- 12 Inferior vena cava
- 13 Colon
- 14 Duodenum
- 15 Pancreas
- 16 Psoas muscle
- 17 Liver
- 18 Pelvis

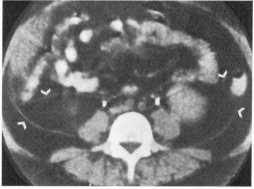

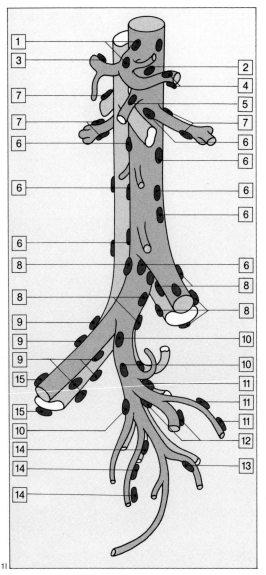
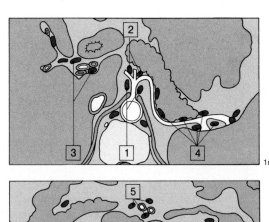
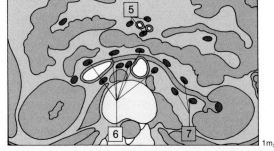
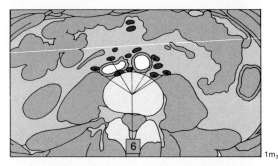
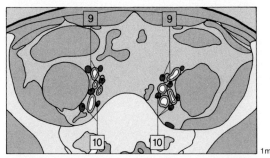
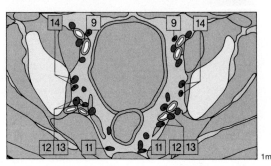

Fig. 86-1 l, m: Topography of the retroperitoneal lymph nodes.

1 l: Location

1 m: In the transverse section

Key
1. Lnn. coeliaci
2. Lnn. gastrici sinistri
3. Lnn. hepatici
4. Lnn. pancreatico-lienales
5. Lnn. mesenterici superiores
6. Lnn. lumbales (peri-aortal, pericaval, subaortal)
7. Lnn. renales
8. Lnn. iliaci communes
9. Lnn. iliaci externi
10. Lnn. iliaci interni
11. Lnn. sacrales laterales
12. Lnn. glutaei superiores
13. Lnn. glutaei inferiores
14. Lnn. obturatorii
15. Lnn. inguinales

Lymph nodes (86-15)
Lymph nodes, which have a cross-section of about 0.5–1 cm, lie at the lower limit of computerized tomographic resolution, which is determined to a decisive extent by the amount of surrounding fatty tissue. Diseases of the lymph nodes can therefore only be detected by computerized tomography when the nodes are enlarged. The **paraaortic lymph nodes** are arranged around the abdominal aorta and the inferior vena cava. The abdominal aorta, which runs axially through the slice, and the inferior vena cava are sharply depicted with their boundary surfaces (see above). Under these favourable scanning conditions, a thin layer of fat is sufficient for demarcation of any enlargement of the paraaortic lymph nodes. However, the anterior edge of the vertebral bodies and the ventrally adjacent structures of the (retro-) peritoneal space can lie against sections of the vascular wall in such a way as to prevent its demarcation. The lateral vascular walls are, on the other hand, usually clearly recognizable. The vascular wall becomes masked, i. e. the fatty tissue is obliterated, on enlargement of the perivascular lymph nodes. The ventral contours of the psoas become increasingly obliterated depending on the degree of lymph node enlargement, giving rise finally to a homogeneous and large prevertebral soft-tissue mass. A paraaortic lymph node can usually be demonstrated by computerized tomography from a diameter of 1 cm, but almost always from a diameter of 2 cm. The **mesenteric lymph nodes**, which are arranged along the mesenteric vessels, can be demonstrated to varying degrees if adequate fat is interposed. Lymph nodes must usually be larger than 3 cm in diameter in this region to be reliably identified, and optimal bowel opacification is essential. Similarly unfavourable scanning conditions also occur in the pelvis. Although the pelvic vessels are recognizable on the psoas muscle, they run obliquely through the CT slice and their demarcation is frequently blurred. The branching tree of the **internal iliac structures** above the piriform muscle normally appears as a nodular structure. Consequently, comparison of the sides assumes particular importance in the search for lymphadenopathy in poorly demonstrable regions (aortic bifurcation, internal iliac structures). Enlarged lymph nodes in the region of organ stems are reliably and sensitively identifiable only in the **region of the renal hilum**. Frequently, only larger lymph node masses with a diameter of more than 2–3 cm can be diagnosed in the region of the **porta hepatis** with its complicated structure and the **splenic hilum**.

In comparison to computerized tomography, **lymphography** can demonstrate both lymph node enlargements and structural changes of normal-sized lymph nodes. The demonstration of infiltrated, non-enlarged lymph nodes, which are present in about 10 % of cases (681, 686, 695) and which escape computerized tomographic detection, therefore remains an indication for lymphography. This method cannot, however, supply any information about unopacified lymph node groups, in particular lymph nodes of the splenic or hepatic hilum and high paraaortic, retrocrural, mesenteric and hypogastric groups. Larger conglomerates of lymph nodes are generally more accessible to computerized tomography (674). Lymphography appears to be dispensable if the histology is confirmed and the CT finding is positive.

Examination technique (86-20)

● **Reduction of intestinal gas** by means of a low residue diet 48 hours before the examination, particularly with 20-second scanners.

● **Intestinal opacification** (4-23): partial or total bowel opacification depending on the anticipated finding. Total bowel opacification in investigations of the entire retroperitoneal space. Particularly important in the region of the lower retroperitoneal space (pelvis).

● **Spasmolytics:** scopolamine-N-butyl-bromide 30–45 mg i.v. or glucagon 1–2 mg i.v. immediately before the examination in the case of 20-second scanners, as required in the case of shorter scanning times.

● **Scanning** with slice thicknesses of 8–10 mm. Adjacent slice sequence in localized processes. Slice intervals of 20 mm, if necessary with intermediate slices, in extensive processes (including systemic diseases).

Scanning area: dependent on the clinical findings and the problem.

● **Intravenous contrast medium administration** (facultative): infusion (4-36) with 250 ml Urovison i.v. (in extensive processes). Guided bolus injection (4-32) in localized processes for further differentiation.

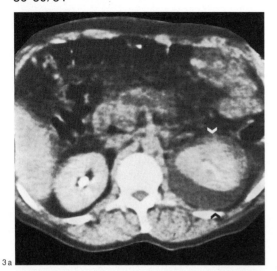

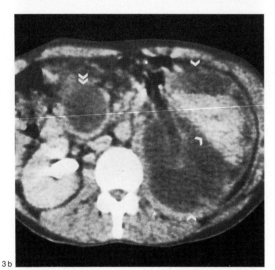

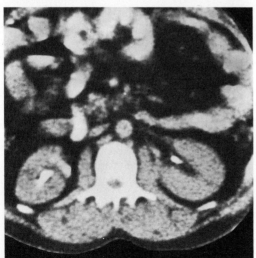

Perirenal and pararenal lesions (86-30)

Exudative haemorrhagic lesions of the perirenal space (86-31)

Most frequently, perirenal abscesses are encountered as a consequence of an inflammatory process of the kidney, e. g. in pyelonephritis, carbuncle or tuberculosis. The perirenal space becomes saturated with the exudate and the fatty tissue finally dissolves. The incorporation of gas formed by bacteria (E. coli, Aerobacter and clostridia), which may already be recognizable in the general film of the abdomen, can also be demonstrated by computerized tomography. Less frequent is the spread of an inflammation from a more distant site. For example, a pseudocyst of the pancreas can discharge into the perirenal space. Not infrequently, fatty tissue necroses and parafascial saturation with fermenting exudate are demonstrable in acute haemorrhagic-necrotic pancreatitis (73-51). Extensive purulent events, which eventually penetrate the fascial space, lead to liquefaction of adjacent organs (psoas muscle, colon).

● CT

The principle sign is the diffuse increase of density of the entire perirenal fatty tissue. The perirenal space dilates depending on the amount of exudate. The renal fasciae, which are normally barely visible, are thickened and usually well demarcated. The entire circumference of the perirenal space is generally involved.

The **radiodensity** depends on the protein content of the exudate and on the age of the process (3-53). Density values of 0–30 HU are usually demonstrable.

Either complete restitution of the fatty tissue (Fig. 86–3c) or organization of the exudate (86-34) can take place following therapy (surgery).

Fig. 86-3 a–c: **Perirenal pseudocyst of the pancreas.** Density increase of the perirenal fatty tissue to 3 HU (a). 18 weeks later considerable enlargement of the perirenal space with ventral displacement of the kidney (>). Also, demonstration of a pseudocyst in the head of the pancreas (b ≫). Following drainage, complete regression of the exudate and regeneration of the fatty tissue (c).

Urinomas (perirenal pseudocysts) (86-32)

Following injury to the urinary tract (traumatic or iatrogenic), urine collects in the perirenal fatty tissue and the renal fascia then forms the wall of the pseudocyst. This can, however, only happen if three situations coincide:

1. In the presence of a functioning kidney.
2. In the presence of a (distal) obstruction of flow.
3. In the presence of sterile urine.

The time interval between trauma and the occurrence of symptoms can range from just a few weeks to years. The clinical symptoms of an abscess develop if the extravasate becomes infected.

● CT

The obstruction of flow – usually with a lack of contrast medium excretion – can be demonstrated directly by the dilation of the renal cavity system. The diagnosis of a perirenal pseudocyst is almost certain if an accumulation of fluid is found within the perirenal space in the presence of a kidney which is usually of normal size and if the case history reveals trauma (accident, gynaecological surgery etc.) (Fig. 86-3d). The level of the ureteral blockage is usually determined by retrograde probing. It is noteworthy that the posterior pararenal space is flattened by the perirenal mass, which is usually considerable. Extravasation of urine can be recognized in the acute stage by the emergence of contrast medium and the increase of density of the fluid collection (518, 614). Abscess of the urinoma can only be assumed initially from the clinical symptoms. Computerized tomography raises the suspicion of an infection if other retroperitoneal spaces, e. g. the psoas space (Fig. 86-3f), are opened. Density values which signal a higher protein content (approx. 30 HU) are a further indication of a purulent process.

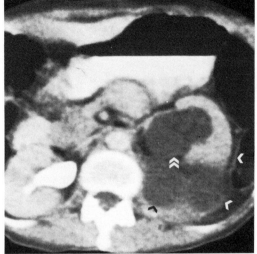

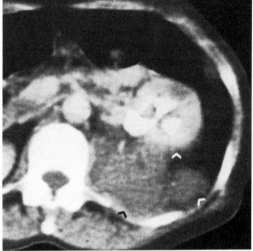

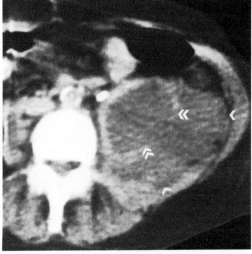

Fig. 86-3 d–f: Urinomas.

3d: 5 months after gynaecological surgery, silent kidney left with dilation of the cavity system (≫). Demonstration of a perirenal mass with density values of 12 HU (extravasation of urine). Ureteral occlusion in the middle third.

3 e,f: Rupture of the ureter near the renal pelvis. Moderate congestion of the cavity system. Extravasation of urine into the perirenal space with ventral displacement of the kidney (>). Opening of the bed of the psoas muscle (≫) as a sign of superinfection. Density value of the liquid mass: 26 HU.

Perirenal haematoma (86-33)
(Pathogenesis cf. 81-61)

● **CT**

The haematoma usually fills the entire perirenal space, although local haematomas are also possible (Fig. 86-3g, i).

The radiodensity is dependent on the age and the configuration of the haematoma (compact accumulation of blood, suggilation). Fresh, compact haematomas can remain hyperdense in comparison to unenhanced muscle or renal tissue for a few days. As avascular lesions they do not change their density after enhancement and usually appear hypodense in comparison to the enhanced renal parenchyma.

Solid perirenal lesions (86-34)

It is exceptional for the perirenal space to be the site of origin of a local neoplasm. Neighbouring processes such as malignant growth of the kidney, haematomas with connective-tissue organization or abscesses are the main causes of solid perirenal lesions.

Hypernephromas obliterate the perirenal fatty tissue and expand up to the renal fascia, which they finally penetrate. If connective-tissue organization of the entire circumference of the perirenal space has taken place, the cause of a solid perirenal mass is probably a **haematoma** or **exudate**, since accumulations of fluid completely saturate the compartment. Because the fatty tissue has a high potential for regeneration, however, extensive perirenal fibrosis is rare. Frequently, the only indications of a past perinephritis are thickening and stretching of the renal fascia. Calcifications are found both in organized haematomas and abscesses and in most renal neoplasms.

● **CT**

A solid mass in the perirenal space must be differentiated primarily from expanding renal tumours. This does not represent a problem as long as the site of origin and the destruction in the renal parenchyma are visible. In doubtful cases the vascularity of the mass should be checked by a guided contrast medium injection (Fig. 86-3l), since masses with connective-tissue organization are very poorly vascularized in comparison to the solid parts of a renal carcinoma. The renal fascia does not restrain malignant growth, but tends to form a barrier for accumulations of fluid, which become organized in the absence of absorption (Fig. 86-3k). The adipose capsule of the kidney remains conserved in localized processes and

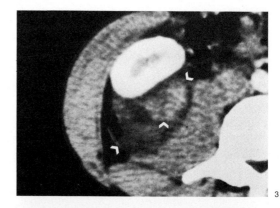

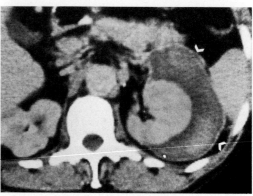

Fig. 86-3g–i: Perirenal haematoma.

3g, h: Dorsal to the right kidney, demonstration of an increase of density with hyperdense areas (g ><). Extensive haematoma with complete filling of the perirenal space (renal fascia >). Inhomogeneous density of 35/55 HU (h).

3i: Organized perirenal haematoma. Demonstration of a mass of soft-tissue density (>) ventral to the right lower renal pole. The perirenal fatty tissue is conserved. Thickened and intact Gerota's fascia (≫).

Fig. 86-3k: **Perirenal fibrosis.** Demonstration of a mass of soft-tissue density with ventral displacement of the left kidney, which is delimited by the Gerota's fascia (>).

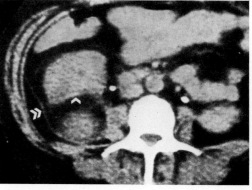

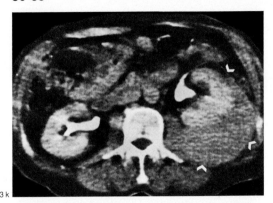

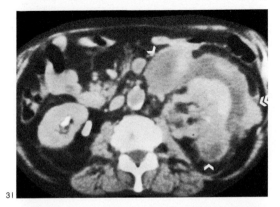

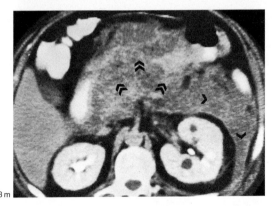

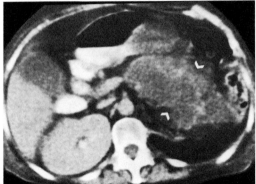

merely becomes displaced (encapsulated perirenal haematoma Fig. 86–3i). Thickening of the renal fascia is the expression of an inflammatory or absorptive reaction. It is nonspecific and should be considered in the differential diagnosis only in association with other signs.

Lesions in the anterior pararenal space
(86-35)

In 60% of cases, exudative-haemorrhagic processes in the anterior pararenal space are the result of extraperitoneal perforations of the gastrointestinal tract following inflammation and tumour disease. Disease of the pancreas (20% of cases) and kidneys are comparatively rare. Damage to the large vessels following blunt abdominal trauma, rupture of an aneurysm and iatrogenic vascular puncture can lead to extensive retroperitoneal haematomas. The admixture of gas following perforation can be caused both by emerging intestinal gas and by bacteria.

● CT

Exudations and haemorrhages can remain local or saturate the entire retroperitoneal space (618). In circumscribed fluid accumulations, differentiation between a haematoma and an abscess is only possible when high densities as in fresh haematomas (3-52) or gas bubbles are demonstrated due to an infection. If blood or exudate infiltrates fatty tissue, mixed CT values are recorded and it is impossible to make a definitive diagnosis. The case history, clinical symptoms and any follow-up studies (83) must be used for the differentiation of abscesses from haematomas.

Fig. 86-3 l: **Hypernephroma** with penetration of the Gerota's fascia as a sign of infiltration (≫).

Fig. 86-3 m, n: **Pararenal lesions.**

3 m: Extensive exudative zones in acute pancreatitis. Typical expansion into the paracolic space (>) and the root of mesentery (≫).

3 n: Pararenal abscess formation consequent on perforation of a diverticulum with expansion to the tail of the pancreas. No demonstration of gas bubbles within the septate mass, the density of which is 24 HU.

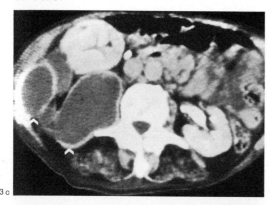

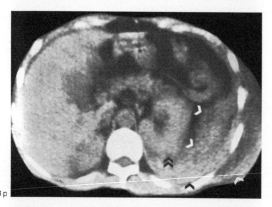

Lesions in the posterior pararenal space (86-36)

Fluid collections in the posterior pararenal space are usually caused by haemorrhages (traumatic or spontaneous in coagulopathies). Inflammatory processes spread secondarily to this compartment. They take place usually as part of a complication following surgery and less frequently as a consequence of spondylitis. The exudations of acute pancreatitis enter the posterior pararenal space after moving round the lower pole of the fascial cone of the kidney (32). Less frequently, in aggressive forms, the exudates penetrate the lateroconal fascia. Lymphatic extravasation or a lymphocele must be considered in cystic masses.

● **CT**

A pararenal mass causes ventral displacement of the perirenal space. The properitoneal fatty tissue becomes involved in the process, i. e. the radiodensity also increases in that region. The CT image provides only limited differential-diagnostic aspects (86-35). However, the anterior renal space (pancreatitis), which is simultaneously depicted, together with the perirenal space and the patient's clinical history and symptoms usually provide clear indications of the etiology of the lesion.

Iliopsoas muscle (86-37)

The iliopsoas muscle is rarely the site of origin of a pathological process (e.g. rhabdomyosarcoma, haematogenous abscess). Exudative haemorrhagic lesions of the retroperitoneal space and spinal column usually have fascial barriers to overcome before they reach the psoas muscle. If a process does penetrate the fascia of the muscle, it can spread within the muscle space as far as the groin. The incidence of tuberculosis is now very much lower than that of pyogenic abscesses of the kidney, pancreas, spinal column and bowel.

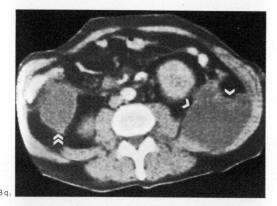

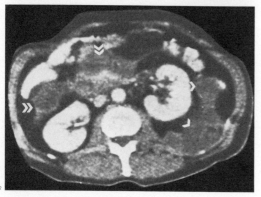

Fig. 86-3 o: **Abscesses** in the region of the perirenal and posterior pararenal space including the psoas muscle. The cystoid zones of reduced density (19 HU) display distinct marginal enhancement.

Fig. 86-3 p: **Haemorrhage** into the posterior pararenal space following perforation of the inferior vena cava. Displacement of the kidney in a ventral direction (≫). Density of the haemorrhage: 61 HU.

Fig. 86-3 q: **Exudative, non-purulent pancreatitis.** Demonstration of exudate zones (13 HU) in the posterior pararenal space (>) and anterior pararenal space (≫).

CT

The computed tomogram contains the typical signs of muscle abscesses (92-40), the clinical classification of which is usually simple in association with other retroperitoneal processes (Fig. 86-3r,s). Haematomas of the psoas muscle occasionally occur under anticoagulant therapy; the clinical symptoms are disorders of neurological function. CT signs cf. 92-50.

Neoplastic infiltration is caused by malignant growths of the retroperitoneal space and spinal column (86-50, 86-60, 81-41). Unless it is accompanied by a clear muscular defect, however, obliteration of the muscle contours does not automatically signify infiltration. Administration of contrast medium improves the differentiation of neoplasms from the muscle tissue.

Lesions in the subperitoneal space (86-38)

As in the other retroperitoneal spaces (86-31 to 86-37), exudative haemorrhagic lesions develop in the subperitoneal space along the fascial boundaries, which are created mainly by the holding apparatus of the uterus. Further details cf. 85-50.

Retroperitoneal fibrosis (86-40)

The estimated incidence of retroperitoneal fibrosis in the normal population is 1 : 200,000. The mortality rate is 10–20% (52). There are two distinct forms – one idiopathic, the other secondary. The secondary form is induced by adjacent inflammatory foci, drugs (methysergide), trauma, aneurysms, radiation injury or carcinoma. Overall, men are affected more frequently than women (ratio 3 : 1).

Inadequate fibrinolysis in response to inflammatory stimulation resulting in connective-tissue organization of the unabsorbed exudate (fibrin) is held pathogenetically responsible for **idiopathic retroperitoneal fibrosis (IRF)**.

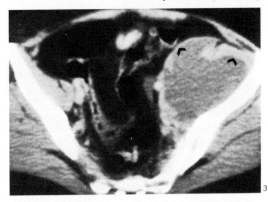

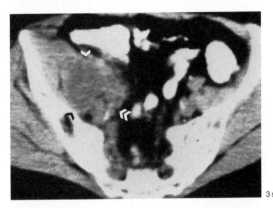

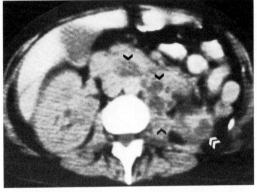

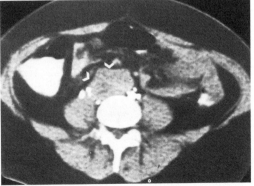

Fig. 86-3r: **Liquefied haematoma of the iliopsoas muscle.** 11 months after hysterectomy, demonstration of a hypodense (17 HU), smoothly bordered mass with flattening of the surrounding iliopsoas muscle (>).
Fig. 86-3s: **Abscess of the iliopsoas muscle.** Demonstration of a moderately hypodense zone with swelling of the iliopsoas muscle and enlargement of adjacent lymph nodes (≫).
Fig. 86-3t: **Psoas abscesses** (>) in extensive renal abscesses (≫).
Fig. 86-4a: **Idiopathic retroperitoneal fibrosis.** Mass of soft-tissue density at the level of the 4th and 5th lumbar vertebrae encircling and masking the aorta and inferior vena cava.

Vasculitis of the vasa vasorum, which spreads to the surrounding fatty tissue and which would explain the perivascular development of the fibrosis as well as local vascular stenosis, has been suggested as regards the etiology. A constant finding in IRF is a sclerotic connective-tissue layer ranging in thickness from a few millimeters to 2 (max 6) centimeters and which extends most frequently from the 4th lumbar vertebra to the first sacral vertebra. The fibrotic plate expands laterally and asymmetrically and envelops the inferior vena cava, the ureters and the lymphatic vessels as well as the aorta. The longitudinal extension is also variable, ranging in length from cords the thickness of a finger to more than 20 cm and possibly affecting all levels of the retroperitoneal space. Reports have been published of (amorphous) calcifications within the fibrotic zones (52).

● **CT**

The tentative diagnosis of retroperitoneal fibrosis is usually made by means of urography. Urinary stasis resulting from segmental ureteral stenosis and ventrolateral displacement of the ureters are the guiding roentgenological signs. In most cases, the critical region can therefore be demonstrated specifically by computerized tomography. The sharply demarcated soft-tissue zone around the large vessels leads to obliteration of their contours (Fig. 86-4a). An aneurysm-like effect can develop, albeit without its relatively typical circular calcification. Since the geometrical scanning conditions at the aortic bifurcation are already unfavourable, demarcation from lymph nodes can be difficult. The differential diagnosis can be narrowed down by the circumscribed finding and the absence of retroperitoneal lymph nodes together with the urographic signs. Of further assistance in doubtful cases is a rapid injection of contrast medium, which can lead to distinct enhancement of the tissue zone ($\sim$ 50 HU [604]), something which cannot be achieved in lymphadenopathy or within aneurysm thrombi. Marked concomitant stenosis of large vessels can also be demonstrated by computerized tomography if the bolus technique is used.

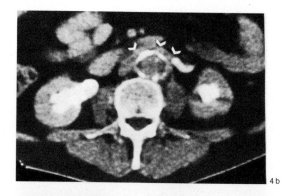

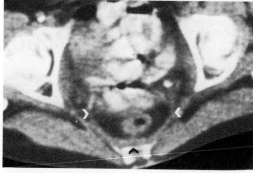

Fig. 86-4c: **Secondary retroperitoneal fibrosis.** In post-radiation status, demonstration of distinct thickening of perirectal fasciae (c_1>). Fibrosis in status following abdomino-perirenal proctectomy (c_2>) with presacral soft-tissue zones and displacement of the ureters (c_2≫) in a medial direction.

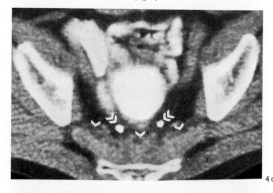

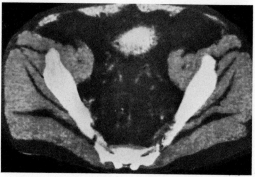

Fig. 86-4b: **Retroperitoneal fibrosis.** Narrow soft-tissue zone around the aorta with adherence of the left ureter (>) in moderate, bilateral urinary stasis.

Fig. 86-4d: **Pelvic fibrolipomatosis.** Extensive fatty tissue in the entire minor pelvis with compression and displacement of intrapelvic organs.

Secondary retroperitoneal fibrosis (86-41)

Fibrotic zones are often discovered by chance without any typical clinical symptoms being manifest. For example, thickening of individual fascial membranes (perirenal, perirectal) is frequently found after irradiation (Fig. 86-4c). Perirenal fibrosis (86-34) is usually a chance finding. Circular fibrosis which also includes the ureters and which can give rise to the clinical picture of IRF is occasionally found in the vicinity of aneurysms – usually those caused by arteriosclerosis (Fig. 86-4b). Enhancement can be demonstrated to varying degrees – probably depending on the extent of the inflammation – following administration of contrast medium (626).

Presacral fibrosis following proctectomy has achieved diagnostic importance (Fig. 86-4c). Depending on wound care (drainage), delayed healing and retention of secretions can be expected (in 10–60 % of cases [52]) which, following organization, progress to fibrotic zones. These processes must be considered in postoperative controls and in the search for tumour recurrence (74-31).

Pelvic fibrolipomatosis (86-42)

Individual authors assume a close etiological association between pelvic fibrolipomatosis and retroperitoneal fibrosis. In pelvic fibrolipomatosis, the fibrous component is not as prominent as the fatty tissue component. Since the entire pelvis is filled with fatty tissue, impression of the bladder, ureters and the rectosigmoid occurs. The main clinical symptoms are pain in the sides of the abdomen, constipation, dysuria and cystitis. Cystography reveals typical pear-shaped deformation of the urinary bladder and it is this which, together with the signs of displacement of the terminal ilium, leads to the tentative diagnosis. Since, however, this picture can also be caused by malignant growths (598), further diagnostic measures are indicated.

● CT

The entire pelvis is filled in with fatty tissue and offers good scanning conditions. The pelvic organs are symmetrically compressed (Fig. 86-4d). A retroperitoneal lipoma causes asymmetrical displacement of the viscera (Fig. 86-6c).

Lymph node diseases (86-50)

Malignant lymphomas (86-51)
(cf. also 61-30)

Hodgkin's disease is differentiated from non-Hodgkin's lymphoma by the different pattern of involvement and the prognosis. Non-Hodgkin's lymphomas are also subdivided histopathologically into a nodular and a diffuse form. The probability of abdominal involvement in suprahrenic manifestation of Hodgkin's disease (15 %–45 % of cases) is about half as great as with the other malignant lymphomas (75 % of cases). As Fig. 86-5a shows, the mesenteric and paraaortic lymph nodes are the preferred sites of involvement in cases of non-Hodgkin's lymphoma. The spleen, which is affected least of all by the diffuse type of non-Hodgkin's lymphoma, is the main site of involvement in the abdominal pattern of Hodgkin's disease. Splenic involvement is highly probable if splenomegaly is present in non-Hodgkin's lymphoma. In contrast, splenomegaly can be demonstrated in only 50 % of cases of Hodgkin's disease (683). Hepatic organ involvement is a rare finding (5 % in Hodgkin's disease, 15 % in non-Hodgkin's lymphoma).

Localization	Hodgkin's disease %	Non-Hodgkin's lymphoma %
Spleen	37	41
Liver	8	14
Marrow	3	15
Paraaortic nodes	25	49
Mesenteric nodes	4	51

Fig. 86-5a: **Anatomical distribution of malignant lymphomas** in untreated patients (in > 100) after Harell (683).

● CT

The characteristic sign is lymph node enlargement, usually resulting in homogeneous conglomerates (Fig. 86-5f). Displacement of the adjacent organs is dependent on the size of the mass and can be considerable. The contours of the individual lymph nodes are frequently still recognizable. Due consideration must be given to the fact that moderate lymph node enlargement can be caused by reactive hyperplasia (677) or non-specific lymphadenitis (686).

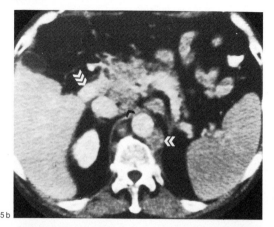

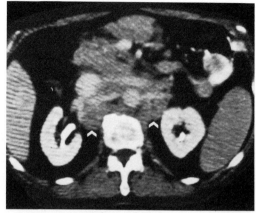

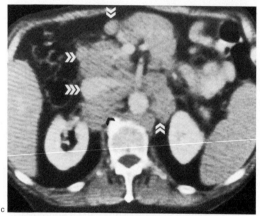

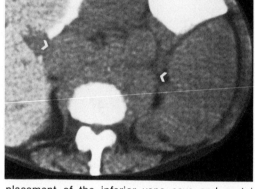

Fig. 86-5 b–g: **Malignant lymphomas.** If the disease is extensive, the vascular structures can be demarcated from the lymph node structures following administration of contrast medium, revealing considerable displacement of the vessels.

b: Retrocrural (≫) and hepatoduodenal (>) lymphomas. Portal vein (≫), splenomegaly.

5 c: Retrocaval and retroaortic (>) peripancreatic (≫) lymphomas. Distinct ventral displacement of the retroperitoneal vessels (inferior vena cava ≫).

5 d: Retrocaval and retroaortic (>) peripancreatic (≫) and splenic (≫) lymphomas. Distinct ventral displacement of the inferior vena cava and portal vein.

5 e: Retroaortic, renal (>) and mesenteric lymphomas. The contours of the pancreas are masked in Figs. 5 b–e.

5 f: Massive lymphomas retropancreatic and retrocrural and in the region of the porta hepatis. The retroperitoneal vessels cannot be identified without contrast administration. Splenomegaly.

5 g: Lymphomas in the region of the minor pelvis. Involvement of the internal iliac and obturator groups.

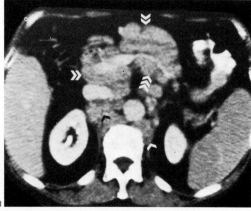

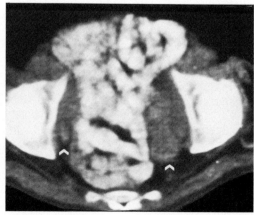

At the level of the diaphragm, special attention must be paid to the retrocrural space (86-12) and the contours of the abdominal aorta. An exact comparison of the sides is essential in the pelvis. Since lymphomas are frequently fused with the psoas muscle, differences between the two sides of this muscle must also be considered, especially when the boundary to the iliac muscle is abolished or filled in. In highly malignant forms, infiltration of the retroperitoneal fasciae and other organs including bones is demonstrable (Fig. 86-5k).

The **radiodensity** of lymphatic neoplasms is the same as that of muscle tissue (40–60 HU). Reduction of the density frequently occurs under therapy and leads to the reappearance of the contours of the psoas muscle. It is noteworthy that there is almost complete restitution of retroperitoneal fatty tissue in the case of complete remission (comp. with 86-31, 86-52).

The **liver** and **spleen** must, without fail, be assessed at the same time. Enlargement alone is an important indication that these two organs are involved. Parenchymatous changes can be demonstrated in only a few cases (Fig. 76-4a), and frequently only after a guided bolus injection (686, 677, 693). The porta hepatis and the region of the splenic hilum must also be scanned in a narrow slice sequence. Polycyclic protrusions, perhaps with displacement of the (enhanced) organ vessels, are further indications of organ involvement. The finding that the spleen and liver are of normal shape and size does not exclude organ involvement, particularly in Hodgkin's disease.

The mesentery, which can only be assessed following optimal bowel opacification, must be closely inspected for mesenteric lymphomas (Fig. 86-5h). Distinctly thickened intestinal walls (by more than 1 cm) can be recognized and indicate gastrointestinal involvement (74-30).

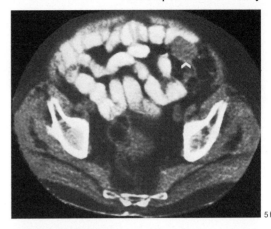

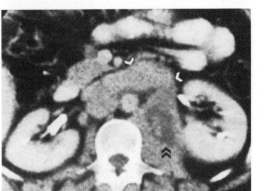

Fig. 5h–k: Malignant lymphomas.

5h: Lymphomas near the root of the mesentery of the small bowel (>).

5i: Hodgkin's disease with sharply delineated lymph node enlargements (>), partly with hypodense areas (≫) as a sign of regressive changes.

5k: Mesenteric involvement (>) and osseous destruction (here of the sacrum ≫).

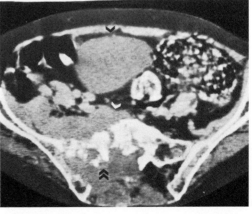

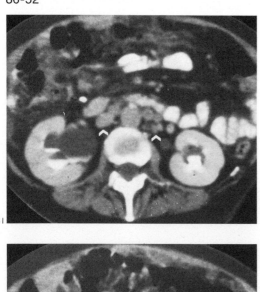
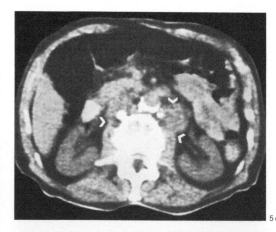
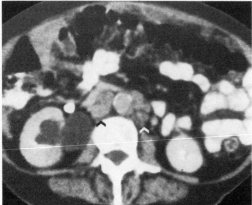
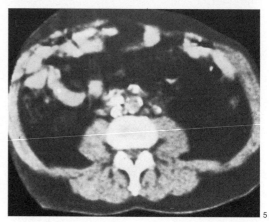

Fig. 86-5 l–q: Lymph node metastases.

5 l, m: Well demarcated nodular structures (diameter 0.5–2.5 cm) paraaortic and retrocaval (>). Lymph node metastases from metastatic carcinoma of the cervix. Congestion kidneys bilateral, right more pronounced than left, with contrast medium substratification phenomenon.

5 o, p: Paraaortic lymph node metastases from a malignant tumour of the uterus. Masking of the psoas contours (>). In status after lymphography, opacification of the smaller lymph nodes which have not yet been destroyed.

5 n, q: Metastases from a seminoma. Homogeneous soft-tissue masses paraaortic with displacement of the kidney to the left and of the pancreas in a ventral direction (>). Following irradiation (q) virtual normalization of the finding. Demonstration of a thickened Gerota's fascia (≫) resulting from irradiation.

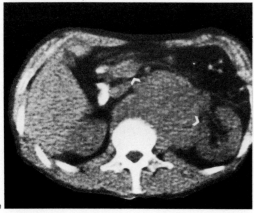
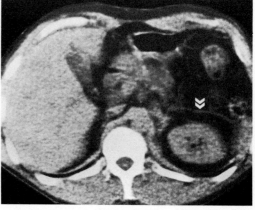

Lymph node metastases (86-52)

The lymphatic dissemination of a malignant lesion is determined by the position and the flow of lymph from the organ concerned. Consequently, metastases should be sought first of all in the closer and then in the further groups of lymph nodes to determine the full extent of tumour spread. In the case of testicular, ovarian and extensive uterine tumours it must be borne in mind that direct drainage pathways exist from the ovaries and testes to the renal hilum. In the epigastrium, malignant tumours of the pancreas, kidneys and stomach are the cause of regional lymph node enlargement which can also extend caudalward to below the renal stem. The predilection sites for seminomas and ovarian carcinomas are the paraaortic lymph node groups, and for colonic carcinoma the root of mesentery. Tumours in the pelvis (uterus, prostate and bladder) metastasize first of all regionally to the iliac regions and, not infrequently, to the presacral lymph nodes as well, and enlargement of these can readily be identified in the computed tomogram.

● CT

A nodular structure is a fairly frequent but not regular finding in lymph node enlargement, although confluence of metastatic tissue – particularly in larger seminoma metastases – is not unusual (Fig. 86–5n). In contrast to malignant lymphomas, a generalized pattern of involvement is rare. Unless other signs of lymphatic organ involvement (e.g. splenomegaly) are present, however, differentiation can be impossible in the individual case. Bone destruction is more an indication of metastasis than of a malignant lymphoma. However, since the primary tumour is usually known in practice, differential diagnosis is frequently unnecessary.

The **radiodensity** is the same as or less than that of the psoas muscle. Marked fusion with liquefaction can reduce the density values to within the range of those of water, resulting in a cystic appearance. Lymph nodes are usually poorly vascularized and consequently display little enhancement.

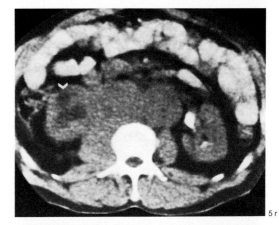

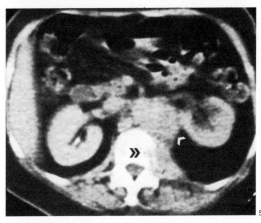

Fig. 86-5r–t: **Lymph node metastases.**

5r: Metastases from a testicular teratocarcinoma. Homogeneous soft-tissue masses retroperitoneal with masking of the great vessels and right psoas muscle. Silent kidney right with dilated cavity system (>).

5s: Metastases from a uterine carcinoma. Demonstration of a homogeneous soft-tissue mass (>), vertebral destruction (») and a hydronephrotic atrophic kidney left.

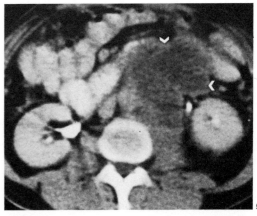

5t: Metastases from a seminoma with teratoid components. Polycyclic mass with hypodense areas (>) as a sign of tumour necrosis.

Benign lymphadenopathies (86-53)

Reactive hyperplasias lead only to moderate enlargement of the lymph nodes with harmonic internal structures. In immunity-deficient patients, the reactive hyperplasia – which usually causes intramural nodes of the gastrointestinal tract 2–5 mm in size – can assume the appearance of a malignant retroperitoneal lymphoma (pseudolymphoma [676]).

Primary retroperitoneal tumours (86-60)

Primary retroperitoneal tumours are defined as neoplasms of the various kinds of tissue of the retroperitoneal space, but not of the organs embedded within it (including lymphomas). They are encountered very rarely, accounting for 0.1–3‰ (47) of all tumours in man, and display signs of malignancy in 85 % of cases (1). Most of the different kinds of tumour are moderately vascularized – only haemangiomas, angiosarcomas and phaeochromocytomas are usually highly vascularized. The differentiated tumour forms

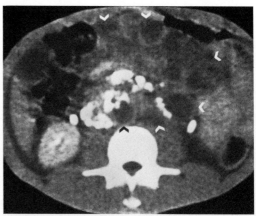

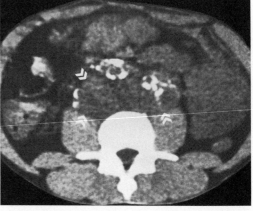

Fig. 86-5 u, v: **Abdominal lymph node tuberculosis.** Demonstration of roundish hypodense (40 HU) areas retroperitoneal and intraabdominal (>). In status after lymphography, only partial opacification of the lymph nodes. Caseous lymph node conglomerates were found at laparoscopy. 10 weeks after therapy (v), decrease mainly of the hypodense areas. Also, demonstration of fused, homogeneous lymph node conglomerates (≫).

		Beningn forms	Malignant forms
Mesodermal tumours	50 % (40–60%)	Lipoma Leiomyoma Rhabdomyoma Myxoma Fibroma Lymphangioma Haemangioma Haemangiopericytoma Mesenchymoma	Liposarcoma Leiomyosarcoma Rhabdomyosarcoma Myxosarcoma Fibrosarcoma Lymphangiosarcoma Angiosarcoma Malignant haemangiopericytoma **Malignant mesenchymoma**
Neurogenous tumours	30 % (15–50%)	Ganglioneuroma Paraganglioma **Phaeochromocytoma** **Neurofibroma** Neurolemmoma	Neuroblastoma (<6th year) Phaeochromoblastoma Malignant schwannoma
Remnant tumours	10 % (5–25%)	Teratoma (in infancy) Dermoid cyst Chordoma	Malignant teratoma Malignant chordoma
	10 % (5–11%)	Adenoma Epithelial cyst	Carcinoma

Fig. 86-**6 a:** Relative frequency of **primary tumours of the retroperitoneum** (6, 47).

Fig. 86-**6 d, g: Retroperitoneal sarcomas.**

6 d: Polymorphcellular sarcoma. Smoothly bordered soft-tissue zone with invasion of the psoas muscle and erector muscle of the spine and destruction of the right transverse vertebral process. No demonstration of regional lymph node metastases.

6 g: Spindle-cell sarcoma. Bulbous swelling lying against the psoas muscle right. No demonstration of regional lymphomas.

Retroperitoneal cavity

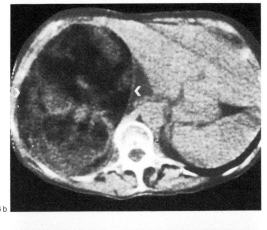

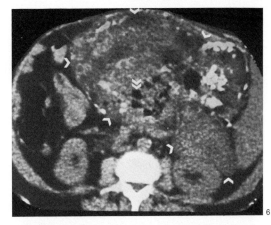

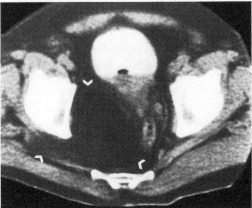

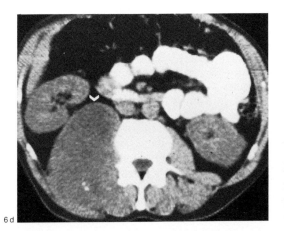

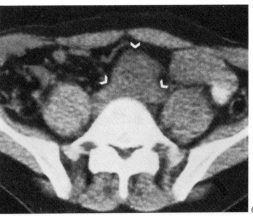

Fig. 86-6 b–g: Primary retroperitoneal tumours.

Fig. 86-6 b, c: Lipoid tumours.

6 b: Liposarcoma. Smoothly bordered zone with inhomogeneous density pattern consisting of fat-equidense and soft-tissue structures.

6 c: Lipoma. Homogeneous, fat-equidense zone with displacement of the organs in the minor pelvis and herniation through the ischiadic foramen.

Fig. 86-6 e, f: **Mesenchymoma.** In the upper and lower abdomen, demonstration of an extensive mass displaying lipoid, soft-tissue and myxomatous components. Demonstration of calcium and cartilage formations and gas bubbles (≫) corresponding to necrobiotic processes but not abscess formation.

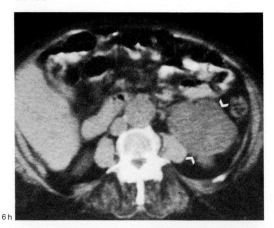

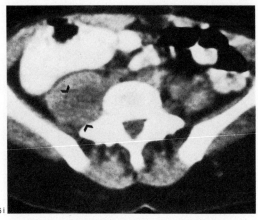

Fig. 86-**6h–k: Primary retroperitoneal tumours.**
6h: Myxoma of the retroperitoneal space with relatively smooth borders and slight hypodensity (19 HU) compared to muscle tissue. Tumour recurrence.
6i: Neurofibroma impressing and displacing the psoas muscle from behind right as a hypodense soft-tissue structure.

6k: Polymorphcellular sarcoma. Polycyclic solitary, soft-tissue mass. Demonstration of hypodense areas as a sign of tumour necrosis (≫).

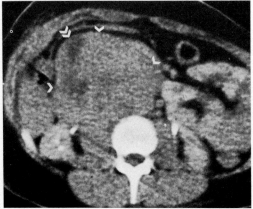

normally resemble the tissue from which they originate. Intratumorous calcifications are found to an increased extent in neuroblastomas, ganglioneurinomas, haemangiomas and haemangiopericytomas. Larger tumours, and particularly leiomyosarcomas, undergo cystic degeneration (625).

● **CT**

The computed tomogram frequently reveals a solid mass which, on enlargement, can be multilocular and bilateral. It lies preferably in front of the spinal column and in front of the psoas muscle (625).

Clear **demarcation** – due to conserved peritumorous fatty lamellae – and the absence of metastases indicate a localized process, but do not rule out malignancy. On the other hand, invasive growth which shows no respect for the pertinent anatomical boundaries can be taken as a criterion of malignancy, as can the demonstration of metastases and bone destruction. As known from angiography, vascular erosion is a rare event.

The **radiodensity** is about the same as that of the tissue of origin, i. e. soft tissue or muscle tissue. Lipomas display a density value of -80 to -90 HU – identical to that of retroperitoneal fatty tissue. The density of liposarcomas, and particularly of differentiated liposarcomas, lies within the negative range. The radiodensity of water is frequently exceeded in isolated parts of the tumour and is due to myxomatous tissue components and fibrous tissue zones, which give the tumour an inhomogeneous structure. It is always possible for even a smoothly bordered and normally septated lipoma to undergo malignant degeneration. Myxomatous tissue displays reduced density which can be homogeneous or localized. Cystic degeneration occurs to an increased extent in leiomyosarcomas (625) and becomes clearly demarcated following administration of contrast medium.

Bolus injections can provide information about the degree of vascularity (phaeochromocytoma [82-42]). The overall incidence of calcifications, which are demonstrated mainly in neurogenic tumours, is very low. Their structure is usually amorphous, but sometimes shell-like (608), creating the impression of a calcified aneurysm, abscess or haematoma. Lymphoceles appear as a cystic formation.

Vascular lesions (86-70)

Aneurysms (86-71)

The large arteries of the retroperitoneal space are visible even in the plain scan, while some of the smaller ones appear after a guided bolus injection (86-11). Although arteriosclerotic calcifications further facilitate the demarcation of vessels in the plain scan, they must be differentiated from aneurysmal calcifications, which display a larger diameter than the supplying vessel. In comparison to aortic aneurysms, aneurysms of the organ arteries are rare and occur mainly in the splenic artery (40% of cases) and the renal artery (20% of cases).

Aneurysms of the abdominal aorta (86-72)

In 98.5% of cases, aneurysms of the abdominal aorta are caused by arteriosclerosis. Syphilitic, mycotic and traumatic forms have become rare. Only 5% of arteriosclerotic but 70% of syphilitic aneurysms are localized cranially of the points of departure of the renal arteries. Infrarenal forms frequently continue into the pelvic arteries. Dissecting aneurysms in the abdominal region are rare and, in the majority of cases, represent a continuation of the dissection of the thoracic aorta. Some authors consider a non-ruptured aneurysm to be an indication for surgery once it has exceeded a diameter of 5 cm and make it dependent on the clinical finding (18).

● CT

Dilation of the aortic lumen is readily identifiable in the computed tomogram. Even the plain scan frequently reveals a slightly hypodense annular figure close to the vascular wall and corresponding to the thrombotic layers. The free vascular lumen and the departing renal arteries can be opacified following a guided bolus injection, providing adequate information for surgery (702). A ruptured aneurysm can sometimes be recognized by the periaortic haematoma, which masks or displaces the retroperitoneal structures. The pelvic arteries should always be included in the investigation so as to determine the full extent of the aneurysm. A mycotic aneurysm can sometimes be recognized by the incorporation of gas in the vascular wall (363). Erosion of vertebral bodies, which can be sensitively demonstrated by computerized tomography, can occur in extensive and long-standing vascular dilation (725).

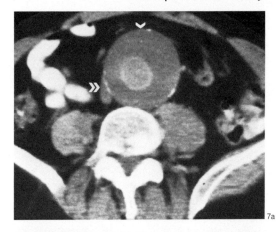

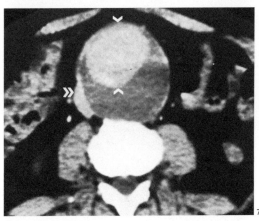

Fig. 86-**7a–c**: Aneurysms.

7a: Mass with a diameter of 7 cm and a central residual lumen of 2.5 cm. Inferior vena cava (≫).

7b: Extensive aneurysm with excentric residual lumen (>). Inferior vena cava (≫).

7c: Aneurysms of the common iliac arteries. Broad thrombotic deposit with wide central, excentric lumina. Common iliac veins (≫).

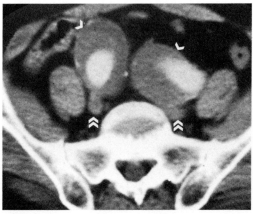

Trauma of the aorta (86-73)

Blunt trauma, rupture of an aneurysm and iatrogenic puncture of vessels can give rise to extensive pararenal haematomas. CT signs 86-34.

Periaortic haematomas of varying size are found in the majority of patients following **translumbar puncture** (704). Depending on the level of the puncture site, the haematoma can fill the retrocrural space (86-12) and displace the crura of the diaphragm (704).

Anomalies of the inferior vena cava (86-74)

The inferior vena cava is formed embryonally from the rudiments and obliteration of the three pairs of cardinal veins. Variations of caval anomalies — the overall incidence of which is rare — are therefore understandable. The azygos vein takes over venous drainage of the abdominal cavity if the hepatic segment of the inferior vena cava fails to develop. The hemiazygos vein also becomes involved in the case of dual development of the cava (707).

● CT

An anomaly of the inferior vena cava must be considered in dilation of the azygos and hemiazygos veins, which is demonstrated most reliably in the retrocrural space. Longitudinal cords next to the abdominal aorta must initially always be regarded as vessels. The administration of contrast medium is a simple way to confirm this assumption. However, differentiation from lymph node enlargement is difficult if a network of veins has developed (Fig. 86-7g). Vascular structures are usually more sharply demarcated than lymph nodes. Diagnostic demarcation is achieved by the administration of contrast medium. An azygos vein continuation syndrome can be diagnosed in the plain scan if the caval contours in the caudate lobe of the liver are absent and the azygos vein is dilated (709).

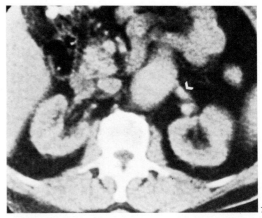

Fig. 86-7 d–f: Aneurysms.

7 d: Infrarenal aneurysm. Enhancement of the entire lumen including the renal artery left (>) following administration of contrast medium.

7 e: Dissecting aneurysm. False lumen ventral (>) and thrombotic deposits (≫).

7 f: Ruptured aneurysm with haematoma in the right perirenal space (>). Residual lumen (≫).

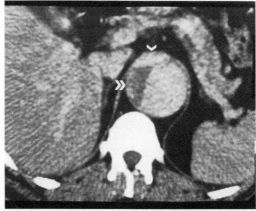

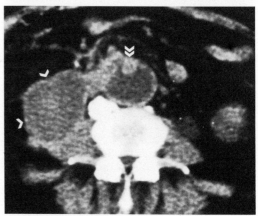

Retroperitoneal cavity

Thrombosis of the inferior vena cava (including pelvic veins) (86-75)

Thrombosis of the inferior vena cava is caused by external compression, invasion by tumour thrombi, or by expanding pelvic vein thrombi. Primary caval thromboses, e. g. in antithrombin deficiency, are rare events. In renal carcinoma, a tumour thrombus grows first of all into the renal vein and partially blocks the inferior vena cava, the lumen of which dilates increasingly. A similar mechanism is found in adrenal carcinoma which, like hepatocellular carcinoma (703), can also lead to caval thrombosis by direct infiltration. The thrombus, which becomes organized from its borders only 4 days after its development, can become softened in the centre and liquefy.

● **CT**

In thrombosis, the vascular lumen is frequently dilated and sharply contrasted towards the outside (727). The lumen can be less dense than the accompanying artery even in the plain scan (563). In the case of partial occlusion, the thrombus can be demarcated from the vascular lumen following administration of contrast medium. In complete thrombotic occlusion, there is no enhancement throughout the vascular lumen, which stands out from the surrounding enhanced tissue as a hypodense zone. Since fresh thrombi display the density of blood or even higher values (3-52), they cannot always be depicted by computerized tomography at this stage (727). The administration of a sufficiently high dose of contrast medium, if necessary by infusion via a leg vein, can assist the diagnosis in such cases.

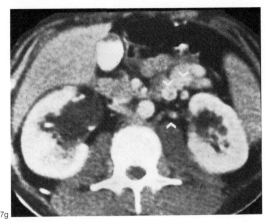

Fig. 86-7 g–i: **Venous lesions.**

7 g: Missing inferior vena cava with extensive venous plexus at the level of the renal hila (>) with involvement of the azygos vein system.

7 h: Extensive constriction of the inferior vena cava due to tumour thrombosis in hypernephroma. Enhancement of the tumour masses including the adrenal metastases (>) following bolus injection.

7 i: Partial thrombosis of the inferior vena cava in hypernephroma. The (opacified) lumen is constricted in the shape of a sickle (>).

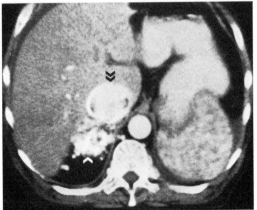

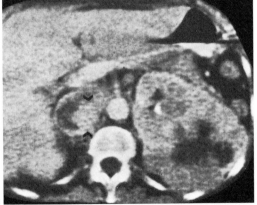

Skeleton
and soft tissues (90-00)

Fig. 91–1a: Histological classification of soft-tissue tumours (modified from Anderson [4], WHO [Enzinger] and Armed Forces Institute of Pathology [1980]).

Type of tissue	Benign tumours	Malignant tumours
Fibrous tissue	Fibroma (fibroma molle, fibroma durum, elastofibroma etc.)	Fibrosarcoma (differentiated, nonmetastasizing fibrosarcoma, poorly differentiated)
	Fibromatosis (cicatricial, irradiation, keloid, desmoid, nodular fasciitis etc.)	
Mesenchyme (undifferentiated, pluripotential)	Myxoma Mesenchymoma	Myxosarcoma Malignant mesenchymoma
Adipose tissue	Lipoma Lipomatosis Hibernoma Lipoblastomatosis	Liposarcoma (differentiated, myxoid, undifferentiated)
Muscle	Rhabdomyoma	Rhabdomyosarcoma (embryonal-botryoid type, spindle cell type) (undifferentiated adult)
	Leiomyoma (superficial, deep)	Leiomyosarcoma
Blood vessels Lymph vessels	Haemangioma (capillary, cavernous, arterial, venous, arteriovenous) Haemangioendothelioma	Angiosarcoma Malignant haemangioendothelioma
	Lymphangioma (capillary, cavernous, cystic) Lymphangiomatosis	Lymphangiosarcoma
Mesothelial tissue	Mesothelioma (epithelial, fibrous)	Malignant mesothelioma (diffuse) (epithelial, spindle cell, pleomorphic, and mixed-cell)
Synovial tissue	Giant cell tumour (of synovial sheath)	Malignant giant cell tumour Synovial sarcoma
Other tissues (partially heterotopic)	Chondroma Osteoma Benign xanthogranuloma Neurofibroma Neurofibromatosis Neurilemoma Myositis ossificans	(Extraosseous) chondrosarcoma Osteosarcoma Malignant xanthogranuloma (Histiocytoma) Neurofibrosarcoma Malignant schwannoma Myeloblastoma

Soft-tissue tumours (of the extremities) (91-00)

Pathology of soft-tissue tumours (91-10)

Lipomas are the most frequent kind of benign soft-tissue tumour. They are found primarily in the region of the shoulder, neck and back and, but less frequently, in the extremities. In contrast, **liposarcomas** are encountered in the extremities in more than 50 % of cases (4). Most lipomas originate from subcutaneous tissue. Intramuscular and intermuscular expansion and even local infiltration are possible if the site of origin is deeper. Cellular atypias, which are found in well-differentiated liposarcomas consisting mainly of mature fatty tissue, cannot be demonstrated in the histological section of lipomas.

Depending on their degree of differentiation, liposarcomas contain varying proportions of myxomatous and mucous tissue. Fibrous components can become prominent, giving rise to the aspect of a fibrosarcoma.

Fibromas originate from diverse connective-tissue structures (Fig. 91-1a) and are named accordingly. Musculoaponeurotic fibromatosis can assume considerable proportions and invade the adjacent tissue (including bones) without metastasizing (aggressive fibromatosis). Differentiation from a **fibrosarcoma** may be difficult because the features overlap.

Rhabdomyosarcomas in soft tissue follow liposarcomas and fibrosarcomas in order of frequency. Apart from embryonal botryoid rhabdomyosarcomas (83-52), the other kinds are found primarily in the extremities. In the adult form, necrosis, haemorrhage and cystic transformation can predominate over the features of the tumour. Benign **rhabdomyomas** are an extremely rare finding.

Leiomyomas not originating in the uterus arise within various intraabdominal organs and in soft tissue, where they are usually situated subcutaneously. **Leiomyosarcomas** are numerically superior to the benign variants in the deeper layers of muscle.

In contrast to lymphangiomas, lymphangiosarcomas and angiosarcomas, **haemangiomas** (capillary and cavernous form) are not an infrequent finding in the soft tissues of the extremities.

Examination technique (91-20)
- No preparation of the patient is required.
- **Scanning** at slice intervals of 10–25 mm, if necessary intermediate slices.

Scanning area: entire lesion including the adjacent tissue.
- **Administration of contrast medium** in special cases.

CT of soft-tissue tumours (91-30)

Diagnosis of the extremities demands comparison of the two sides, since the shape, size and septation of the muscles are subject to individual variations. The signs of a mass are hypodense zones and enlargement of the muscle bed. The amount of **interposing fat** determines the extent to which the muscular fascial planes can be demarcated and, in particular, determines whether large vessels and nerves can be demonstrated as separate punctiform structures (743).

Sharp boundaries and homogeneity of the tumorous density values are indications of benignity. The main representative is the lipoma, which is marked by its unequivocal density values. Necroses, oedema and haemorrhagic permeation, which occur primarily in rapidly growing kinds of tumour, are marked by inhomogeneity of the density pattern. In association with **poorly defined demarcation** from the vicinity, this inhomogeneity must therefore be interpreted as a sign of malignancy. These criteria are indirect and must be applied with caution. In contrast, destruction of the adjacent osseous tissue and invasion of adjacent organs are unequivocal signs of malignant growth – apart from metastases, which occur rarely and late in malignant soft-tissue tumours.

In liposarcomas, mottled or funicular tissue zones (fibrous, myxomatous and mucinous components) displaying higher **radiodensity** than fat lend the tumour a streaky and inhomogeneous appearance. The tissue density of a fat-containing tumour can exceed the density of water (735). Lipomas differ from liposarcomas by virtue of their uniform density (−80 to −100 HU). They also have thin walls and uniform septations.

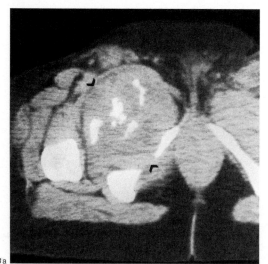

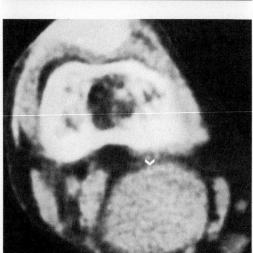

Myxomatous tissue is hypodense because of its sparse vascularity and its higher water content in comparison to muscle tissue. Necrosis, oedema and haemorrhagic permeation lead to circumscribed reductions of density and can produce cystic formations with density values similar to those of water. **Phleboliths** are found to an increased extent within haemangiomas, which can display an increase of density due to enhancement (71-43) following administration of contrast medium, particularly in the cavernous forms. **Calcifications** are frequently the consequence of irradiation (735). The **administration of contrast material** usually results in better demonstration of the mass. A soft-tissue tumour which is isodense in the plain scan can – although rarely (7 % of cases [741]) – only be demarcated following a normal-dose infusion. Enhancement of the tumour depends on its degree of vascularity.

Since the histology can usually be obtained by puncture, computerized tomography offers the possibility of exact **localization** of a deeper-lying tumour. Since it can be difficult to establish the identity of a soft-tissue tumour even by histology (4), computerized tomographic assessment of the extent and invasiveness can make a major contribution to the diagnosis. Computerized tomography therefore has a considerable influence on the therapeutic procedure (741, 752).

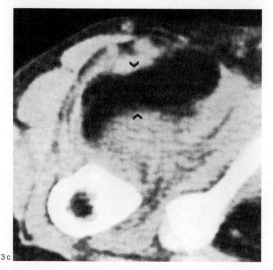

Fig. 91-3 a–c: Benign connective tissue tumours.

3a: Desmoid in the region of the adductors of the right thigh with calcareous deposits (>).

3b: Ganglion in the region of the right popliteal space. Smoothly bordered mass, slightly hypodense (40 HU) compared to muscle tissue. Histologically, tight collagen-rich connective tissue with mucinous areas.

3c: Lipoma in the region of the right thigh with homogeneous density values (–95 HU).

Soft-tissue tumours (of the extremities)

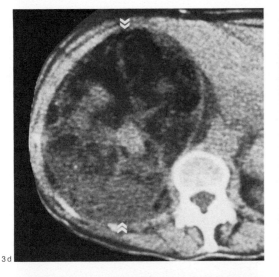

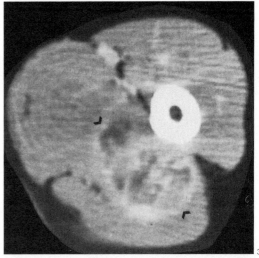

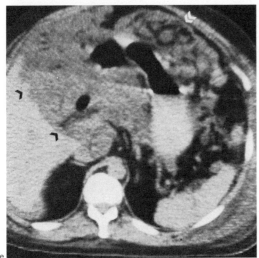

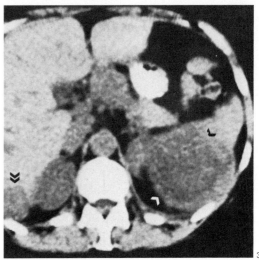

Fig. 91-3 d–f: Liposarcomas.

3 d: Retroperitoneal liposarcoma with fatty (−85 HU) and distinct connective tissue components.

3 e: Mesenteric liposarcoma with generally reduced tissue density (18 HU) with relatively sharply demarcated, narrow fat-equivalent areas (≫).

3 f: Abdominal liposarcoma with myxomatous components. Inhomogeneous density pattern with density values of 10–28 HU, reflecting the varying fatty tissue areas.

Fig. 91-3 g: Malignant fibrous histiocytoma (malignant xanthogranuloma) of the right thigh, inflammatory type. Following contrast medium administration, distinct enhancement and demonstration of tumour necroses, simulating the CT appearance of abscess formation.

Fig. 91-3 h: Metastases from a uterine leiomyosarcoma, which appear as inhomogeneous (18–34 HU) hypodense areas within the spleen (>) and liver (≫).

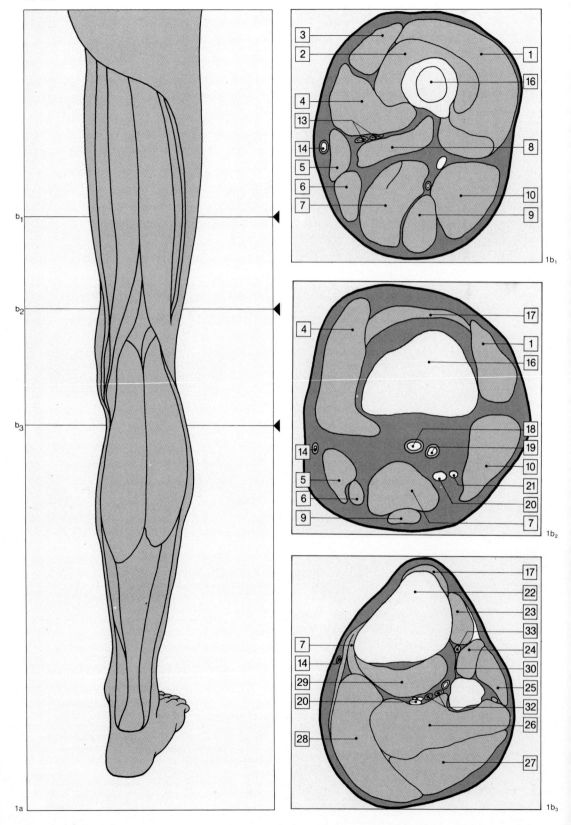

Muscle tissue (92-00)

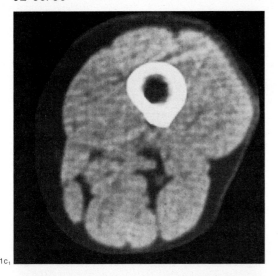

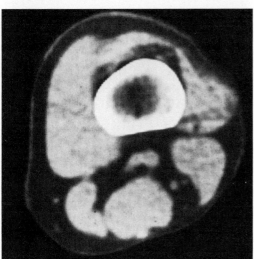

Fig. 92-1 a–c: Anatomy of the leg.
Key
1 M. vastus lateralis
2 M. vastus intermedius
3 M. rectus femoris
4 M. vastus medialis
5 M. sartorius
6 M. gracilis
7 M. semi-membranosus
8 M. adductor longus
9 M. semitendinosus
10 M. biceps femoris (caput longum)
11 M. biceps femoris (caput breve)
12 A. femoralis
13 V. femoralis
14 V. saphena magna
15 N. ischiadicus
16 Femur
17 Lig. patellae
18 A. poplitea
19 V. poplitea
20 N. tibialis
21 N. fibularis
22 Tibia
23 M. tibialis anterior
24 M. extensor dig. longus
25 M. peronaeus longus
26 M. soleus
27 M. gastrocnemius (caput laterale)
28 M. gastrocnemius (caput mediale)
29 M. popliteus
30 Membrana interossea
31 N. fibularis (prof.)
32 A. V. fibularis
33 A. tibialis anterior

Examination technique (92-10)
(cf. 91-20)

Atrophy (92-20)
Muscle tissue decreases during periods of inactivity, steroid medication and denervation, and the diameter of the individual muscle cords diminishes. Moderate interposition of fat between the septa of the muscles can be found in relation to the constitution of the patient. In denervation of a muscular fascicle, the muscle tissue is replaced by fatty tissue.

● CT

Computerized tomography permits only a rough assessment of the atrophy, since it varies greatly depending on the physical fitness of the individual patient. Circumscribed atrophy (e. g. following injury) can be assessed exactly by comparing the sides.

Progressive muscular dystrophy (92-30)
The vast majority of cases of progressive muscular dystrophy are of the Duchenne type, in which the muscles of the pelvic girdle are affected first of all. Pseudohypertrophy of the calves is present in 80 % of cases. In contrast, pseudohypertrophy of the affected muscles is found less frequently in the limb girdle type and only by way of exception in the fascioscapulohumeral type. Histologically, the various forms differ from each other only in the extent and intensity of the tissue changes. Focal necroses of a muscle fibre – initially reversible by restorative processes – are compensated for by hypertrophy of the unaffected elements. On progression of the disease, the muscle tissue is gradually replaced by fat and connective tissue until it has almost disappeared.

● CT

The fatty-tissue transformation is recognizable in the computed tomogram, the muscular septa usually standing out clearly as a matrix. Both homogeneous involvement of a muscle or muscle group and patchy permeation of fatty tissue can be demonstrated. At the present time it is still unclear what diagnostic or prognostic value attaches to these different patterns of dystrophy. In the calves, the more centrally situated muscle cords are affected last of all (746).

Inflammatory muscle changes (92-40)

Purulent myositis (muscular abscess) (92-41)

Purulent myositis develops either as a result of trauma or metastatic-embolically via the usual pus-forming organisms, which can lead to liquefaction and encapsulation of the muscle tissue and, hence, to an abscess. In infections caused by Streptococcus pyogenes, the liquefaction can contain gas and develop into a gas phlegmon.

● **CT**

The computed tomogram reveals a hypodense zone which masks the muscular septa and the surrounding fatty tissue and usually leads to swelling of the affected region. A hyperdense ring, the CT equivalent of granulation tissue, can frequently be demonstrated following the administration of contrast medium, particularly in chronic processes. Gas within the hypodense zones is regarded as pathognomonic for a bacterial process.

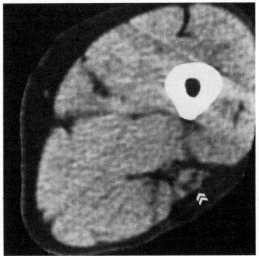

Sarcoidosis (92-42)

The muscle tissue is affected in more than 50% of cases of generalized sarcoidosis. Muscular atrophy can develop (rarely) primarily as a result of direct granulomatous involvement of the muscle fibre or indirectly via alteration of the motor nerves.

● **CT**

Atrophy cannot be demonstrated by computerized tomography until the muscle fibres have been replaced by fatty tissue.

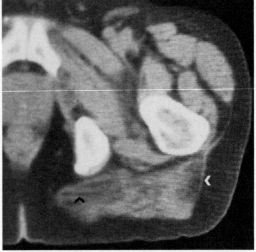

Polymyositis (92-43)

In 80% of cases, polymyositis manifests itself as a feature of dermatomyositis. The acute form is marked by extensive and rapidly developing muscular necrosis which can display fine, plaque-like calcifications. Depending on the extent of muscle tissue necrosis, primarily chronic polymyositis displays liposclerotic transformation more frequently than the secondarily chronic form.

● **CT**

The extent of both fatty-tissue incorporation and atrophy can be assessed by computerized tomography. No differential-diagnostic criteria in respect of progressive muscular dystrophy have yet been reported.

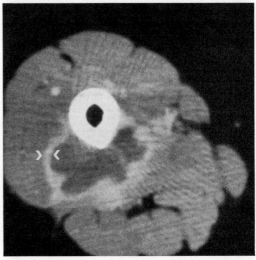

Muscle haematoma (92-50)

Following (blunt) trauma, particularly in haemophilia or anticoagulent therapy, the haematoma leads to swelling of the muscle and is enclosed by the muscle fasciae. Clinical signs of vascular and neurological deficiency can occur as a result of the displacement. In the further course, the haematoma can be absorbed, liquefy or become organized. Calcifications are regressive changes of longstanding connective-tissue organization.

● **CT**

In the fresh stage of localized haematomas the computed tomogram reveals hyperdense patches which can, however, also be absent on saturation of the muscle tissue. Frequently, only swelling of a muscle is recognizable, and this must be distinguished diagnostically from hypertrophy. This can normally be done by studying the case history and the clinical findings (posture of the spinal column).

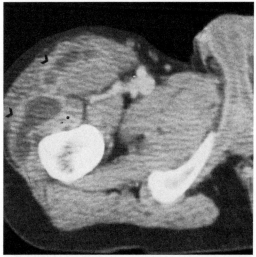

4b

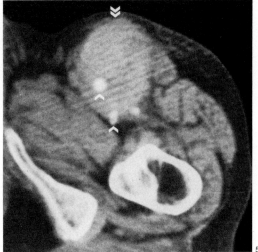

5a

Fig. 92-2 a, b: Muscular atrophy.
2a: In status after a war injury, atrophy of the semimembranous muscle, which can best be evaluated by a comparison of the sides.
2b: Senile atrophy of the gluteal muscles, demonstrable by the patchy incorporation of fat within the muscle (>).

Fig. 92-4 a, b: Muscle abscess.
Demonstration of hypodense areas (>) surrounded by granulation tissue which displays ring-shaped enhancement following contrast medium administration (><).

Fig. 92-5 a, b: Muscle haematoma.
5a: Haematoma consequent to deep plastic surgery (false aneurysm). Within the haematoma, demonstration of patent femoral vessels following a bolus injection (>).
5b: Liquefied haematoma of the iliopsoas muscle. Demonstration of septate hypodense (17 HU) areas within the iliac and psoas muscles (11 months after hysterectomy). Rim enhancement after contrast medium administration (><) as a sign of extensive absorptive granulation tissue, making CT differentiation from an abscess impossible.

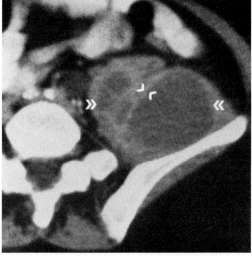

5b

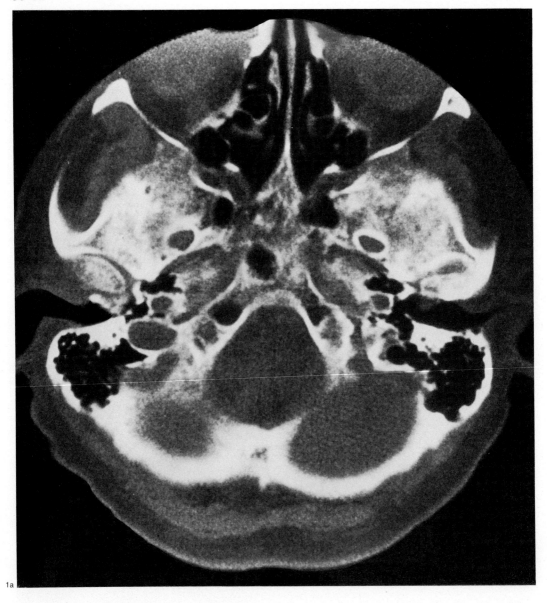

Fig. 93-1a: **Computed tomogram of the base of the skull.** The image, which is devoid of superimposition and disturbing shadows, permits detailed evaluation of the bone structures and foramina.

Skeleton (93-00)

Anatomy and imaging (93-10)

Conventional radiological techniques (including pluridimensional tomography) have already made competent differential diagnosis of the skeleton possible. The high contrast of the calcareous, osseous structures and the resultant plethora of detail were an essential part of this. Due to the breaking-up of the image into volume elements, the partial volume effect and the rigid slice geometry, computerized tomography has limited spatial resolution although it can now be increased considerably on certain scanners by the use of special computer programs. The CT-technique is successfully employed in skeletal diagnosis for the following reasons:

● The axial projection depicts certain osseous structures better.

● In dense (osteosclerotic) processes and in marked overshadowing, computerized tomography is superior to conventional tomography because there is no blurring of the image.

● Adjacent soft-tissue structures can be assessed in detail.

● The density values permit quantitative conclusions regarding mineralization.

Parts of the skeleton which run axially, e. g. the spinal column, can be demonstrated clearly. However, the physiological curvature means that only a few of the end-plates of the vertebral bodies and the discs run parallel to the sectional plane. For optimal demonstration, the gantry must therefore be aligned individually with the respective angular position of a vertebral body, a procedure which has been made possible by the scoutview technique (cf. CT terminology [97-00]). The anterior surface of the sacrum, which lies obliquely in the sectional plane, can be demonstrated by appropriate tilting of the gantry — likewise parallel to the sectional plane. The contours of the osseous pelvis and the entire circumference of the hip joints, the thighs and lower legs can be scanned easily without tilting the unit. The medullary spaces of the thigh and lower leg in particular are highly accessible.

Narrow, horizontal fissures, particularly the intervertebral spaces, are best demonstrated — without partial volume effects — when the chosen slice thickness is thinner than the height of

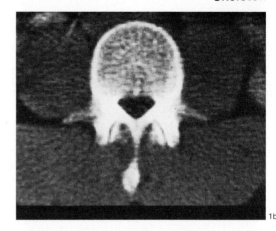

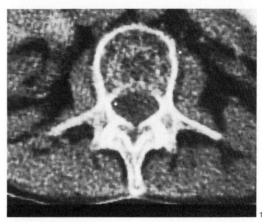

Fig. 93-**1 b, c: Mineralization of bone.**
1 b: Normal bone structure of a lumbar vertebra (22-year old male). Radiodensity of the spongy substance: 212 HU (median value).
1 c: Osteoporosis. Radiodensity of the spongy substance: −12 HU (median value).

Fig. 93-**3 a: Vertebral plasmocytoma.** Irregular and coarse-grained bone structure, with some disintegration of compact bone.

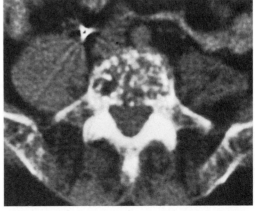

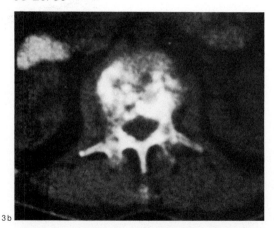

Fig. 93-3b: **Metastatic destruction.** Mixed type metastases in mammary carcinoma. Osteoplastic and osteolytic components are demonstrated in detail.

Fig. 93-3c: **Osteogenic sarcoma** of the thigh. The soft-tissue scan reveals tumour invasion of the thigh muscles (>). A change of window setting permits evaluation of the osseous structures including involvement of the fat-containing medullary space without any disturbing shadows.

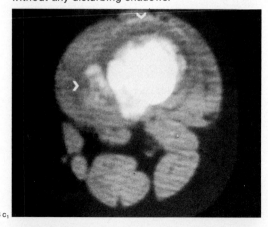

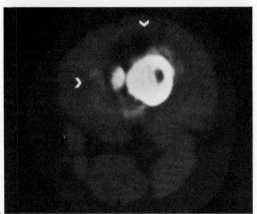

the fissure. Slice thicknesses of 2 mm are available on some scanners.

If partial volume effects are avoided, the horizontal spatial resolution in the computed tomogram is usually adequate — depending on the picture matrix — for analysis of the spongy structure (Fig. 93-1b). This situation does not obtain in the case of the curved, flat bones of the pelvis and ribs, which run obliquely through the slice.

Examination technique (93-20)

- Positioning of the extremities (long bones) vertical to the sectional plane.
- **Scanning** with slice thicknesses of 8–13 mm. Slice interval and scanning area dependent on the problem (extent of the process).
- **Contrast medium** (guided bolus injection) in special cases (see below).

Cf. 93-52 for examination technique for the vertebral column.

Mineralization of bone (93-30)

Senile involution of bone tissue, hypogonadism, Cushing's disease, haemochromatosis, sclerodermia, inflammatory bone disease, and atrophy due to inactivity lead to reduction of the osseous substance, i. e. to osteoporosis. Disorders of vitamin D metabolism cause osteomalacia. Depending on the severity of the disease, chronic renal failure can result in both a decrease and an increase of osseous substance (osteosclerosis).

- **CT**

Changes of bone density can be assessed quantitatively by computerized tomography. The scanning object is the spongy (trabecular) bone, which reacts most sensitively to metabolic chances. The measuring sites are radius and ulna (85, 101, 107) or the vertebral body (76, 109, 120). When measuring the density it is essential to ascertain that the measuring volume lies within the spongy bone tissue. To avoid undesired partial volume effects, the effect of physiological lordosis of the spinal column can be counteracted by tilting the gantry (scoutview) or by mathematical calculations (81). Using special methods (88) it appears to be possible to differentiate between an increase of mineralization and an increase of organic bone substance, but this has not been confirmed in a large enough population of patients. However, certain methodological limitations (120) restrict the accuracy and sensitivity of the measurement.

Bone tumours (93-40)

Osteomas, osteoblastomas, chondromas, osteochondromas and **chondromyxoid fibromas** are benign bone tumours which, because they are localized within the skeleton and because of their radiological morphology, lend themselves almost perfectly to differential diagnosis with the X-ray film. Since their boundaries are visible and they are unlikely to be surrounded by a soft-tissue component, computerized tomography cannot offer any additional diagnostic information.

The only tumour which has aroused any interest as regards computerized tomography is the **osteoid osteoma** (750, 752), which can lead to inflammatory reactions of the surrounding osseous and periosteal tissue. Because of disturbing shadows, the nidus cannot always be optimally demonstrated by conventional tomography in pronounced periosteal reactions. This limitation does not exist in computerized tomography.

In expansive or invasive, usually malignant tumours, computerized tomography supplies information which assists both the diagnosis and therapy-planning. It also permits assessment of the **medullary space** and early detection of **penetration through the cortical bone** and **invasion of adjacent tissue** in primarily central tumours. This goes in particular for parts of the tumour which do not contain any calcareous structures. Conversely, the computed tomogram can also reveal medullary expansion in primarily parosteal malignant lesions. Tumour tissue can be assumed in Ewing's sarcomas and reticulosarcomas on the basis of an increase of density of the fat-containing medullary space in the contralateral comparison (730), although discrete periosteal changes escape computerized tomographic detection. The expansion of parosteal, non-calcifying soft-tissue tumours (e. g. parosteal fibrosarcoma, solitary myeloma, aneurysmal bone cysts and peripheral chondrosarcoma) can be assessed better by computerized tomography than with other methods.

Following surgery, it is possible despite the altered topography to detect a recurrence by means of a detailed comparison – if possible with an initial postoperative finding – even in the absence of typical calcifications of the osteoid or cartilage within the malignant lesion, which are demonstrable in the general X-ray film.

The **administration of contrast medium** has not produced any distinct enhancement even in highly vascular bone tumours (741, 750). It is, however, of use in the demarcation of non-calcified tumour tissue from normal soft tissue.

Type of tissue	Age (years)	Benign tumours	Age (years)	Malignant tumours
Cartilage	10–25	Chondroblastoma		
	10–25	Chondromyxoid fibroma	30–60	Chondrosarcoma (primary, secondary)
	10–30	Osteochondroma		
	10–40	Chondroma	20–60	Mesenchymal chondrosarcoma
Bone	40–50	Osteoma		
	10–30	Osteoid osteoma	10–25	Osteosarcoma
	10–30	Osteoblastoma	30–60	Parosteal osteosarcoma
Marrow elements			40–60	Plasma cell myeloma
			5–20	Ewing's sarcoma
			30–60	Reticulum cell sarcoma (histiocytic malignant lymphoma)
		(Lipoma)		(Liposarcoma)
Vessels	20–50	Haemangioma Glomus tumour Lymphangioma		Angiosarcoma
Fibrous tissue	20–30	Desmoplastic fibroma	20–60	Fibrosarcoma
Neurogenous tissue		Neurofibromatosis Neurilemoma Ganglioneuroma		
	20–40	Giant cell tumour	20–40	Giant cell tumour Adamantinoma
			40–60	Chordoma

Fig. 93–**4a: Classification of primary bone tumours** (modified from Anderson [4] and Spjut et al.).

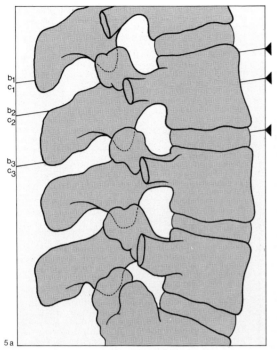

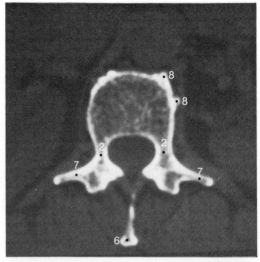

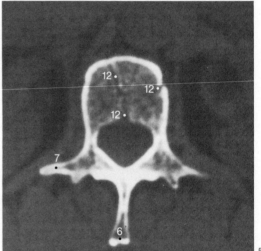

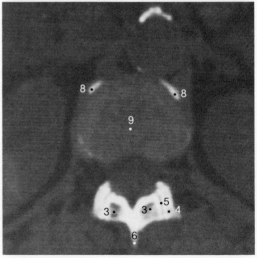

Fig. 93-5 a–c: Lumbar vertebral column.

5 a: Lateral view.

5 b: Transverse sections in bone scan (window setting + 500 HU).

5 c: The same transverse sections in the soft-tissue scan (window setting + 60 HU). Cf. 5a for level of section.

Key
1 Vertebral body
2 Root of arch
3 Superior articular process
4 Inferior articular process
5 Facetal joint
6 Spinous process
7 Transverse process
8 Spondylophytes
9 Disk
10 Flaval ligament
11 Epidural space
12 Basivertebral vessel
13 Nerve routes
14 Paravertebral veins (external vertebral venous plexus including the intervertebral vein)

Skeleton

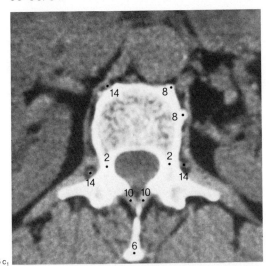

5 c₁

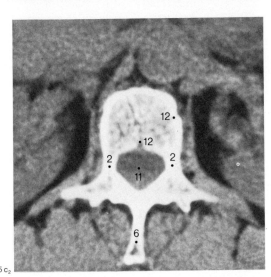

5 c₂

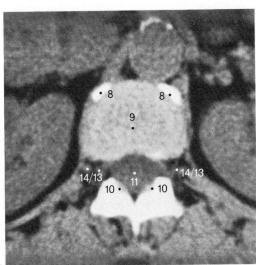

5 c₃

Vertebral column and vertebral canal (93-50)

Anatomy and imaging (93-51)

As stated in 93-10, the vertebral body should always be scanned parallel to its terminal plates. Depending on the problem, thin slices (up to 2 mm) should be used to minimize the partial volume effect. However, diagnostic information can frequently be obtained even with the usual slice thickness of 10–13 mm (650).

The spongy **vertebral body** can be imaged centrally, i. e. without partial volume effects from other structures if it is scanned in the plane of the pedicles (at the exact level of the site of entry of the basivertebral vessels) (Fig. 93-5b). The upper edge of the spinal process is just touched in this sectional plane.

The osseous **spinal canal** is not a cylindrical tube. It is narrowest at the upper limit of the lamina because of the roofing tile configuration of the vertebral arches and widens slightly caudalward. At the level of the intervertebral joints, the spinal canal is closed by the flaval ligaments, which are 2–4 mm thick. The interspinal and supraspinal ligaments are denser than the surrounding connective tissue and can therefore be demonstrated by computerized tomography. The posterior longitudinal ligament is relatively thick in the cervical region and becomes thinner caudalward. It is fixed to the intervertebral discs and, because of the inserting vertebral vessels, lies up to 3–4 mm from the posterior vertebral surface at the level of the vertebral bodies, making it sometimes demonstrable as a separate entity in the computerized tomogram. The width of the epidural space between the dura and the periosteum, which is filled with fatty tissue and the internal venous plexus, varies because of the wavy edges of the dorsal osseous vertebral canal and the continuously straight contours of the dura mater. The amount of epidural fatty tissue increases caudalward and can be demonstrated in quantity particularly in the region of the cauda equina and the sacrum.

In adults, the **spinal cord** extends to the level of L 1/2 and can be demarcated from the subdural space unter certain technical conditions (HR-CT) if the width of the latter exceeds 2 mm. With some scanners (662), this anatomical differentiation is possible only in the cervical region. The dimensions of the spinal cord, which displays its greater diameters in the region of

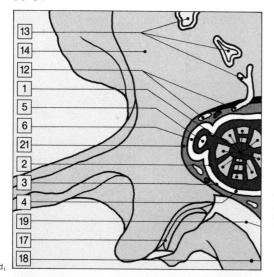
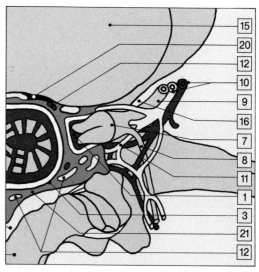

Fig. 93-5d: Soft-tissue structures of the lumbar canal.

5d₁: Diagramatic representation through the intervertebral space (L 2/L 3 right) and through the middle of the third lumbar vertebra (left).

Key

1 Subarachnoid space (with spinal nerve)
2 Arachnoidea
3 Spinal dura mater
4 Subdural space
5 N. lumbalis III
6 Radicular pouch
7 Spinal ganglion
8 Ramus dorsalis N. lumbalis II
9 Ramus ventralis N. lumbalis II
10 A. V. lumbalis
11 V. intervertebralis
12 Plexus venosus vertebralis internus
13 V. basivertebralis
14 Vertebral body
15 Disk
16 Intervertebral foramen
17 Facetal joint L 2/L 3
18 Spinous process
19 Flaval ligament
20 Posterior longitudinal ligament
21 Epidural space

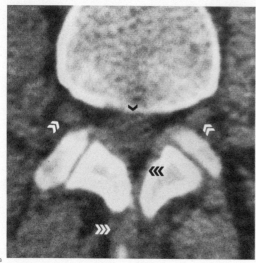
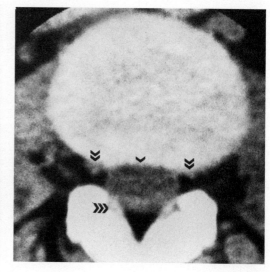

the lower cervical and thoracic segments, are well known (44).

The **spinal nerves** leave the vertebral canal in the upper section of the intervertebral foramen directly beneath the pedicles, where the spinal ganglion and the dural sheath form a fusiform bulge. Overall, the diameter of the roots and nerves varies from patient to patient, but usually increases in an individual patient from cranial to caudal. Under good scanning conditions (particularly with HR-CT), the nerve roots and the extradural section of the filum terminale in the lumbosacral region can be directly depicted in the computed tomogram because of the greater amounts of epidural and juxtavertebral fatty tissue.

The internal **vertebral venous plexus,** which passes through the epidural space, has relatively wide veins which can achieve a calibre of 5 mm. The four longitudinal (anterior and posterior) cords can frequently be identified even without administration of contrast medium if they display a diameter of more than 3 mm.

Examination technique (93-52)
● Parallel adjustment of the **sectional plane** to the intervertebral space.
This can only be done accurately with the scoutview technique (97-00). If the gantry cannot be tilted, adduction of the thighs to compensate for lumbar lordosis.

● **Slice thickness**
a) Slice thicknesses of 8 mm are usually sufficient to demonstrate osseous changes (tumours, fractures etc.).
b) Slice thicknesses of 2 mm (max. 4 mm) are required to demonstrate the intervertebral space and for multiplanar reconstruction.

● **Interval between slices:** depending on the problem (extent of the process).
● **Intrathecal administration of contrast medium** (metrizamide myelography) in suspected intraspinal processes.
Primary CT myelography
Administration of small amounts of metrizamide (4-25) at the site of the suspected tumour.
Secondary CT myelography
Examination of the spinal canal 30–120 minutes after conventional metrizamide myelography with the usual dosage of contrast media.
● **Reduction of movements** of superimposing organs, particularly of cervical soft tissue organs (swallowing act, respiratory movements etc.).

In the abdominal region: 1–3 mg glucagon i. v. or 30 mg scopolamine-N-butyl-bromide i. v., scanning during breath holding.

◄
$5d_2$: CT section through the middle of lumbar vertebra 3. Demonstration of the point of entry of the basivertebral vein (≫), the radicular pouches (>) and the epidural space.
$5d_3$: Same patient. Level of section 6 mm deeper than d_2. Demonstration of the spinal ganglion (≫), the epidural space (>) and the interspinal flaval ligament (≫).
$5d_4$: CT section through the disk L3/L4 with physiological dorsoconcave shape of the posterior surface (>). Demonstration of the anterior internal vertebral veins (≫) and the flaval ligament (≫). The generally homogeneous dural sack is demarcated by fatty tissue, as are also the vascular and nerve structures emerging in the intervertebral foramen.

Fig. 93-**5e: Computer-guided puncture** of a vertebral metastasis.

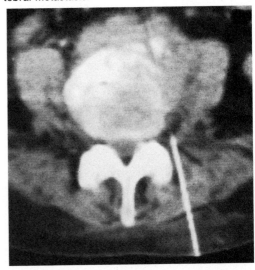

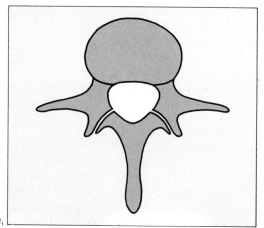

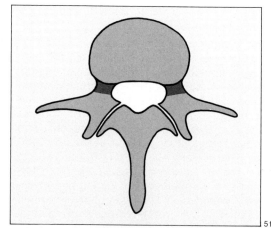

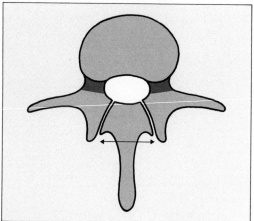

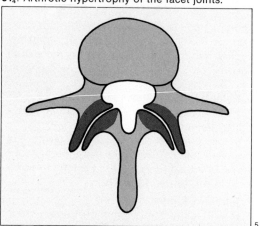

Fig. 93-5f: The narrow lumbar canal.
5f$_1$: Normal width of the lumbar canal.
5f$_2$: Concentric constriction of the lumbar canal. Shortening of the roots of the arch and horizontal closing-in (medialization) of the facet joints.
5f$_3$: Decreased anterior-posterior distance of lumbar canal as a result of shortening of roots of arch.
5f$_4$: Arthrotic hypertrophy of the facet joints.

Fig. 93-**5g: Dimensions of the lumbar canal.**
AP = sagittal diameter, anterior-posterior distance
IPD = interpedicular distance
IFD = distance between the facet joints
PH = height of the roots of the arch
(after Lee [650]).

Fig. 93-**5h: Jones-Thomson Quotient,** defined as A x B / C x D, is normal between 1/2 and 1/4.5. Denominators greater than 4.5 signify a narrow lumbar canal. R = width of the radicular canal or of the antero-lateral recess (51).

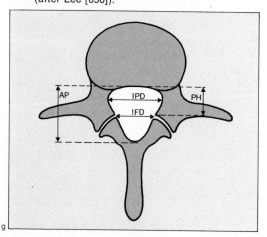

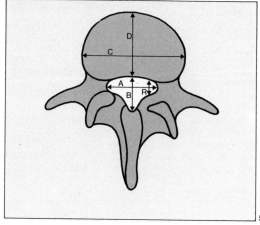

(Lumbar) spinal stenosis (93-53)

The Verbiest classification (49, 51) lists the following forms:

● **Congenital forms** (achondroplasia and other chondrodysplasias, severe malformations of the spinal column, meningoceles, spina bifida, vertebral dysgenesis and the like).

● **Developmental forms** (usually dysplasias of the neural arch, e. g. excessively short roots and the like).

● **Acquired forms** (arthrosis of the facetal joints, spondylolisthesis, sequelae of trauma and surgery, severe kyphosis or scoliosis, Paget's disease, discopathy and the like).

(Lumbar) spinal stenoses lead to typical neurological deficiency symptoms as a result of compression of the neurogenic structures concerned (narrow lumbar canal syndrome, narrow radicular canal syndrome).

● **CT**

Because the vertebral bodies are demonstrated axially, the canal can be measured accurately by computerized tomography provided that the dorsal posterior surface of the vertebral bodies is aligned in a strict axial direction (scoutview – cf. CT terminology, 97-00). Tilting by a mere 10° leads to an illusory enlargement of the sagittal diameter of 0.8 mm (51). The measurement should be made with a wide window setting and a medium window position (97-00). It is also advisable to measure the distances on an electronically enlarged display, since the interactive display is frequently inaccurate (51).

Computerized tomography can provide quite an amount of morphometric data (Fig. 93-5i, k), the most important of which from a clinical point of view is shortening of the median anteroposterior distance (Verbiest) (Fig. 93-5f). From a diameter of 12 mm it is regarded as relative stenosis, from a diameter of 10 mm as absolute stenosis. Special attention must be paid to the lateral recess, which is bounded cranially by the medial contour of the superior articular facet and the lamina, laterally by the pedicles and caudally by the vertebral body and the adjacent intervertebral space. The spinal canal usually has a transverse oval shape at the level of L1 and assumes more of a triangular or deltoid configuration caudalward, which increases to a clover-leaf shape in pathological cases. The extent of the indentation due to intervertebral arthrosis can be described by the distance to the dorsal wall of the vertebral body (Fig. 93-5g). Similarly, constrictions of the spinal canal due to spondylotic drawing-out of the posterior edge of the vertebral body or to increased segmental mobility (as a result of a narrowed intervertebral space) can be demonstrated with a high degree of accuracy by computerized tomography. Scoliosis frequently makes it difficult to compare the sides and thus accurately to measure or assess an asymmetrical canal.

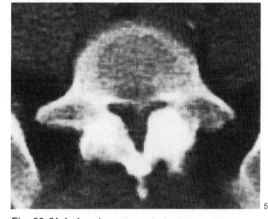

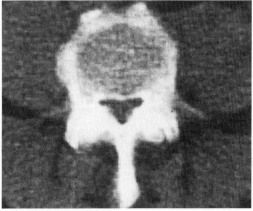

Fig. 93-**5i, k: Lumbar stenosis** in the computed tomogram due to intervertebral arthrosis.

Disc herniation (93-54)

A normal intervertebral disc is 5–15 mm in height. The density of the nucleus pulposus is said to contrast slightly with that of the anulus fibrosus when a high-resolution scanner is used (641). In a healthy person the disc projects only slightly above the adjacent contours of the vertebral body. On marked dehydration it loses height and bulges out a bit more in all directions but, overall, symmetrically. Herniation is marked by isolated, dorsoconvex protrusion in front of the ventroconvex configuration of the posterior surface of the vertebral canal.

● **CT**

In the computed tomogram the difference in density from the lumen of the spinal canal is so small in the case of a well hydrated disc that discrete prolapses of the disc cannot be detected in all cases (647). Demonstration is, however, more certain with increasing degeneration of the anulus fibrosus, which is usually accompanied by an increase of density or by calcifications. In these cases, computerized tomography is superior to myelography in that the entire circumference of the disc and herniated masses can be scanned in one slice. Overall, comparative studies show that computerized tomography is at least equal to the invasive method of myelography.

Difficulties are encountered with both methods in the demonstration of a recurrent prolapse, the density of which cannot be distinguished from that of postoperative scar tissue. The value of contrast medium administration in these cases has not yet been clearly established.

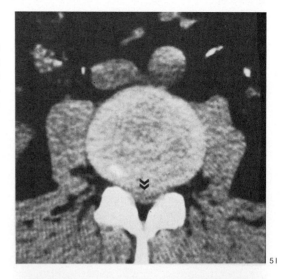

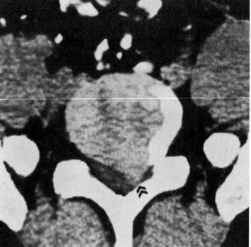

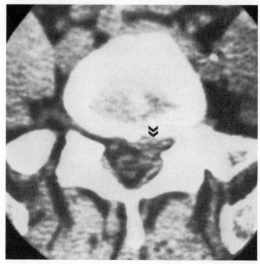

Fig. 93-5l–n: Disc herniation.
5 l = medial herniation
5 m = lateral herniation (L 5/S 1),
5 n = lateral herniation (L 4/L 5).

Skeleton

Vertebragenic tumours and tumour-like lesions (93-55)

Apart from **haemangiomas, primary tumours** of the vertebrae, e. g. myelomas, chordomas, giant cell tumours, osteomas, osteoblastomas, osteoid osteomas, osteogenic fibromas, osteochondromas, chondro-, osteo-, fibrosarcomas, Ewing's sarcomas, are rare in comparison to **metastatic tumours.** The extent within the vertebral arch, the constriction of the vertebral canal, marginal erosions of the vertebral body and discrete circumscribed destructions of the vertebral arch and its processes can usually be detected better by computerized tomography than by conventional methods (662). In particular, computerized tomography permits evaluation of intraspinal and paravertebral tumour invasion of the surrounding tissue in the case of **soft-tissue tumours** (myelomas, giant cell tumours, neurofibromas, fibrosarcomas etc.). Narrowness of the vertebral canal in **tumour-like lesions** (Paget's disease, fibrous dysplasia) can also be reliably assessed (93-53). The differential-diagnostic criteria are based on the usual radiological signs.

In the search for lytic **metastases,** attention must be paid to the continuity of the cortical bone in addition to localized destruction of the structure of the trabecular substance. Osteoplastic metastases must be differentiated from compacta islands, which can be seen in increased numbers in the computed tomogram. Bone islands are sharply demarcated and are devoid of contour defects and local destruction.

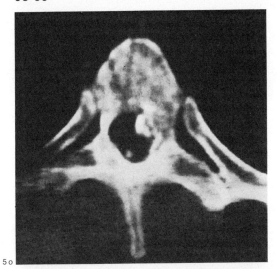

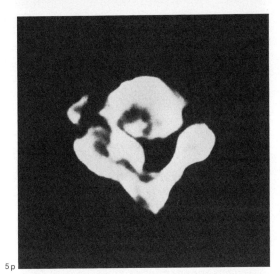

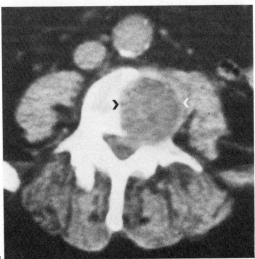

Fig. 93-5 o–q: **Vertebragenic tumours.**

5 o: Osteogenic giant cell tumour at the level of cervical vertebra 2–3 with constriction of the spinal canal.

5 p: Osteochondroma of the root of the left arch at the level of thoracic vertebra 3.

5 q: Giant cell tumour of lumbar vertebra 4 with destruction of the vertebral body and incipient infiltration of the spinal canal (>).

Intraspinal masses (93-56)

A. Congenital masses

Congenital tumours include lipomas, dermoids, epidermoids, teratomas, meningoceles and myelomeningoceles.

Lipomas are usually discovered in children below 15 years of age and are normally accompanied by defects of the neural arch (including the sacral canal), diastematomyelias and other vertebral malformations. Lipomas are usually extramedullary lesions, or they are situated secondarily within the medulla. They occur with almost equal frequency in all segments of the vertebral canal. Extradural tumours can assume an hourglass shape if an intraspinal and an extraspinal part communicate through the intervertebral foramen.

Dermoids are usually well-encapsulated, round or oval masses with walls of varying thickness and, likewise, are frequently combined with dysrhaphias. They are found primarily in the lumbosacral segment as intra- or extramedullary tumours.

Epidermoid tumours occur somewhat less frequently than dermoids and do not become manifest until later in life. They are usually found as intradural and extramedullary masses.

Teratomas are the most frequent sacrococcygeal tumours. The benign forms, which are observed primarily in children and adolescents, can achieve a considerable size and are then situated within and outside the osseous pelvis. Malignant teratomas, on the other hand, do not become clinically apparent until later in life, and then usually in men. They are usually highly invasive and display regional lymph node metastasis.

(Myelo-)meningoceles are congenital malformations of the neural tube ranging from an open neural plate to a closed spinal canal and are found most frequently in the lower lumbar segment. Sacral meningoceles usually protrude ventrally or laterally through the sacral foramina and are accompanied by osseous malformations of the sacrum of varying severity. (Myelo-)meningoceles are usually recognized immediately after birth, whereas the so-called occult meningoceles, which lead to widening of the spinal canal, do not become clinically manifest until later. A bony spur in the middle of the widened spinal canal is typical of a **diastematomyelia**. The separation of the spinal cord can also consist of a chondral or connective-tissue septum.

B. Acquired masses

The most frequent intraspinal masses are **intradural-extramedullary** tumours (about 55–60% of cases), of which **meningeomas** and **neurofibromas** are the most important group. Meningeomas – which, like the intracranial form, occasionally display psammomatous calcifications – are situated in the thoracic segment in 80% of cases. Neurofibromas, which occur with almost equal frequency, have no predilection for any particular segment of the spine. About 15% of meningeomas and 30% of neurofibromas are found extradurally. The usually small intraspinal masses do not lead to osseous usurpation until later, on expansion of the tumours, while the peripheral neurofibromas situated in the radicular canal extend the narrow osseous borders of the intervertebral foramen early on.

The second most frequent group of intraspinal masses are **extradural tumours,** which usually invade the vertebral canal from the immediate vicinity. They are represented primarily by metastases of the vertebral column (bronchial and mammary carcinoma), and penetrate the dural sac on increasing infiltration. Primary extradural metastasis without bone destruction is rare. Sarcomas and caudal chordomas are an occasional finding, the preferred site being extradural.

Intramedullary masses

The main **solid** masses are gliomas or paragliomas **(ependymomas** in 60–65% of cases, **astrocytomas** in 25–30% of cases and, less frequently, **oligodendrogliomas, melanomas, glioblastoma multiforme** and **haemangioblastomas).** While the predilection site of astrocytomas is the thoracic and cervical region, ependymomas develop most frequently beneath the medullary cone in the region of the filum terminale, although they can also occur in the other segments of the spinal canal. Depending on their size, ependymomas lead to erosion of the vertebral bodies and to thinning and protrusion of the vertebral arch, which can eventually be perforated.

The **syringomyelia** is a **cystic** mass based on a prenatal developmental disturbance and produces clinical symptoms between the age of 25 and 40 years. It consists patho-anatomically of cylindrical widening of the central canal

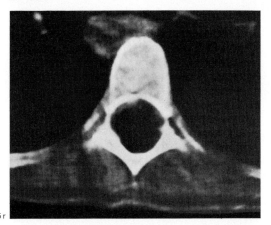

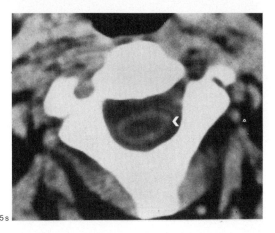

Fig. 93-5r–t: Intraspinal lesions.

5r: Intraspinal lipoma with dilation of the vertebral canal and fat-equidense density values.

5s: Cystic cervicothoracic astrocytoma with reduced density values within the cervical medulla giving rise to a ring-shaped appearance (>).

5t: Cervical syringomyelia with reduced density values within the cervical medulla, giving rise to a ring-shaped appearance.

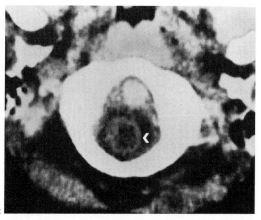

(hydromelia) which occurs either symmetrically or as a protrusion; the cystic formations do not always communicate with each other. The widening of the spinal cord is usually fusiform and can lead secondarily to local widening of the vertebral canal. This is generally not the case in other cystic intramedullary masses which are regarded as the sequelae of **myelomalacia** and necroses due to trauma or ischaemia. The latter must be differentiated from intratumoral necroses in ependymomas and gliomas (Fig. 93-5s).

● **CT**

In analogy to the plain X-ray examination, **widening of the vertebral canal** is an important if insensitive radiological sign. The extent of the osseous defects in dysrhaphias can usually be demonstrated without difficulty and in detail (spina bifida [occult], os sacrum bifidum etc.). Like constriction, widening of the spinal canal must also be measured exactly parallel to the posterior surface of the vertebral body (93-53). Thinning and convex deformity of the laminae become evident at an early stage in the computed tomogram and suggest an expansive intraspinal process.

In **congenital tumours with dysrhaphia** the diagnosis can be made clinically in the majority of cases. However, computerized tomography can be used to determine the extent of the osseous changes. The size and extent of the lipomatous component (lipomeningocele) can be determined in comparison to the fluid-filled (water-equidense) parts. The demonstration of a low-placed medullary cone or a tethered (usually thickened) filum terminale is frequently successful in dysrhaphias with few external signs, e. g. in occult spina bifida (646). Ventrally and laterally protruding meningoceles and the bony spurs of diastematomyelia are readily accessible to computerized tomography (Fig. 93-5w).

The demonstration of **intraspinal masses without widening of the vertebral canal,** and particulary of areas of tissue containing calcium, water and fat, frequently succeeds in the plain scan via visualization of distinct differences of density in the spinal canal. A meningeoma, for example, can be detected very sensitively by means of psammomatous calcifications, concentric and, more frequently, circumscribed unilateral forms being demonstrable. Central cystic changes of the spinal cord can be demarcated in the cervical region by high-resolution computerized tomography,

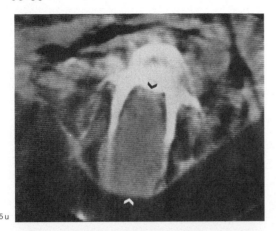

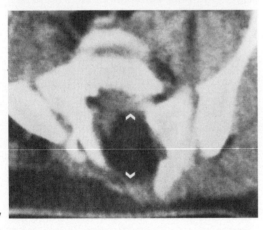

Fig. 93-5u–w: **Dysrhaphias.**

5u: Meningocele at S1. Open sacral canal with protruding soft-tissue mass displaying moderately reduced density values in the centre.

5v: Lipomeningocele. Open sacral canal from L5–S3. Density values within the mass in the region of those of fat.

5w: Diastematomyelia. Demonstration of a median osseous lamella within the spinal canal.

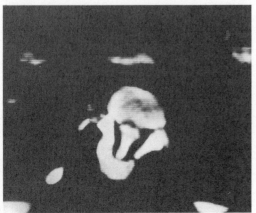

making the diagnosis of syringomyelia in this segment of the spine (under certain technical conditions) highly successful. The differentiation from other medullary cystic masses must be narrowed down by the case history and clinical data. Although circumscribed areas of fatty tissue density can correspond to a lipoma, they must be differentiated from epidural fatty tissue. This demarcation frequently presents difficulties and, consequently, a lipoma is frequently only discovered in the plain scan by expansive growth with widening of the vertebral canal (Fig. 93-5r). The value of intravenous contrast medium administration has not yet been clearly defined. So far it has been found to be of some assistance only in the diagnosis of angioblastomas and arteriovenous anomalies, which are marked by positive enhancement.

Since the subarachnoid space cannot be reliably demonstrated by the present generation of scanners, the relationship of an intramedullary mass to the spinal marrow cannot be clarified by computerized tomography. This space with its branches and pouches can, on the other hand, be demarcated in detail by **myelography,** so that even very small masses situated within the space can be demonstrated. Computerized tomography can frequently complement myelography to a decisive degree, particularly when epidural and paravertebral lesions are present.

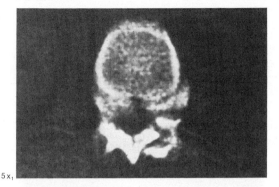

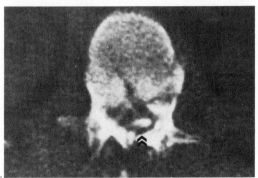

Fig. 93-**5x**: **Fracture of lumbar vertebra 1.** Dislocation of the facetal joint and disruption of continuity within the vertebral body. Demonstration of a fragment within the vertebral canal (x_2 ≫).

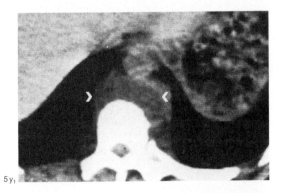

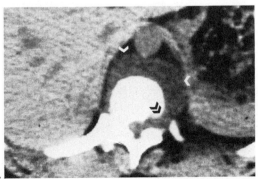

Trauma of the vertebral column (93-57)

The classical X-ray examinations of the traumatized vertebral column are not replaced by computerized tomography, but rather complemented by it to resolve special problems.

As in classical radiodiagnosis, the disruption of osseous continuity can only be demonstrated when the rays cut it tangentially. Fracture lines running almost vertically to the horizontal CT slice and which are not always visible on frontal and anteroposterior X-ray films can be clearly depicted within the slice (663). Because of the partial volume effect, only a translucent zone can be identified in gaping fractures which run obliquely through the CT slice. The computed tomogram — particularly when made with the usual slice thicknesses of 8 to 13 mm — is less informative than conventional radiological techniques in compression fractures of the vertebral bodies. The vertebral arch or canal, on the other hand, is depicted with particular clarity, permitting detailed identification of infractions of the laminae, divulsions of the vertebral bodies, dislocations of the pedicles and fragments within the spinal canal. In most cases, the facetal joints are also clearly depicted in the computed tomogram. Luxation fractures in whiplash traumas (distraction traumas) can be recognized by the absence of articular surfaces (naked facet). The concomitant haematoma and traumatic changes of the adjacent soft tissues are demonstrated and diagnosed with the same slice (particularly after contrast medium administration), while the intraspinal haematoma cannot yet be reliably depicted because of inadequate absorption resolution at the present time.

Inflammations of the vertebral column (93-58)

Inflammations of the vertebral column primarily involve the discs and the adjacent parts of the vertebral bodies — regions which are accessible to computerized tomography only under certain conditions, particularly when the intervertebral space is already deformed. The **paravertebral abscess** is, however, an important indication for CT, since its extent and route of expansion can be determined with a high degree of accuracy (86-37).

Fig. 93-**5y**: **Tuberculous spondylitis** with paravertebral abscess (>) and inflammatory liquefaction of the root of the left arch (y_2 ≫). Density of the abscess: 21 HU.

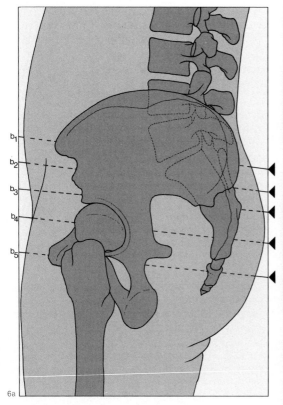

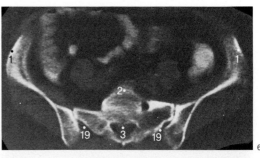

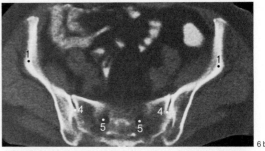

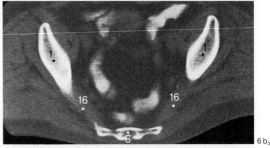

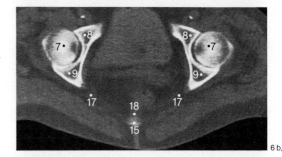

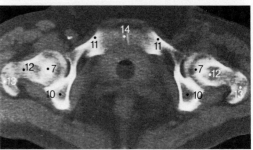

Fig. 93-6a, b: Osseous pelvis.

6a: Lateral view.

6b: In the transverse section. Cf. 6a for level of section. (Bone scan: window setting 500 HU.)

Key
1. Wing of ilium
2. Promontory
3. Sacral canal
4. Iliosacral joints
5. Sacral foramina of the pelvis
6. Sacrum
7. Head of the femur
8. Anterior pillar of the acetabulum
9. Posterior pillar of the acetabulum
10. Tuber ossis pubis
11. Superior pubic ramus
12. Neck of the femur
13. Greater trochanter
14. Symphysis
15. Coccyx
16. Ischiadic foramen
17. Sacrospinal ligament
18. Anococcygeal ligament
19. Retroauricular space

Osseous pelvis (93-60)

Anatomy and imaging (93-61)

Because of its convex surfaces, the osseous pelvis offers the standard projections of radiodiagnosis only a few tangential and thus demonstrable boundary surfaces. The third – transversal – plane of computerized tomography can depict additional contours, in particular those of the wing of ilium, the sacroiliac joints and the hip joints. With the patient in supine position, the anterior surface of the sacrum runs for the greater part obliquely through the CT slice. Because of the partial volume effect, it therefore appears as a poorly defined structure.

Osteogenic tumours (93-62)

In analogy to the discussion under 93-40, the differential diagnosis of pelvic **bone tumours** is narrowed down and decided by standard radiographs. Although the extent of osteogenic tumours is recognizable in the absence of soft-tissue components, signs of displacement in exophytic forms can arouse clinical interest – unlike in the case of the extremities. In tumours with soft-tissue components **(metastases, myelomas, aneurysmatic bone cysts, sarcomas, malignant lymphomas, chondromatoses, giant cell tumours, chordomas etc.),** the bone destruction is frequently only the tip of the iceberg.

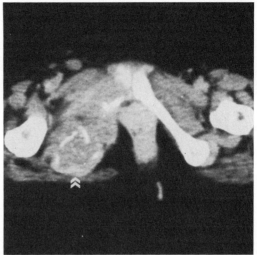
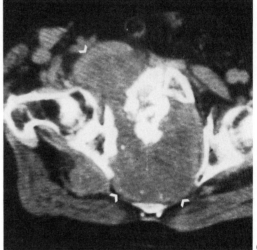
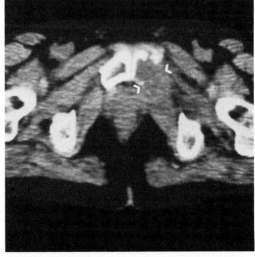

Fig. 93-6 c–e: Osteogenic tumours of the pelvis.
6 c: Chondrosarcoma of the right ischium.
6 d: Osteogenic sarcoma of the right pubic bone with virtual occupation of the minor pelvis.
6 e: Giant cell tumour of the left pubic bone (>).

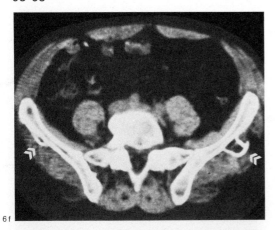

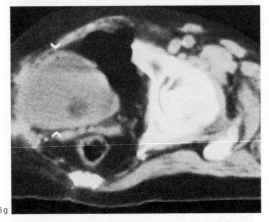

Fig. 93-**6f–h: Tumours of the osseous pelvis.**
6f: Cartilaginous exostosis (≫).
6g: Osteogenic sarcoma. Recurrence in status following hemipelvectomy.

6h: Metastatic destruction of the wing of ilium left and of the sacrum in metastatic cervical carcinoma (≫).

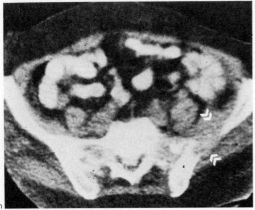

● CT

The indication for computerized tomography in tumours of the osseous pelvis is therefore the determination of the extent of a previously diagnosed mass. Infiltration of the soft tissues of the pelvic cavity, the gluteal muscles and critical nerve regions is usually readily demonstrable, although total oral opacification of the bowel is recommended in extensive processes. Frequently, the computed tomogram is also of assistance in the differential diagnosis – namely when an intrapelvic or extrapelvic soft-tissue component of the tumour is demonstrated, which must be regarded as malignant until the opposite is proven. It is not always possible to differentiate between primary bone tumours of soft-tissue density and retroperitoneal masses invading the bones secondarily. Apart from osteogenic tumours, neurogenic (neurofibromas, ganglioneurinomas) and congenital tumours (dermoid cysts, teratomas, chordomas, meningoceles) must also be considered in the differential diagnosis of primary neoplasms in the region of the sacrum and coccyx.

Bone injuries (93-63)

In bone injuries, the transversal plane can provide important additional information which complements that from the usual X-ray projections (anteroposterior, ala and obturator films [605]). In fractures of the acetabulum the horizontal circumference of the articular space is reproduced in detail, providing for sensitive demonstration of injuries to the anterior and posterior pillar, intraarticular fragments and divulsions of the head of the hip joint. Fractures of the sacrum and wing of ilium and slight divulsions and subluxations of the sacroiliac joints can also be diagnosed without difficulty in most cases – even with marked superimposition of intestinal gas and suboptimal positioning of the patient. The concomitant haematoma in the region of the fracture and other intrapelvic soft-tissue injuries can be discovered with the same examination. Certain constellations call for open revision of the acetabulum fracture, particularly when the dislocated dorsal pillar leads to instability, when fragments have entered the articular space and when divulsions of the head of the femur or complex fractures of the medial articular surface are present. In these cases, the computed tomogram can provide important diagnostic information for planning surgery (621).

The sacroiliac joints (93-64)

The sacroiliac joints have convex articular surfaces which — apart from the caudal section — can be clearly depicted in the axial plane. The space which can be seen in the computed tomogram between the sacrum and the wing of ilium corresponds ventrally to the articular surfaces of the sacroiliac joints and dorsally to the retroarticular space, which is filled by the interosseous sacroiliac ligaments (dorsal capsular apparatus).

In **loosening of the pelvis** (sacrolisthesis), computerized tomography can reveal slight shifts of the sacrum in relation to the ilium which can otherwise only be detected by specific functional X-ray films (732).

In **luxations of the sacroiliac joints,** computerized tomography depicts not only the degree of dislocation, but also the concomitant haematoma. Calcifications of the dorsal capsular apparatus (pelvic rigidity) are clearly depicted in the computed tomogram. In contrast, the practically important question of sacroiliitis can be answered no sooner by computerized tomography than by conventional pluridimensional tomography. The same applies to iliitis condensans and the accessory sacroiliac joints (732).

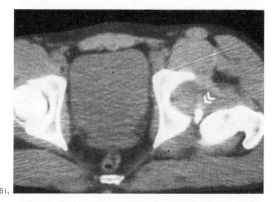

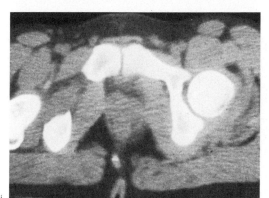

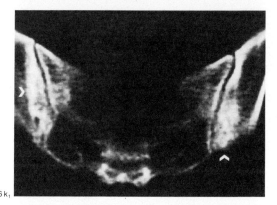

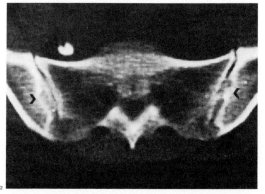

Fig. 93-**6i: Luxation of the left hip joint** with splintering of the dorsal acetabular margin (i_1). Status after reposition (i_2).

Fig. 93-**6k: Iliosacral arthritis** with sclerosis and erosion on both sides of the iliosacral interarticular space.

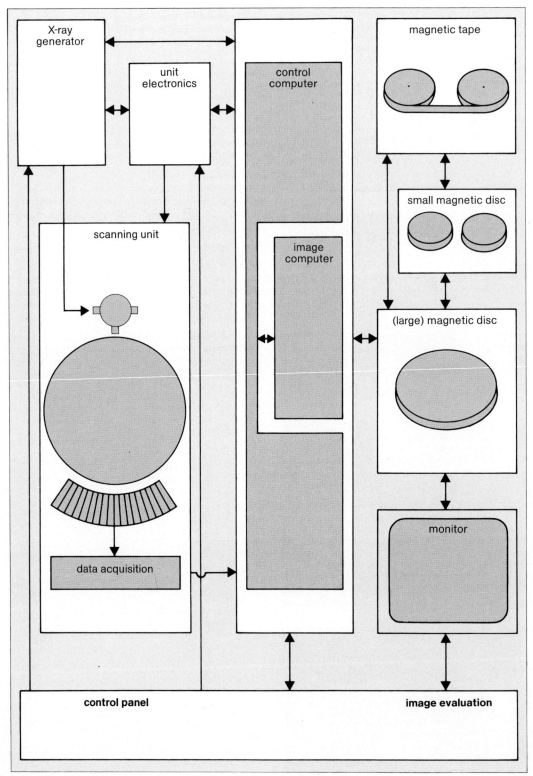

Fig. 97-1: **Block diagram of the CT unit.**

CT terminology (97-00)
(alphabetical)

Absorption of X-rays → attenuation of X-rays

Absorption profile: A curve of detector readings from one angle (view, projection) of the scanning movement.

Absorption resolution (= density resolution): This is limited by the image noise (3-10) described by the standard deviation of the density values from the mean value (→ image evaluation, histogram analysis). The smaller the standard deviation, the better the absorption resolution. Depending on the radiation dose, it can be less than 0.3% ($\triangleq$ 3 HU).

Addition of image slices → image evaluation

Algorithm = a rule of (procedure for the) computation

Archival storage = long term storage → image filing

Artifacts: Artifacts (artificial products) are errors in the reconstructed image. There are many different types in computerized tomography because of the complex imaging system. Since data acquisition and electronic processing are related to projections (→ image reconstruction), an error in the reconstructed image frequently leads to adulteration of linear or streaky zones of density which run through the entire computed tomogram. In the case of movement artifacts (cf. Fig. 97-2), which are of clinical importance, the several projections of the object detail moved during scanning cannot be brought to congruence in the reconstructed image. The result is therefore not local blurring due to movement, but a streaky, star-shaped pattern from the disturbed projections which pass tangentially through the object moved. This property must be taken into account when analysing the image.

Attenuation of X-rays takes place as the rays pass through the material. Depending on the radiation energy, it occurs as a photoelectric effect (absorption), scattering or pair production (the latter is irrelevant for diagnostic work). The attenuation is described quantitatively by the law of attenuation:

Law of attenuation: $I = I_0 e^{-\mu d}$
I_0 = intensity on entry
I = intensity on exit
μ = linear attenuation coefficient
d = path length

Back-projection → image reconstruction

Beam hardening: A heterogeneous beam traversing an absorbing medium becomes richer in higher energy X-rays.

Centre → image reproduction, window level

Collimation = shaping of the X-ray beam. There are two kinds of collimation – primary (on the tube side) and secondary (on the detector side). Collimation affects the thickness and geometry of the slice (→), the absorption resolution (→) and the radiation dose (→) for the patient.

Convolution → image reconstruction

Convolution core → image reconstruction

Convolution function → image reconstruction

Coordinates → image matrix

Density profile → image evaluation

Density resolution → absorption resolution

Detector: A measuring chamber which detects incoming X-rays and indicates them quantitatively. Materials used for the detectors in computerized tomography are highly compressed gasses (e.g. xenon) or solid matter (e.g. iodide or germanate crystals).

Digital X-ray picture (topogram, scoutview, radiogram): With the tube detector system fixed, the patient is advanced successively and longitudinally through the scanning unit. This gives rise to a digital X-ray picture. It consists of an image matrix (→), the rows of which correspond to the slice thickness. The number of picture elements (→) of each row is determined by the number of detectors used in the measurement. Lateral, antero-posterior and oblique projections can be achieved depending on the angular position of the tube. The level of the slice in the body can be reproducibly set before the scan. The inclination of the scanning unit to the body axis can be controlled in the lateral projection (important for examinations of the spinal column).

Directory: Display (list of contents) of the occupied storage places (files) for recalling an individual computed tomogram.

Disc store → equipment, image store

Display = reproduction unit

Distance measurement → image evaluation

Cause of artifacts			
Physical artifacts	**Patient-related artifacts**		
Beam hardening	Movement of patient	Metallic foreign bodies	Transgression of scan field
Name			
Hardening artifacts (shading, dishing)	Movement artifacts	Streak artifacts (high-density streaking)	
Appearance			
Shadowy adulteration of density in surrounding area and within dense structures.	Streaky shift of density, the extent of which depends on the contrast of the structure moved. The streaks run (tangentially) through the centre of movement.	Streaky, high (positive, negative) density adulteration of density proceeding from the metal object (cf. loss of measured value).	Areal increase of density in the areas of the image adjacent to the parts of the organ transgressing the scan field. The entire level of density of the computed tomogram is usually shifted at the same time.
a, b: Teflon rod in water. The high radio-density of teflon produces shadowy adulteration of density in the vicinity (a) and within the rod (b). **c:** Density gradient within a large renal cyst due to dense adjacent structures.	Streak artifacts **a:** In short linear, **b, c:** in oscillating movement during the scanning process. **Contrast: a, b:** air in water **c:** Contrast medium solution (+ 150 HU) in water.	Streaking **a:** Due to a hip joint prosthesis with the density of metal. **b, c:** Due to metal clips.	**a:** Oval water phantom exceeding the scan field laterally: general increase of density by 14 HU and lateral (>), visible adulteration of density. **b, c:** Analogous adulteration of density in the patient.

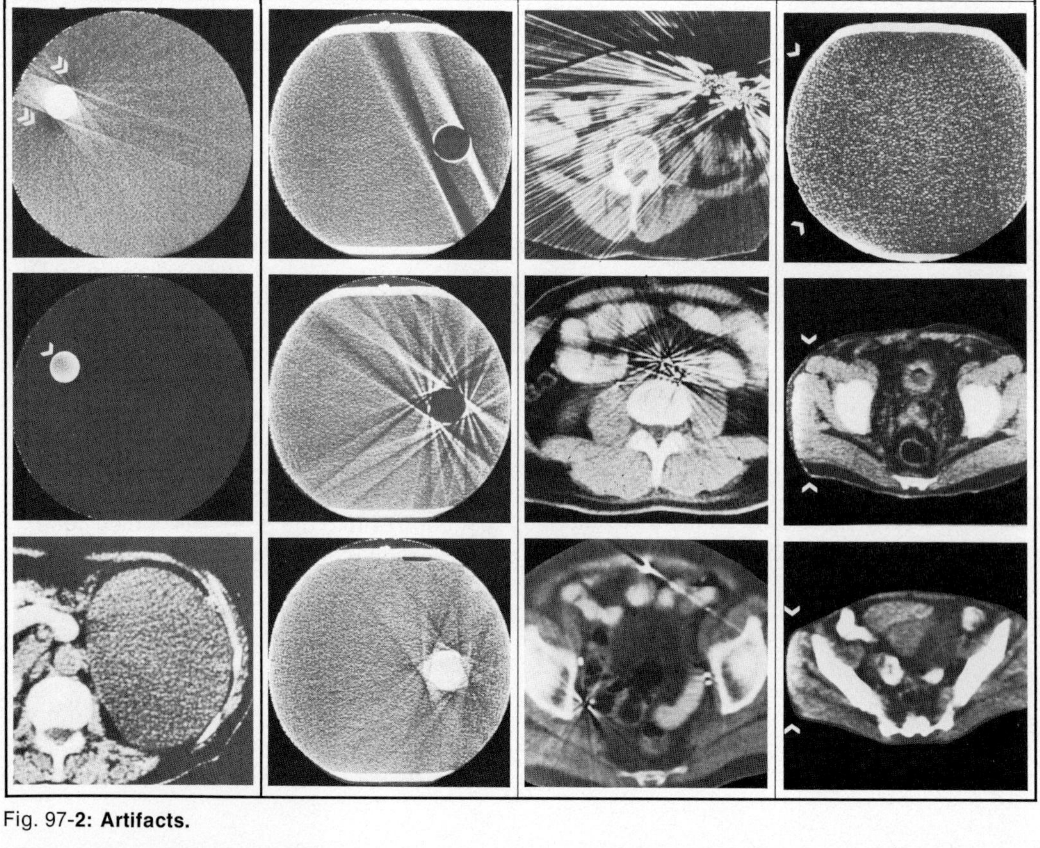

Fig. 97-2: **Artifacts.**

CT terminology

Cause of artifacts

Scanner-related artifacts

Reconstruction filter	Overloaded data acquisition	Maladjusted detectors (3rd generation scanners)	Loss of measured value due to scanner defect
Name			
Edge effects	Overrange artifacts	Ring artifacts	e.g. line artifacts
Appearance			
Overshooting of edges occurring at organ boundaries of great contrast (e.g. lung, bone).	Plateau-shaped shift of density within and in the vicinity of parts of organs which were not measured linearly by the overloaded detector-amplifier system.	Fine, circular figures running around the centre of the image.	The missing projection appears in the computed tomogram as a diametric, trilinear structure.
Edge effects **a:** Simulation of a subarachnoid space. **b:** Simulation of pleural calcifications.	**a:** Streaky artifacts in the lung phantom due to overranging. **b:** Areal reduction of density in ventral areas of the abdomen due to overloading of the measuring system.	**a, b:** Disturbing circular figures due to maladjustment of the detectors.	**a, b:** Loss of measured values from a single projection (trilinear structure). **c:** Loss of measured values from several projections of the same direction.

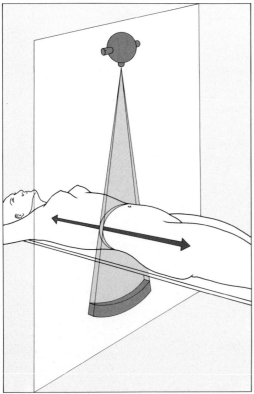

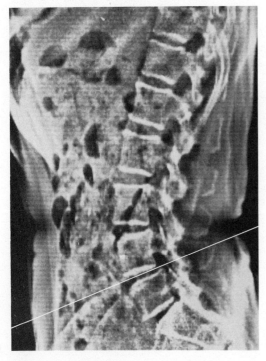

Fig. 97-**3, 4**: **Digital X-ray image.** Summation images result when the scanning system is fixed and the patient is moved longitudinally. The slice plane can be positioned exactly by fading in the tilt of the gantry (white line, Fig. 4).

Dose → radiation dose

Edge enhancement → artifacts

Equipment: A computerized tomographic machine consists of

● the **computer,** which controls all partial functions of the system and reconstructs the image (→ image reconstruction)

● the **scanning unit** (gantry), which consists of the tube, detector system and data-acquisition system

● the **X-ray generator** and the **equipment electronics,** which are assigned to the scanning unit

● the **control console** (control panel) and **image evaluation unit,** with which the individual functions can be recalled in dialogue with the computer

● facilities for **image storage:** a magnetic disc for temporary storage of the computed tomograms (intermediate store, disc store). Long-term storage (magnetic tape, floppy disc) → image filing.

Fan-beam = fan-shaped emission of rays (1-20)

File → image filing

File = storage place

Filter → image reconstruction, → image filtration

Floppy disc = small magnetic disc → image filing

Gantry = scanning unit (→ equipment)

Gonadal dose → radiation dose

Highlighting: In highlighting, selectable ranges of density are made to appear light, as a result of which they stand out clearly from the grey shades of the computed tomogram – regardless of the window setting.

HR/CT = high-resolution CT. The picture elements in areas of the image (usually central) can be diminished in size by reducing the scan field or narrowing the distance between the detectors, i.e. the spatial resolution can be improved. At present, picture element diameters of 0.2 mm can already be achieved. Diminishing the size of the picture or volume element leads to an increase of image noise, so that particularly high-contrast structures, e.g. bones, can be clearly demonstrated by HR/CT. For the same reason, longer scanning times must be chosen for soft-tissue structures. Since small measuring fields are usually employed, this is also referred to as a **sector scan**.

HU = Hounsfield unit

Image evaluation: Objective data can be gained from the computed tomogram by simple mathematical operations. The evaluation of an image is facilitated by an interactive display (→).

• Area and volume measurement: The area content of an ROI (→) is calculated from the number of picture elements contained (1-40), while the volume is calculated from the number of volume elements contained (1-30).

• Distance measurement: The distance between two structures in the body can be determined by marking two points in the image. **Measurement of an angle** to the coordinate system (x, y axis) can be performed in a similar way.

• Density measurement, histogram analysis: The histogram is the distribution of the frequency of a variable, in this case the density values. The frequency distribution of the density values of an ROI (→) is usually presented as a columnar diagram above the density scale. **Normal distribution** appears in the histogram as a symmetrical (Gaussian) bell-shaped curve, **the standard deviation (SD)** of which can be calculated via the half-value width. The distribution of the density values of a homogeneous medium (water phantom) is usually normal and, hence, unequivocally described by the **mean value** and standard deviation. The standard deviation is displayed directly by the evaluation units and represents primarily the **image noise** i.e. the statistical variation of the photon flow during scanning (quantum noise). Inhomogeneous media (tissues) usually display (asymmetrical) widening of the histogram curve. Different tissue components can appear in the histogram as additional peaks (plurimodal histogram). Formation of mean values is not permissible (and inaccurate) in such cases.

• Subtraction, addition, density profile: The density values of two computed tomograms of the **same slice** are **subtracted** from each other. Subtraction is particularly suitable for contrast medium studies, where the precontrast values are subtracted from the contrasted computed tomogram and the accumulation of contrast medium can be visualized directly. By means of **addition** of adjacent slices it is possible to construct larger slice thicknesses in retro-

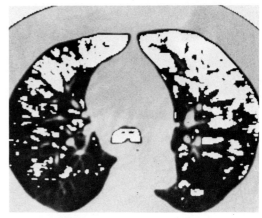

Fig. 97-**5: Highlighting.** All the points of the image which appear white lie within a (freely selectable) density range (here: −850 to −1000 HU).

Fig. 97-**6,7: Density measurement.** The density values of the picture elements lying within the region of interest (here circular areas) display symmetrical curves (6) in homogeneous media and asymmetrical (7) or irregular density curves in inhomogeneous media (e.g. pulmonary tissue).

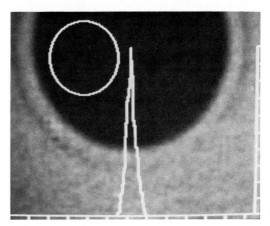

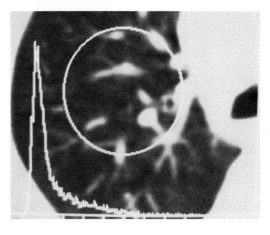

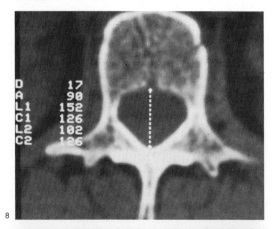

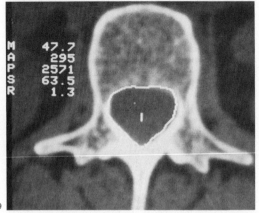

Fig. 97-8: **Distance measurement.** Marking of two points in the image (+). Distance here (D) expressed in mm.

Fig. 97-9: **Area measurement.** The area of interest is circumscribed with a light pencil. The sum of the picture elements contained represents the transverse area, here in mm² (A). The circumscribed area serves simultaneously as a region of interest for the density measurement (cf. Fig. 97-6,7).

Fig. 97-10: **Density profile.** The density values of the picture elements lying on the chosen stretch of the image are reproduced not in grey tones, but in scale units related to the location.

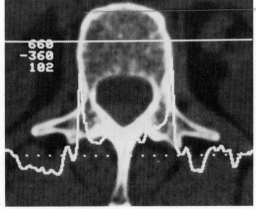

spect. In the case of **density profiles,** the density values of selectable stretches or diameters depicted in the computed tomogram as different shades of grey are represented (analogously) as a density curve, whereby the y axis corresponds to the density scale.

Image filing: The computed tomogram contained in the temporary disc store can be recalled to the monitor and recorded **photographically.** This permanently fixes the window level and width (→ image reproduction) of the computed tomogram. The **magnetic tape** and the **floppy disc** (small magnetic disc) are long-term electronic (digital) storage media on which the entire information pertinent to a computed tomogram is stored. This means that, on later recall of an image, the window level and width can be set and other processes of image evaluation (→) performed.

Image filtration: Each individual point of an image can be subjected to a computing operation which takes account of the extent and importance of the surrounding points. Image noise, definition and contours can be optically altered by different image filters. Image filtration, which takes the already computed tomogram as its basis and can be repeated at will (secondary image filtration), should not be confused with the primary filtration of image reconstruction (→).

Image matrix: Depending on the type of scanner, the image matrix may be composed of 80 x 80, 160 x 160, 256 x 256 or 512 x 512 picture elements, or pixels, arranged in rows and columns, and is usually quadratic. The individual pixels are unequivocally defined by the **coordinate system.** By general agreement, pixels on the axes (x, y) are counted from the top left-hand corner of the matrix. A picture element (x_1, y_1) is defined by the pair of numbers making up the intercept (in this case $x_1 = 10$ and $y_1 = 21$). x_1 is also denoted as the 10th **column,** y_1 as the 21st **row.**

Image noise: Statistical inaccuracy of the density value of an individual pixel caused by the statistical variation in the photon flow (histogram analysis → image evaluation).

Image reconstruction: Image reconstruction is a process of computation which produces the computed tomogram from the data acquired. The algebraic methods (1–10) have now been replaced by faster convolution algorithms. These involve subjecting the absorption profiles to a **filtering function** (convolution core) and then superimposing them in the direction from which they were measured (back-projection). The filtering function (core) is necessary to suppress the blurring which occurs at the boundaries of the object on back-projection. It can be applied in various ways and be adapted to certain problems. The impression of the image alters as a result. **Edge enhancement** (edge effects) at absorption boundaries may resemble artifacts.

Image reproduction: The computed tomogram consists of a grid of numerical values covering a scale of, for instance, 2,000 units. Since, under normal evaluation conditions, only 15–20 **shades of grey** can be distinguished with the naked eye, each shade would have to represent about 50 HU if the grey scale is to be extended over the entire density scale. The **image window** was introduced so that fine differences in density can be recognized while allowing evaluation of high-contrast structures. Using the window, the grey scale can be extended over selectable density ranges (25–1000 HU) **(window width). The window level (centre)** within the density scale determines which density value will be represented by the middle shade of grey. The choice of window setting (Fig. 97-14) depends on the diagnostic query. Narrow window settings involve the risk of structures outside the frame not being seen and thus of being excluded from the diagnosis. Wide window settings homogenize and mask slight differences in density.

Interactive display: Individual pixels of the image matrix can be marked on the monitor screen by means of **light pencils (joy stick, roller ball).** The site of the pixels is recorded visually, which obviates the need to note the coordinate intercepts (x_1, y_1) ($\rightarrow$ image matrix). The marked pixels may represent the mid-points of circular areas and rectangles, the surface areas of which can be varied (regular ROI $\rightarrow$). Freely selectable areas are recorded by drawing around the corresponding areas of the image with the light pencil (irregular ROI $\rightarrow$).

Joystick $\rightarrow$ interactive display

Light pencil $\rightarrow$ interactive display

Linear attenuation coefficient $\rightarrow$ attenuation of X-rays

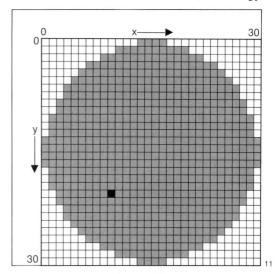

Fig. 97-**11: Coordinates of the image matrix.**

Fig. 97-**12, 13: Image noise.** The image noise limits the density resolution.

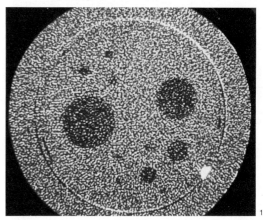

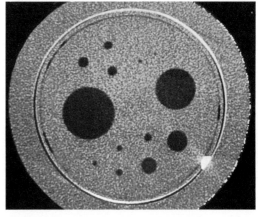

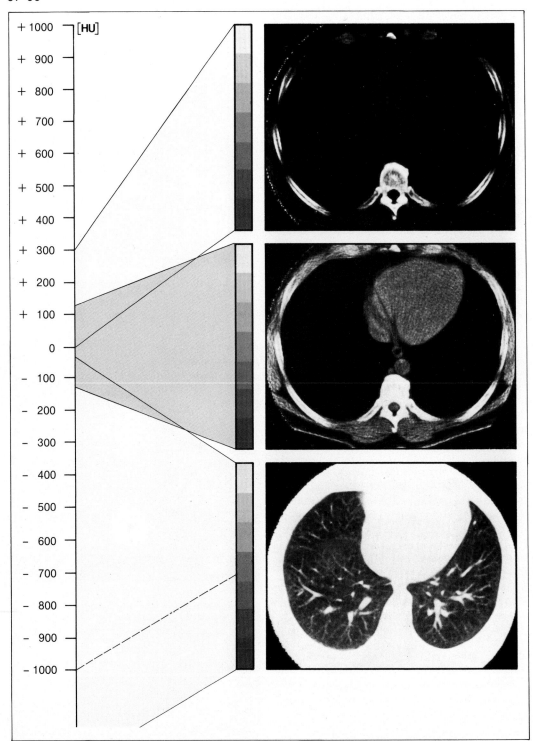

Fig. 97-14: **Window setting** of the computed tomogram. The limited number of grey values (cf. grey tone key left in the computed tomogram) is allocated by the evaluator to a certain density range of the Hounsfield scale by selection of the window level and width. Body tissues of varying density thus become accessible to image evaluation. At the same time, the impression of the image in the same computed tomogram changes considerably.

Magnetic disc → equipment, image store

Matrix: An array of numbers arranged in two dimensions (→ image matrix).

Measurement of angle → image evaluation

Monitor: TV screen used to display the CT image

Noise → image noise

Picture element: The smallest unit of the computed image matrix (→)

Pixel = **pic**ture **el**ement (1-30)

Profile → absorption profile, → image evaluation (density profile)

Projection → absorption profile

Radiation dose:

● **Somatic radiation dose:** With well-collimated scanners, the (somatic) radiation dose **for the trunk of the body** is 2–3 rad. It is therefore of the order of that of other examination methods (urography, colonic contrast enema).

Collimation of the X-rays restricts the dose to the slice of the body to be demonstrated. According to McCullough (758), the maximum surface dose is
3–13 rad per single slice for examinations of the skull
1.5–3.5 rad per single slice for examinations of the trunk,
although doses of more than 10 rad are also possible in the trunk if slower scanning times (low noise scan) are used.

With a series of scans, the formation of half-shadows and scattering cause a 1.2–1.9-fold increase in the dose received in a single slice (pile-up factor, multiple/single ratio). The total dose received during an examination of the whole body is therefore at least 2 rad. A clearer way of describing the radiation stress on the patient is to state the area-dose product, which also permits indirect conclusions about the integral dose of an examination. With most CT examinations, the entire field of entry of a scan series corresponds to the radiographic field of a conventional X-ray film, i.e. the irradiated volume of a scan series and that of a large-format X-ray film are comparable. It is not permissible to multiply the dose values of the single slice by the number of slices scanned and to regard this as the total dose because, although the volume dose increases as the number of slices increases, the energy absorption per volume element (= rad) hardly changes.

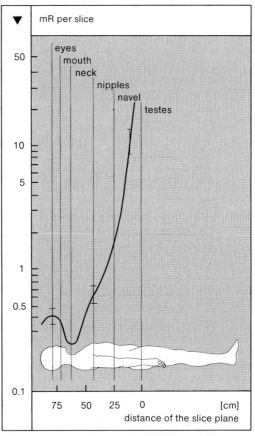

Fig. 97-**15: Gonadal dose** caused by scattered rays in relation to the distance of the scanning plane from the gonads (from 753).

Fig. 97-**16: Increase of the radiation dose** by scattered rays and penumbra formation with an adjacent sclice sequence (pile-up factor) (758).

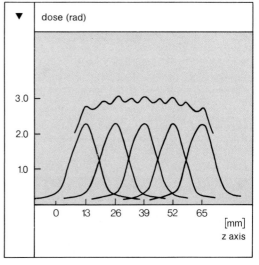

- **Gonadal dose:** If they are not within the slice being scanned, the gonads receive a varying dose of scattered radiation which decreases considerably with increasing distance of the gonads from the slice plane. However, the scattered and leakage radiation within the scanner is greater than that within the body (758).

Region of interest → ROI

ROI = region of interest: An area of the image which can be freely selected during image evaluation by entering the coordinates (→ image matrix) or by means of the interactive display (→).

Scan (scan field, time, area) → scanning

Scanner → equipment

Scanning: Measuring process of the tube-detector system revolving around the patient. The quality of the computed tomogram is determined by a number of (selectable) parameters (scan modes, scan parameters):

- **Scan time:** Shortening the scan times reduces movement artifacts (→ artifacts). Because the capacity of the tube determines the radiation dose which can be used during the scan time, the extent to which the times can be shortened is limited. There is a direct association between the radiation dose and image noise (→) or absorption resolution (→).
- **Scanning area:** A region of the body measured in a longitudinal direction and covered by a series of slices. There is a choice of slice sequences: adjacent (table advance = slice thickness), overlapping (table advance < slice thickness) and non-adjacent (table advance > slice thickness).
- **Scanning field:** A circular field of measurement traversed by the tube-detector system. Parts of the object lying outside the scanning field falsify the density values of the computed tomogram (→ artifacts).

The scanning field chosen should therefore be of an adequate size. The size of the scanning field determines the size of the picture element (1-30) for a given image matrix (→).

(Diameter of scanning field [mm]/number of picture elements of a matrix row = width of the picture element [mm]).

- **Slice thickness:** The width of the X-rays (in the z axis) can be varied by collimation. Narrow collimation restricts the photon flow and, consequently, increases image noise, so that longer scan times may become necessary.
- **Tube voltage:** The tube voltage produced by the generator determines the energy of the

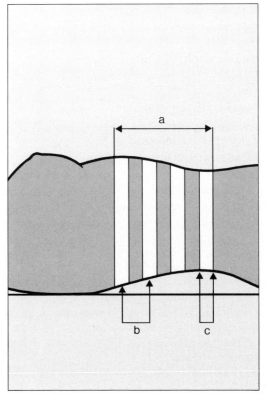

Fig. 97-**17: Scanning area** (a), **slice interval** (b), **slice thickness** (c).

emitted X-radiation. A higher X-ray voltage leads to a greater photon flow due to reduced attenuation of the X-rays in the object and reduces the image noise. Higher tube voltages reduce the tissue contrast (reduced density resolution) and hardening artifacts (→ artifacts). A tube voltage of 120 kV to 140 kV is used for whole-body examinations on most scanners.

Scattering of X-rays → attenuation of X-rays

Scoutview → digital X-ray picture

SD = standard deviation → image evaluation, histogram analysis

Secondary slices: If a series of adjacent slices is performed, the column created by stacking the individual slices on top of each other represents a body volume gridded continuously in volume elements. The analogous picture elements of the adjacent slice can be located and reproduced on the monitor for every diameter and every row and column of the image matrix (→). This results in the production of secondary frontal or sagittal slices which

CT terminology

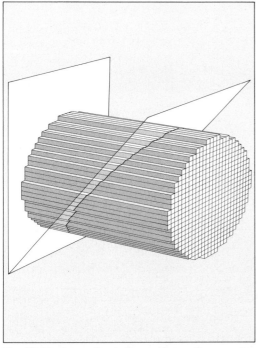

Fig. 97-**18: Secondary slices.** Depending on the evaluation programme, freely selectable slices can be constructed (multiplanar reconstruction) by interpolation of the orthogonally arranged volume elements.

Fig. 97-**19: Slice, designation of the plane.**
a = horizontal, transverse plane, **b** = sagittal plane, **c** = frontal plane.

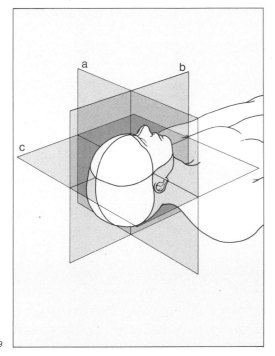

can only be assessed visually if thin slices (2–5 [max. 8] mm) are chosen. Complicated interpolation programmes are required if slice planes are chosen which deviate from the orthogonal coordinates (x, y, z) (multiplanar reconstruction in the narrow sense).

Sector scan → HR/CT

Slice, slice geometry: The measured data acquired by means of the various scanning principles (1–20) originate from a largely flat cross-sectional area of the body. The divergence of the rays after they leave the X-ray tube means that

● the CT slice does not run parallel, i.e. the slice thickness is not constant,

● the measuring sensitivity varies within the slice thickness (along the z-axis), i.e. the medial plane of the slice is measured most sensitively,

● half-shadows form which do not provide an image but contribute to the radiation dose.

Plane-parallel slices are best achieved by moving the scanner through 360° around the object. The other factors which influence the slice geometry can be reduced (to varying degrees) by concentrating the rays in a certain way (primary and secondary collimation). Because of the varying geometry, the **slice thickness** is expressed as the half-value width of the measuring sensitivity profile (on the z-axis) in the centre of the scanning field. The **slice plane** is usually set vertical to the body axis (transverse slice, horizontal slice). Some slight deviation from the vertical to the body axis can be achieved by tilting the gantry. In cranial CT, slices in the **frontal plane** can be achieved by means of hyperreflection of the head and tilting of the gantry. In whole-body CT, frontal and sagittal slices can be obtained by means of secondary slices (→).

Standard deviation → image evaluation, histogram analysis

Table advance → scanning

Topogram → digital X-ray picture

View → absorption profile

Volume measurement → image evaluation

Voxel = **vo**lume **el**ement (1-30)

Window, window level, window width → image reproduction

x, y coordinates → image matrix

z-axis: A coordinate (axis) vertical to the slice plane which usually runs parallel to the body axis.

Literature (98-00)

	No.		No.
General references	1	Liver	374
CT monographies	59	Bile ducts	426
Densitometry	74	Pancreas	443
Contrast media	124	Stomach, bowel	491
General CT literature	163	Urogenital tract	503
Orbit	183	Adrenals	573
Facial skull, neck	221	Retroperitoneum, pelvis	597
Thorax	257	Vertebral column	628
Mediastinum	271	Lymphatic system (spleen)	674
Heart, pericardium	296	Large vessels	698
Lung, pleura	318	Muscles, skeleton	728
Abdomen	338	Technique	753

General references

1. Abrams, H. L. (Ed.): Angiography. Little, Brown and Co., Boston 1971.
2. Anacker, E. (Ed.): Efficiency and limits of radiologic examination of the pancreas. Georg Thieme Publishers, Stuttgart 1975.
3. Anacker, H., Weiss, H. D., Kramann, B.: Endoscopic retrograde pancreatico-cholangiography (ERPC). Springer-Verlag, Berlin – Heidelberg – New York 1977.
4. Anderson, W. A. D., Kissane, J. M.: Pathology. C. V. Mosby Co., St. Louis 1977.
5. Becker, V. (Ed.): Bauchspeicheldrüse, Inselapparat ausgenommen. Springer-Verlag, Berlin – Heidelberg – New York 1973.
6. Bosniak, M. A., Siegelmann, S. S., Evans, J. A.: The adrenal, retroperitoneum and lower urinary tract. Year Book Medical Publishers Inc., Chicago 1976.
7. Diethelm, L., Heuck, F., Olsson, O., Strnad, F., Vieten, H., Zuppinger, A. (Eds.): Handbuch der medizinischen Radiologie. Vol. IX. Springer-Verlag, Berlin – Heidelberg – New York 1978.
8. Dodd, G. D., Jing, B. Sh.: Radiology of the nose, paranasal sinuses and nasopharynx. Williams & Wilkins Co., Baltimore 1977.
9. Doerr, W.: Spezielle pathologische Anatomie. Springer-Verlag, Berlin – Heidelberg – New York 1970.
10. Doerr, W.: Organpathologie, Vol. 1–3. Georg Thieme Verlag, Stuttgart 1974.
11. Edeiken, J., Hodes, Ph. J.: Roentgen diagnosis of diseases of bone. Williams & Wilkins Co., Baltimore 1967.
12. Emmett, J. L., Witten, D. M.: Clinical urography. An atlas and textbook of roentgenologic diagnosis. W. B. Saunders Co., Philadelphia – London – Toronto 1971.
13. Epstein, B. S.: The vertebral column. Year Book Medical Publishers Inc., Chicago 1974.
14. Fraser, R. G., Paré, J. A. P.: Diagnosis of diseases of the chest. W. B. Saunders Co., Philadelphia – London – Toronto 1979.
15. Fuchs, W. A., Triller, J.: Ultraschall – Computertomographie des Abdomens. Verlag Hans Huber, Bern – Stuttgart – Wien 1978.
16. Gambill, E. E.: Pancreatitis. C. V. Mosby Co., St. Louis 1973.
16 a. Hatfield, Ph. M., Wise, R.: The radiology of the gallbladder and the bile ducts. Williams and Wilkings, Baltimore 1976.
17. Haubrich, R. (Ed.): Klinische Röntgendiagnostik innerer Krankheiten. Springer-Verlag, Berlin – Göttingen – Heidelberg 1963.
18. Heberer, G., Rau, G., Schoop, W.: Angiologie – Grundlagen, Klinik und Praxis. Georg Thieme Verlag, Stuttgart 1974.
19. Heitzman, E.: The mediastinum. Radiologic correlations with anatomy and pathology. C. V. Mosby Co., St. Louis 1977.
20. Henderson, J. W.: Orbital tumors. W. B. Saunders Co., Philadelphia – London – Toronto 1973.
21. Huvos, A. G. (Ed.): Bone tumors – diagnosis, treatment and prognosis. W. B. Saunders Co., Philadelphia – London – Toronto 1979.
22. Johnsrude, I. S., Jackson, D. C.: A practical approach to angiography. Little, Brown and Co., Boston 1979
23. Kepp, R., Staemmler, H. J.: Lehrbuch der Gynäkologie. Georg Thieme Verlag, Stuttgart 1971.
24. Lloyd, G. A. S.: Radiology of the orbit. W. B. Saunders Co., London – Philadelphia – Toronto 1975.
25. Löhr, E. (Ed.): Renal and adrenal tumors. Pathology, radiology, ultrasonography, therapy, immunology. Springer-Verlag, Berlin – Heidelberg – New York 1979.
26. Margulis, A. R., Burhenne, H. J. (Eds.): Alimentary tract radiology. Vol. 3: Abdominal imaging. C. V. Mosby Co., St. Louis – Toronto – London 1979.
27. McAfee, J. G., Donner, M. W.: Differential diagnosis of calcifications encountered in abdominal radiographs. Amer. J. Med. Sci. 243 (1962) 609–659.
28. McNulty, J. G.: Radiology of the liver. W. B. Saunders Co., Philadelphia – London – Toronto 1977.
29. Meiisel, P., Apitzsch, D. E. (Eds.): Atlas der Nierenangiographie. Springer-Verlag, Berlin – Heidelberg – New York 1978.
30. Meschan, I. (Ed.): Analysis of roentgen signs in general radiology. W. B. Saunders Co., Philadelphia – London – Toronto 1973.
31. Meschan, I. (Ed.): Synopsis of radiologic anatomy with computed tomography. W. B. Saunders Co., Philadelphia – London –Toronto 1978.
32. Meyers, M. A.: Dynamic radiology of the abdomen. Normal and pathologic anatomy. Springer-Verlag, New York – Heidelberg – Berlin 1976
32 a. Olsson, O., Weiland, P. O.: Renal Fibrolipomatosis. Acta Radiol. Diagn. 1 (1963) 1061–1070.
33. Parker, B. R., Castellino, R. A.: Pediatric oncologic radiology. C. V. Mosby Co., St. Louis 1977.
33 a. Pernkopf, E.: Atlas der topographischen und angewandten Anatomie des Menschen. Ed.: Ferner, H. Urban und Schwarzenberg, München 1980.
34. Piepgras, U.: Neuroradiologie. Georg Thieme Verlag, Stuttgart 1977.
35. Preger, L.: Asbestos-related disease. Grune & Stratton, New York – San Francisco – London 1979.
36. Sarles, H., Sarles, J. C., Camatte, R., Muratore, R. et al.: Observations on 205 confirmed cases of acute pancreatitis, recurring pancreatitis, and chronic pancreatitis. Gut 6 (1965) 545–559.
37. Sarles, H., Martin, M., Camatte, R., Sarles, J.: Le démembrement des pancréatites: les pseudokystes des pancréatites aiguës et des pancréatites chroniques. Presse méd. 71 (1963) 237–240.
38. Scherer, E. (Ed.): Strahlentherapie. Radiologische Onkologie. Springer-Verlag, Berlin – Heidelberg – New York 1976.
39. Schinz, H. R., Baensch, W. E., Frommhold, W., Glauner, R., Uehlinger, E., Wellauer, J. (Eds.): Lehrbuch der Röntgendiagnostik. Band IV/Teil 2: Pleura, Mediastinum und Lunge. Georg Thieme Verlag, Stuttgart 1973.
40. Sobotta, I., Becher, H.: Atlas der deskriptiven Anatomie des Menschen. Urban & Schwarzenberg, München – Berlin 1960.
41. Steinbach, H. L., Minagi, H.: The endocrines. Year Book Medical Publishers Inc., Chicago 1969.
42. Stevens, G. M. (Ed.): The female reproductive system. Year Book Medical Publishers Inc., Chicago 1971.
43. Sussman, M. L., Newman, A.: Urologic radiology. Williams & Wilkins, Baltimore 1976.
44. Taveras, J. M., Morello, F.: Normal neuroradiology, an atlas of the skull, sinuses and facial bones. Year Book Medical Publishers Inc., Chicago – London 1979.
45. Taveras, J. M., Wood, E. H.: Diagnostic neuroradiology. Williams & Wilkins Co., Baltimore 1976.
46. Teschendorf, W., Anacker, H., Thurn, P.: Röntgenologische Differentialdiagnostik. Vol. 1: Thoraxorgane. Georg Thieme Verlag, Stuttgart 1975.
47. Teschendorf, W., Wenz, W.: Röntgenologische Differentialdiagnostik. Vol. 2: Erkrankungen der Bauchorgane. Georg Thieme Verlag, Stuttgart 1978.
48. Triller, J., Fuchs, W. A.: Abdominale Sonographie. Indikation – Information – Integration. Georg Thieme Verlag, Stuttgart – New York 1980.
49. Verbiest, H. (Ed.): Neurogenic intermittent claudication – with special reference to stenosis of the lumbar vertebral canal. North-Holland Publishing Co., Amsterdam – Oxford, American Elsevier Publishing Co., Inc., New York 1976.
49 a. Voegeli, E.: Die Pathogenese der Fibrolipomatose. Radiologe 11 (1971) 209–215.
50. Vogler, E. (Ed.): Radiologische Diagnostik der Harnorgane. Georg Thieme Verlag, Stuttgart 1974.
51. Wackenheim, A., Babin, E.: The narrow lumbar canal. Radiologic signs and surgery. Springer-Verlag, Berlin – Heidelberg – New York 1980.
52. Wagenknecht, L. V. (Ed.): Retroperitoneale Fibrosen. Symptomatik – Diagnostik – Therapie – Prognose. Georg Thieme Verlag, Stuttgart 1978.
53. Whalen, J. P.: Radiology of the abdomen. Lea & Ferbiger, Philadelphia 1976.
54. White, T. T., Sarles, H., Benhamou, I. P.: Liver, bile ducts, and pancreas. Grune & Stratton, New York – San Francisco – London 1977.

55. Wintrobe, M. M. et al. (Eds.): Harrison's principles of internal medicine. McGraw-Hill Book Co., New York – St. Louis 1974.
56. Wise, R. E., O'Keeffe, A. P.: The accessory digestive organs. Year Book Medical Publishers Inc., Chicago 1975.
57. Wood, E. H., Taveras, J. M., Tenner, M. S.: The brain and the eye. Year Book Medical Publishers Inc., Chicago 1975.
58. Zollinger, H. U. (Ed.): Pathologische Anatomie. Georg Thieme Verlag, Stuttgart 1975.

CT monographies

59. Baert, A., Jeanmart, L., Wackenheim. A. (Eds.): Clinical computer tomography. Head and trunk. Springer-Verlag, Berlin – Heidelberg – New York 1978.
60. Baert, A. L., Wackenheim, A., Jeanmart, L. (Eds.): Abdominal computer-tomography. Springer-Verlag, Berlin – Heidelberg – New York 1980.
61. Caillé, J. M., Salamon, G. (Eds.): Computerized tomography. Springer-Verlag, Berlin – Heidelberg – New York 1980.
62. Du Boulay, G. H., Moseley, I. F. (Eds.): The first European seminar on computerized axial tomography in clinical practice. Springer-Verlag, Berlin – Heidelberg – New York 1977.
63. Felson, B. (Ed.): Computerized cranial tomography. A seminar in roentgenology reprint. Grune & Stratton, New York – San Francisco – London 1977.
64. Friedmann, G., Bücheler, E., Thurn, P. (Eds.): Ganzkörper-Computertomographie. Georg Thieme Verlag, Stuttgart – New York 1981.
65. Gambarelli, J., Guérinel, G., Chevrot, L., Mattéi, M.: Ganzkörper-Computer-Tomographie. Anatomie – Radiologie – Scanner. Springer-Verlag, Berlin – Heidelberg – New York 1967.
66. Gerhardt, P., van Kaick, G. (Eds.): Total body computerized tomography. International Symposium Heidelberg 1977. Georg Thieme, Stuttgart 1979.
67. Hübener, K. H.: Computertomographie des Körperstammes. Georg Thieme Verlag, Stuttgart – New York 1981.
68. Jacobs, L., Weisberg, L. A., Kinkel, W. R.: Computerized tomography of the orbit and sella turcica. Raven Press, New York 1980.
69. Kazner, E., Wende, S., Grumme, Th., Lanksch, W., Stochdorph, O.: Computertomographie intrakranieller Tumoren aus klinischer Sicht. Springer-Verlag, Berlin – Heidelberg – New York 1981 (in press).
70. Lange, S., Grumme, Th., Meese, W.: Zerebrale Computer-Tomographie. Med.-wiss. Buchreihe, Schering AG, Berlin – Bergkamen 1977.
71. Lanksch, W., Kazner, E. (Eds.): Cranial computerized tomography. Springer-Verlag, Berlin – Heidelberg – New York 1976.
72. Moss, A. A., Goldberg, H. I.: Computed tomography, ultrasound and x-ray: An integrated approach. Masson Publishing USA, Inc., New York, 1979.
73. Sager, W. D., Ladurner, G. (Eds.): Computertomographie. Derzeitige Stellung in Radiologie und Klinik. Symposium Graz 1978. Georg Thieme Verlag, Stuttgart 1979.

Densitometry

74. Banzer, D., Schneider, U., Wegener, O. H., Oeser, H., Pleul, O.: Quantitative Mineralsalzbestimmung im Wirbelkörper mittels Computertomographie. Fortschr. Röntgenstr. 130 (1979) 77.
75. Banzer, D. H., Schneider, U., Wegener, O. H.: Photon absorptiometry and scanning in determination of bone mineral content. In: Total computerized tomography. (Eds.: Gerhardt, P., van Kaick, G. G. Thieme, Stuttgart (1979).
76. Bergström, M., Ericson, K., Levander, B., Svendsen, P. et al.: Variation with time of the attenuation values of intracranial hematomas. J. Comput. Ass. Tomogr. 1 (1977) 57–63.
77. Bradley, J. G., Huang, H. K., Ledley, R. S.: Evaluation of calcium concentration in bones from CT scans. Radiology 128 (1978) 103–107.
78. Brooks, R. A.: A quantitative theory of the Hounsfield Unit and its application to dual energy scanning. J. Comput. Ass. Tomogr. 1 (1977) 487 ff.
79. Bydder, G. M., Kreel, L.: The temperature dependence of computed tomography attenuation values. J. Comput. Ass. Tomogr. 3 (1979) 506–510.
80. Bydder, G. M., Kreel, L.: Attenuation values of fluid collections within the abdomen. J. Comput. Ass. Tomogr. 4 (1980) 145–150.
81. Cann, C. E., Genant, H. K.: Precise measurement of vertebral mineral content using computed tomography. J. Comput. Ass. Tomogr 4 (1980) 493–500.
82. Chiro, G., Brooks, R. A., Kessler, R. M. et al.: Tissue signatures with dual-energy computed tomography. Radiology 131 (1979) 521–523.
83. Cisternino, S. J., Neiman, H. L., Malave, S. R.: Diagnosis of retroperitoneal hemorrhage by serial computed tomography. J. Comput. Ass. Tomogr. 3 (1979) 686–688.
84. Döhring, W., Linke, G.: Die Grundlagen der quantitativen pulmonalen Computertomographie. Fortschr. Röntgenstr. 130, 2 (1979) 133–143.
85. Exner, G. U., Prader, A., Elsasser, U. et al.: Bone densitometry using computed tomography. Part I – Selective determination of trabecular bone density and other bone mineral parameters. Normal values in children and adults. Brit. J. Radiol. 52 (1979) 14–23.
86. Exner, G. U., Prader, A., Elsasser, U., Anliker, M.: Bone densitometry using computed tomography. Part II – Increased trabecular bone density in children with chronic renal failure. Brit. J. Radiol. 52 (1979) 24–28.
87. Fullerton, G. D., Sewchand, W., Payne, J. T., Levitt, S. H.: CT determination of parameters for inhomogeneity corrections in radiation therapy of the esophagus. Radiology 126 (1978) 167–171.
88. Genant, H. K., Boyd, D.: Quantitative bone mineral analysis using dual energy computed tomography. Invest. Radiol. 12 (1977) 545–551.
89. Gerhardt, P., Duwig, M., Kamphues, R.: Density measurements of abdominal organs in CT. Intern. symp. Heidelberg 1977. Eds.: Paul Gerhardt, Gerhard van Kaick. Georg Thieme, Stuttgart (1979) 150–160.
90. Goldstein, A.: A simple buoyancy method for measuring computed tomography phantom material densities. Radiology 128 (1978) 814–815.
91. Guertler, K. F., Buurman, R., Erbe, W.: Computertomographischer Nachweis von Haematomen des Becken- und Bauchraumes. Fortschr. Röntgenstr. 131 (1979) 493–498.
92. Gur, D., Drayer, B. P., Borovetz, H. S., Griffith, B. P. et al.: Dynamic computed tomography of the lung – Regional ventilation measurements. J. Comput. Ass. Tomogr. 3 (1979) 749–753.
93. Hounsfield, G. N.: Potential uses of more accurate CT absorption values by filtering. AJR 131 (1978) 103–106.
94. Hübener, K. H., Schmitt, W. G. H.: Computertomographische Densitometrie des menschlichen Blutes. Einfluß auf das Absorptionsverhalten von parenchymatösen Organen und Ergußbildungen. Fortschr. Röntgenstr. 130, 2 (1979) 185–188.
95. Hübener, K. H., Schmitt, W. G. H.: Die computertomographische Diagnostik von Abszeßbildungen. Fortschr. Röntgenstr. 130, 1 (1979) 53–57.
96. Jensen, P. S., Orphanoudakis, S. C., Rauschkolb, E. N. et al.: Assessment of bone mass in the radius by computed tomography. AJR 134 (1980) 285–292.
97. Joseph, P. M., Spital, R. D.: A method for correcting bone induced artifacts in computed tomography scanners. J. Comput. Ass. Tomogr. 2 (1978) 100–108.
98. Kirschner, H., Burmester, U., Stringaris, K.: CT – Tomometrie. Teil 1 – Gewebeinhomogenitäten – Bestrahlungsplanung. Strahlentherapie 153 (1977) 601–615.
99. Kirschner, H., Burmester, U., Stringaris, K.: CT – Tomometrie. Teil 2 – Diagnostik – Jodhaltige Kontrastmittel. Strahlentherapie 153 (1977) 616–619.
100. Korobkin, M., Moss, A. A., Callen, P. W., Demartini, W. J., Kaiser, J. A.: Computed tomography of subcapsular splenic hematoma. Radiology 129 (1978) 441–445.
101. Lange, S., Weiss, Th., Gahl, G., Golde, G.: Knochendichtemessung mit dem Computertomographen. Fortschr. Röntgenstr. 129,1 (1978) 66–69.
102. Latchaw, R. E., Gold, L. H., Moore, J. S., Payne, J. T.: The nonspecificity of absorption coefficients in the differentiation of solid tumors and cystic lesions. Radiology 125 (1977) 141–144.
103. Long, J. A., Doppman, J. L., Nienhus, A. W. et al.: Computed tomographic analysis of beta-thalassemic syndromes with hemochromatosis – Pathologic findings with clinical and laboratory correlations. J. Comput. Ass. Tomogr. 4 (1980) 159–165.
104. Mategrano, V. C., Petasnick, J., Clark, J., Weinstein, R.: Attenuation values in computed tomography of the abdomen. Radiology 125 (1977) 135–140.
105. New, P. F. J., Aronow, S.: Attenuation measurements of whole blood and blood fractions in computed tomography. Radiology 121 (1976) 635–640.
106. Norman, D., Price, D., Boyd, D. et al.: Quantitative aspects of computed tomography of the blood and cerebrospinal fluid. Radiology 123 (1977) 335–338.
107. Orphanoudakis, S. C., Jensen, P. S., Rauschkolb, E. N., Lang, R., Rasmussen, H.: Bone mineral analysis using single-energy computed tomography. Invest. Radiol. 14 (1979) 122–130.
108. Piekarski, J., Goldberg, H. I., Royal, S. A., et al.: Difference between liver and spleen CT numbers in the normal adult – Its usefulness

in predicting the presence of diffuse liver disease. Radiology 137 (1980) 727–729.
109. Posner, I., Griffiths, H.: Comparison of CT scanning with photon absorptiometric measurement of bone mineral content in the appendicular skeleton. Invest. Radiol. 12 (1977) 542–544.
110. Pullan, B. R., Roberts, T. E.: Bone mineral measurement using an EMI scanner and standard methods – A comparative study. Brit. J. Radiol. 51 (1978) 24–28.
111. Pullan, B. R., Fawcitt, R. R., Isherwood, I.: Tissue characterization by an analysis of the distribution of attenuation values in computed tomography scans – A preliminary report. J. Comput. Ass. Tomogr. 2 (1978) 49–54.
112. Ritchings, R. T., Pullan, B. R., Lucas, S. B., et al.: An analysis of the spatial distribution of attenuation values in computed tomographic scans of liver and spleen. J. Comput. Ass. Tomogr. 3 (1979) 36–39.
113. Robinson, P. J., Kreel, L.: Pulmonary tissue attenuation with computed tomography – Comparison of inspiration and expiration scans. J. Comput. Ass. Tomogr. 3 (1979) 740–748.
114. Rosenblum, L. J., Mauceri, R. A., Wellenstein, D. E., Bassano, D. A., Cohen, W. N., Heitzman, E. R.: Computed tomography of the lung. Radiology 129 (1978) 521
115. Rüegsegger, P.: Knochendichtemessungen mit dem Computertomographen. Fortschr. Röntgenstr. 130 (1979) 497–498.
116. Rutherford, R. A., Pullan, B. R., Isherwood, I.: Measurement of effective atomic number and electron density using an EMI scanner. Neuroradiology 11 (1976) 15–21.
117. Schmitt, W. G. H., Hübener, K. H.: Dichtebestimmung normaler und pathologisch veränderter Lebergewebe als Basisuntersuchung zur computertomographischen Densitometrie von Fettlebern. Fortschr. Röntgenstr. 129, 5 (1978) 555–559.
118. Schmitt, W. G. H., Hübener, K. H.: Computertomographische Densitometrie formalinfixierter und gefrorener menschlicher Gewebe. Fortschr. Röntgenstr. 133 (1980) 531–534.
119. Wegener, O. H., Koeppe, P., Oeser, H.: Measurement of lung density by computed tomography. J. Comput. Ass. Tomogr. 2 (1978) 263–273.
120. Weissberger, M. A., Zamenhof, R. G., Aronow, S., Neer, R. M.: Computed tomography scanning for the measurement of bone mineral in the human spine. J. Comput. Ass. Tomogr. 2 (1978) 253–262.
121. Wittenberg, J., Maturi, R. A., Ferrucci, J. T., Margolies, M. N.: Computerized tomography of in vitro abdominal organs – Effect of preservation methods on attenuation coefficient. Computerized Tomogr. 1 (1977) 95–101.
122. Zatz, L. M., Alvarez, R. E.: An inaccuracy in computed tomography – The energy dependence of CT values. Radiology 124 (1977) 91–97.
123. Zatz, L. M.: The effect of the KVP level on EMI values. Radiology 119 (1976) 683–688.

Contrast media

124. Baldwin, G. N.: Computed tomography of the pancreas – Negative contrast medium. Radiology 128 (1978) 827–828.
125. Bonafé, A., Manelfe, C., Espagno, J. et al.: Evaluation of syringomyelia with metrizamide computed tomographic myelography. J. Comput. Ass. Tomogr. 4 (1980) 797–802.
126. Coin, C. G., Wilson, G. H., Klebanoff, R.: Contrast enhancement by arterial perfusion during computerized tomography. Neuroradiology 11 (1976) 119–121.
127. Coin, C. G., Chan, Y. S.: Computed tomographic arteriography. J. Comput. Ass. Tomogr. 1 (1977) 165–168.
128. Coin, C. G., Keranen, V. J., Pennink, M., Ahmad, W. D.: Evidence of CSF enhancement in the spinal subarachnoid space after intravenous contrast medium administration – Is intravenous computer assisted myelography possible? J. Comput. Ass. Tomogr. 3 (1979) 267–269.
129. Coin, C., Coin, J. T.: Contact enhancement by xenon gas in computed tomography of the spinal cord and brain – Preliminary observations. J. Comput. Ass. Tomogr. 4 (1980) 217–221.
130. Drayer, B. P., Rosenbaum, A. E., Reigel, D. B., Bank, W. O., Deeb, Z. L.: Metrizamide computed tomography cisternography – Pediatric applications. Radiology 124 (1977) 349–357.
131. Dunnick, N. R., Jones, R. B., Doppman, J. L. et al.: Intraperitoneal contrast infusion for assessment of intraperitoneal fluid dynamics. AJR 133 (1979) 221–223.
132. Fuchs, W. A., Vock, P., Haertel, M.: Pharmakokinetik intravasaler Kontrastmittel bei der Computer-Tomographie. Radiologe 19 (1979) 90–93.
133. Galanski, M., Cramer, B. M., Drewes, G.: Möglichkeiten der Kontrastmittelanwendung bei der Computertomographie. Fortschr. Röntgenstr. 132 (1980) 139–144.
134. Gene, C., Chan, Y. S., Keranen, V., Pennink, M.: Computer assisted myelography in disk disease. J. Comput. Ass. Tomogr. 1 (1977) 398–403.
135. Goldman, K.: The blood-brain barrier – Effects of nonionic contrast media with and without addition of a Ca-2+ and Mg-2+. Invest. Radiol. 14 (1979) 305–308.
136. Grabbe, E.: Methodik und Wert der Darmkontrastierung bei der abdominellen Computertomographie. Fortschr. Röntgenstr. 131 (1979) 588–594.
137. Hacker, H., Becker, H.: Time controlled computed tomographic angiography. J. Comput. Ass. Tomogr. 1 (1977) 405–409.
138. Hatfield, K. D., Segal, S. D., Tait, K.: Barium sulfate for abdominal computer assisted tomography. J. Comput. Ass. Tomogr. 4 (1980) 570.
139. Haughton, V., Donegan, J., Walsh, P. et al.: Clinical cerebral blood flow measurement with inhaled xenon and CT. AJR 134 (1980) 281–283.
140. Hayman, L. A., Evans, R. A., Hinck, V. C.: Rapid high dose (RHD) contrast cranial computed tomography – A concise review of normal anatomy. J. Comput. Ass. Tomogr. 3 (1979) 147–154.
141. Hegglin, R., Rutishauser, W., Kaufmann, G., Luethy, E., Scheu, H.: Kreislaufdiagnostik mit der Farbstoffverdünnungsmethode. G. Thieme, Stuttgart 1962.
142. Hübener, K. H.: Computertomographische Densitometrie von Leber, Milz und Nieren bei intravenös verabreichten lebergängigen Kontrastmitteln in Bolusform. Fortschr. Röntgenstr. 129, 3 (1978) 289–297.
143. Hübener, K. H., Klott, K. J.: „Statisches" und dynamisches Kontrastmittelenhancement der Körperstamm-Computertomographie. Fortschr. Röntgenstr. 133 (1980) 347–354.
144. Keller, M. R., Kessler, R. M., Brooks, R. A. et al.: Optimum energy for performing CT iodinated contrast studies. Brit. J. Radiol. 53 (1980) 576–579.
145. Koehler, R. E., Stanley, R. J., Evens, R. G.: Iosefamate meglumine – An iodinated contrast agent for hepatic computed tomography scanning. Radiology 132 (1979) 115–118.
146. Kormano, M., Dean, P. B.: Extravascular contrast material – The major component of contrast enhancement. Radiology 121 (1976) 379–382.
147. Kormano, M., Dean, P., Kivisaari, L.: Experimental studies on tissue identification with contrast enhancement kinetics. Intern. Symp. Heidelberg 1977. Eds.: Paul Gerhardt, Gerhard van Kaick. G. Thieme, Stuttgart (1979) 115–122
148. Kormano, M. J., Dean, P. B., Hamlin, D. J.: Upper extremity contrast medium infusion in computed tomography of upper mediastinal masses. J. Comput. Ass. Tomogr. 4 (1980) 617–620.
149. Lamarque, J. L., Bruel, J. M., Dondelinger, R., Vendrell, B., Pelissier, O., Rouanet, J. P., Michel, J. L., Boulet, J. C.: The use of iodolipids in hepatosplenic computed tomography. J. Comput. Ass. Tomogr. 3, 1 (1979) 21–24.
150. Leppik, I. E., Thompson, C. J., Ethier, R., Sherwin, A. L.: Diatrizoate in computed cranial tomography – A quantitative study. Invest. Radiol. 12 (1977) 21–26.
151. Mancuso, A., Rice, D., Hanafee, W.: Computed tomography of the parotid gland during contrast sialography. Radiology 132 (1979) 211–213.
152. Manelfe, C., Starling-Jadim, D., Touibi, S. et al.: Transsphenoidal encephalocele associated with agenesis of corpus callosum – Value of metrizamide computed cisternography. J. Comput. Ass. Tomogr. 2 (1978) 356–361.
153. Norman, D., Enzmann, D. R., Newton, T. H.: Comparative efficacy of contrast agents in computed tomography scanning of the brain. J. Comput. Ass. Tomogr. 2 (1978) 319–321.
154. Paling, M. R.: Contrast dose for enhancement of computed tomograms of the brain. Brit. J. Radiol. 52 (1979) 620–623.
155. Pillari, G.: Computed tomographic cavo-urography – Lower-extremity contrast infusion simultaneous with computed tomography of the retroperitoneum. Radiology 130 (1979) 797.
156. Roub, L. W., Drayer, B. P., Orr, D. P. et al.: Computed tomographic positive contrast peritoneography. Radiology 131 (1979) 699–704.
157. Schad, N., Schepke, P., Rhode, U., Schepke, H., Schmid, V., Breit, A.: Timing of exposure in angiographic computed tomography. Cardiovasc. Intervent. Radiol. (1981) 59–65.
158. Vermess, M., Adamson, R. H., Doppman, J.L., Girton, M.: Computed tomographic demonstration of hepatic tumor with the aid of intravenous iodinated fat emulsion. Radiology 125 (1977) 711–715.
159. Vermess, M., Chatterji, D. C., Doppman, J. L., Grimes, G., Adamson, R. H.: Development and experimental evaluation of a contrast medium for computed tomographic examination of the liver and spleen. J. Comput. Ass. Tomogr. 3, 1 (1979) 25–31.
160. Vermess, M., Inscoe, S., Sugarbaker, P.: Use of liposoluble con-

trast material to separate left renal and splenic parenchyma on computed tomography. J. Comput. Ass. Tomogr. 4 (1980) 540–542.
161. Vermess, M., Doppman, J. L., Sugarbaker, P. et al.: Clinical trials with a new intravenous liposoluble contrast material for computed tomography of the liver and spleen. Radiology 137 (1980) 217–222.
161a. Wegener, O. H., Muetzel, W., Souchon, R.: Contrast media for computer tomography of the liver. Acta Radiol. Diagn. 21 (1980) 239–247.
162. Young, S. W., Turner, R. J., Castellino, R. A.: A strategy for the contrast enhancement of malignant tumors using dynamic computed tomography and intravascular pharmacokinetics. Radiology 137 (1980) 137–147.

General CT literature

163. Alfidi, R. J., Haaga, J., Meaney, T. F., MacIntyre, W. J. et al.: Computed tomography of the thorax and abdomen – A preliminary report. Radiology 117 (1975) 257–264.
164. Brecht, G., Lackner, K., Janson, R., Thurn, P.: Die Computertomographie in der Notfalldiagnostik. Fortschr. Röntgenstr. 132 (1980) 272–281.
165. Cohen, W. N., Seidelmann, F. E., Bryan, P. J.: Computed tomography of localized adipose deposits presenting as tumor masses. Am. J. Roentgenol. 128 (1977) 1007–1011.
166. Damgaard-Pedersen, K., Edeling, C. J., Hertz, H.: CT wholebody scanning and scintigraphy in children with malignant tumours. Pediatr. Radiol. 8 (1979) 103–107.
167. Damgaard-Pedersen, K.: Neuroblastoma follow-up by computed tomography. J. Comput. Ass. Tomogr. 3 (1979) 274–275.
168. Fiegler, W., Wegener, O. H., Hartmann, K., Felix, R.: Computertomographie und Sonographie-Vergleichsstudie bei Erkrankungen des Oberbauches und des Retroperitonealraumes. Fortschr. Röntgenstr. 132 (1980) 262–271.
169. Fotter, R., Sager, W. D.: CT des Beckens und Abdomens im Kindesalter. Fortschr. Röntgenstr. 131 (1979) 476–479.
170. Fotter, R., Sager, W. D., Justich, E., Nedden, D.: Die Bedeutung der Computertomographie in der pädiatrischen Diagnostik abdomineller und pelviner Tumoren. Röntgen-Bl. 33 (1980) 156–162.
171. Haertel, M., Fuchs, W. A.: Computertomographie nach stumpfem Abdominaltrauma. Fortschr. Röntgenstr. 131 (1979) 487–492.
172. Kollins, S. A.: Computed tomography of the liver, spleen, and pancreas. Sem. Roentgenol. 13 (1978) 227–234.
173. Lackner, K., Koischwitz, D., Felix, R., Frommhold, H., Thurn, P.: Vergleich zwischen Computertomographie und Ultraschall bei abdominellen und renalen Raumforderungen. Röntgen-Bl. 31 (1978) 123–134.
174. Levitt, R. G., Geisse, G. G., Sagel, S. S., Stanley, R. J. et al.: Complementary use of ultrasound and computed tomography in studies of the pancreas and kidney. Radiology 126 (1978) 149–152.
175. MacCarty, R. L., Wahner, H. W., Stephens, D. H. et al.: Retrospective comparison of radionuclide scans and computed tomography of the liver and pancreas. Am. J. Roentgenol. 129 (1977) 23–28.
176. Rosenfield, A. T., Allen, W. E., Curtis, A., Siegel, N. J. et al.: Gray scale ultrasonography, computerized tomography, and nephrotomography in evaluation of polycystic kidney and liver disease. Urology 9 (1977) 436–438.
177. Sheedy, P. F., Stephens, D. H., Hattery, R. R., Muhm, J. R., Hartman, G. W.: Computed tomography of the body – Initial clinical trial with the EMI prototype. Am. J. Roentgenol. 127 (1976) 23–51.
178. Stanley, R. J., Sagel, S. S., Levitt, R.: Computed tomography of the body – Early trends in application and accuracy of the method. Am. J. Roentgenol. 127 (1976) 53–67.
179. Stephens, D. H., Hattery, R. R., Sheedy, P. F.: Computed tomography of the abdomen. Radiology 119 (1976) 331–335.
180. Wegener, O. H.: Die Bedeutung der Computertomographie für Klinik und Praxis. In: Moderne medizinische Erkenntnisse und deren Bedeutung für die Praxis. Ed.: Ärztekammer Kärnten (1978).
181. Whalen, J. P.: Radiology of the abdomen – Impact of new imaging methods. AJR 133 (1979) 585–618.
182. Winter, J.: Efficiency of utilization of a computed tomography scanner. Am. J. Roentgenol. 131 (1978) 89–93.

Orbit

183. Ambrose, J. A. E., Lloyd, G. A. S., Wright, J. E.: A preliminary evaluation of fine matrix computerized axial tomography (EMI scan) in the diagnosis of orbital space-occupying lesions. Brit. J. Radiol. 47 (1974) 747–751.
184. Bernardino, M. E., Danziger, J., Young, S. E., Wallace, S.: Computed tomography in ocular neoplastic disease. Am. J. Roentgenol. 131 (1978) 111–113.
185. Brant-Zawadzki, M., Enzmann, D. R.: Orbital computed tomography – Calcific densities of the posterior globe. J. Comput. Ass. Tomogr. 3 (1979) 503–505.
186. Brismar, J., Brismar, G., Davis, K. R.: Superior ophthalmic vein at computed tomography. Acta Radiologica Diagnosis 18 (1977) 273–277.
187. Byrd, S. E., Harwood-Nash, D. C., Fitz, C. R. et al.: Computed tomography of intraorbital optic nerve gliomas in children. Radiology 129 (1978) 73–78.
188. Cabanis, E. A., Salvolini, U., Rodallec, A., Menichelli, F. et al.: Computed tomography of the optic nerve – Part II. – Size and shape modifications in papilledema. J. Comput. Ass. Tomogr. 2 (1978) 150–155.
189. Claveria, L. E., Sutton, D., Tress, B. M.: The radiological diagnosis of meningiomas, the impact of EMI scanning. Brit. J. Radiol. 50 (1977) 15–22.
190. Damme, W., Kosmann, P., Wackenheim, C.: A standardized method for computed tomography of the orbits. Neuroradiology 13 (1977) 139–140.
191. Danziger, A., Price, H.: Computed tomographic findings in orbital echinococciasis. J. Comput. Ass. Tomogr. 4 (1980) 128–129.
192. Enzmann, D., Marschall, W. H., Rosenthal, A. R., Kriss, J. P.: Computed tomography in Graves' ophthalmopathy. Radiology 118 (1976) 615–620.
193. Enzmann, D. R., Donaldson, S. S., Kriss, J. P.: Appearance of Graves' disease on orbital computed tomography J. Comput. Ass. Tomogr. 3 (1979) 815–819.
194. Forbes, G. S., Sheedy, P. F., Waller, R. R.: Orbital tumors evaluated by computed tomography. Radiology 136 (1980) 101–111.
195. Gyldensted, C., Lester, J., Fledelius, H.: Computed tomography of orbital lesions. Neuroradiology 13 (1980) 141–150.
196. Hesselink, J. R., Davis, K. R., Dallow, R. L. et al.: Computed tomography of masses in the lacrimal gland region. Radiology 131 (1979) 143–147.
197. Hilal, S. K., Trokel, S. L.: Computerized tomography of the orbit using thin sections. Sem. Roentgenol. 12 (1977) 137–147.
198. Huk, W., Schiefer, W.: Computertomographie bei Prozessen der Schädelbasis und der Orbitae – kombinierte Anwendung von Horizontal- und Frontalschnitten. Fortschr. Röntgenstr. 128, 1 (1978) 8–11.
199. Kadir, S., Aronow, S., Davis, K. R.: The use of computerized tomography in the detection of intra-orbital foreign bodies. Computerized Tomogr. 1 (1977) 151–156.
200. Kazner, E., Lanksch, W., Steinhoff, H., Wilske, J.: Die axiale Computer-Tomographie des Gehirnschädels. Anwendungsmöglichkeiten und klinische Ergebnisse. Georg Thieme, Stuttgart (1975) 1–92.
201. Kollarits, C. R., Moss, M. L., Cogan, D. G., Doppman, J. L. et al.: Scleral calcifications in hyperparathyroidism – Demonstration by computed tomography. J. Comput. Ass. Tomogr. 1 (1977) 500–504.
202. Komaki, S., Baba, H., Matsuura, K.: Oblique computed tomography for orbital mass lesions. Radiology 129 (1978) 79–80.
203. Leonardi, M., Barbina, V., Fabris, G., Penco, T.: Sagittal computed tomography of the orbit. J. Comput. Ass. Tomogr. 1 (1977) 511–512.
204. Mödder, U., Friedmann, G., Gode, A.: Computertomographie der Orbita. Röntgen-Bl. 32 (1979) 457–463.
205. Rothman, S. L. G., Allen, W. E., Simeone, J. F.: Direct coronal computerized tomography. Computerized Tomogr. 1 (1977) 157–163.
206. Salvolini, U., Menichelli, F., Pasquini, U.: Computer assisted tomography in 90 cases of exophthalmos. J. Comput. Ass. Tomogr. 1 (1977) 81 ff.
207. Salvolini, U., Cabanis, E. A., Rodallec, A., Menichelli, F. et al.: Computed tomography of the optic nerve. Part I. – Normal results. J. Comput. Ass. Tomogr. 2 (1978) 141–149.
208. Tadmor, R., New, P. F. J.: Computed tomography of the orbit with special emphasis on coronal sections – Part I: Normal anatomy. J. Comput. Ass. Tomogr. 2 (1978) 24–34.
209. Tadmor, R., New, P. F. J.: Computed tomography of the orbit with special emphasis on coronal sections – Part II: Pathological anatomy. J. Comput. Ass. Tomogr. 2 (1978) 35–44.
210. Takahashi, M., Tamakawa, Y.: Coronal computed tomography in orbital disease. J. Comput. Ass. Tomogr. 1 (1977) 505–509.
211. Toledo, E. C. G., Szelagowski, J. C.: Unilateral exophthalmos in orbital echinococciasis. J. Comput. Ass. Tomogr. 4 (1980) 127.
212. Tourje, E. J., Gold, L. H. A.: Leukemic infiltration of the optic nerves – Demonstration by computerized tomography. Computerized Tomogr. 1 (1977) 225–228.
213. Unsöld, R., Newton, T. H., Hoyt, W. F.: CT examination technique of the optic nerve. J. Comput. Ass. Tomogr. 4 (1980) 560–563.
214. Unsöld, R., Degroot, J., Newton, T. H.: Images of the optic nerve. AJR 135 (1980) 767–773.

215. Vermess, M., Haynes, B. F., Fauci, A. S., Wolff, S. M.: Computer assisted tomography of orbital lesions in Wegener's granulomatosis. J. Comput. Ass. Tomogr. 2 (1978) 45 ff.
216. Wackenheim, A., Damme, W., Kosmann, P. et al.: Computed tomography in ophthalmology. Neuroradiology 13 (1977) 135–138.
217. Wende, S., Kazner, E., Grumme, Th.: Computed tomography of orbital lesions. Intern. Symp. Heidelberg 1977. Eds.: Paul Gerhardt, Gerhard van Kaick. Georg Thieme, Stuttgart (1979) 320–324.
218. Wende, S., Aulich, A., Nover, A. et al.: Computed tomography of orbital lesions. Neuroradiology 13 (1977) 123–134.
219. Wing, S. D., Hunsaker, J. N., Anderson, R. E., Dyk, H. J. L., Osborn, A. G.: Direct sagittal computed tomography in Graves' ophthalmopathy. J. Comput. Ass. Tomogr. 3 (1979) 820–824.
220. Zimmerman, R. A., Bilaniuk, L. T.: CT of orbital infection and its cerebral complications. AJR 134 (1980) 45–50.

Facial skull, neck
221. Archer, C. R., Yeager, V. L.: Evaluation of laryngeal cartilages by computed tomography. J. Comput. Ass. Tomogr. 3 (1979) 604–611.
222. Archer, C. R., Yeager, V. L., Friedman, W. H., Katsantonis, G. P.: Computed tomography of the larynx. J. Comput. Ass. Tomogr. 2 (1978) 404–411.
223. Archer, C. R., Friedman, W. H., Yeager, V. L. et al.: Evaluation of laryngeal cancer by computed tomography. J. Comput. Ass. Tomogr. 2 (1978) 618–624.
224. Balan, E. H., Wegener, O. H.,: Neue Erkenntnisse zur Beurteilung der Kieferfragmentstellung nach Progenieoperation durch das Computertomogramm. Dtsch. Z. Mund-Kiefer-Gesichts-Chir. 2 (1978) 95 S–99 S.
225. Baleriaux-Waha, D., Jeanmart, L., Dupont, M. G., Mortelmans, L. L.: CT scanning in extensive tumors of the face and skull base – Preliminary report from a cancer center. Intern. Symp. Heidelberg 1977. Eds.: Paul Gerhardt, Gerhard van Kaick. Georg Thieme, Stuttgart (1979) 338–344.
226. Caillé, J. M., Constant, Ph., Renaud-Salis, J. L., Dop, A.: CT studies of tumors of the skull base, facial skeleton and nasopharynx. Computerized Tomogr. 1 (1977) 217–224.
227. Carter, B. L., Karmody, C. S.: Computed tomography of the face and neck. Sem. Roentgenol. 13 (1978) 257–266.
228. Claussen, C., Lohkamp, F., Spenneberg, H., Glueck, E.: Computertomographie bei frontobasalen Schädelhirnverletzungen. Laryng. Rhinol. 57 (1978) 698–705.
229. Gonsalves, C. G., Briant, T. D. R., Harmand, W. M.: Computed tomography of the paranasal sinuses, nasopharynx, and soft tissues of the neck. Computerized Tomogr. 2 (1978) 271–278.
230. Hammerschlag, S. B., Wolpert, S. M., Carter, B. L.: Computed tomography of the skull base. J. Comput. Ass. Tomogr. 1 (1977) 75 ff.
231. Hesselink, J. R., New, P. F. J., Davis, K. R., Weber, A. L. et al.: Computed tomography of the paranasal sinuses and face. Part I. – Normal anatomy. J. Comput. Ass. Tomogr. 2 (1978) 559–567.
232. Hesselink, J. R., New, P. F. J., Davis, K. R., Weber, A. L. et al.: Computed tomography of the paranasal sinuses and face . Part II. – Pathological anatomy. J. Comput. Ass. Tomogr. 2 (1978) 568–576.
233. Lloyd, G. A. S., Phelps, P. D., Boulay, G. H.: High-resolution computerized tomography of the petrous bone. Brit. J. Radiol. 53 (1980) 631–641.
234. Lohkamp, F., Claussen, C., Spenneberg, H.: Computertomographie des Gesichtsschädels. Teil II – Pathologische Veränderungen. Fortschr. Röntgenstr. 126, 6 (1977) 513–520.
235. Lohkamp, F., Claussen, C.: Splanchnocranial CT (SCCT) – CT diagnosis of lesions and trauma involving the facial skull. Intern. Symp. Heidelberg 1977. Eds: Paul Gerhardt, Gerhard van Kaick. Georg Thieme, Stuttgart (1979) 324–331.
236. Lohkamp, F., Claussen, C., Spenneberg, H.: Computertomographie der Parotis. Laryng. Rhinol. 56 (1977) 104–120.
237. Lohkamp, F., Claussen, C.: Die Bedeutung der Computertomographie für die TNM-Klassifikation der Gesichtsschädelmalignome im Bereich der Nasennebenhöhlen, des Nasopharynx und der Parotis. Laryng. Rhinol. 56 (1977) 740–748.
238. Mancuso, A. A., Hanafee, W. N., Juillard, G. J. F. et al.: The role of computed tomography in the management of cancer of the larynx. Radiology 124 (1977) 243–244.
239. Mancuso, A. A., Hanafee, W. N., Winter, J., Ward, P.: Extensions of paranasal sinus tumors and inflammatory disease as evaluated by CT and pluridirectional tomography. Neuroradiology 16 (1978) 449–453.
240. Mancuso, A. A., Bohman, L., Hanafee, W., Maxwell, D.: Computed tomography of the nasopharynx – Normal and variants of normal. Radiology 137 (1980) 113–121.
241. Manelfe, C., Bonafé, A., Fabre, P., Pessey, J. J.: Computed tomography in olfactory neuroblastoma – One case of esthesioneuroepithelioma and four cases of esthesioneuroblastoma. J. Comput. Ass. Tomogr. 2 (1978) 412–420.
242. Modic, M. T., Weinstein, M. A., Berlin, A. J.: Maxillary sinus hypoplasia visualized with computed tomography. Radiology 135 (1980) 383–385.
243. Mödder, U., Friedmann, G., Tismer, R. et al.: Comparison of computed tomography and conventional tomography of tumors located in the nasopharynx and paranasal sinuses. Intern. Symp. Heidelberg 1977. Eds.: Paul Gerhardt, Gerhard van Kaick. Georg Thieme, Stuttgart (1979) 332–338.
244. Mödder, U., Friedmann, G., Gode, A., Rose, K. G.: Computertomographie des Gesichtsschädels und des pharyngealen Raumes. Fortschr. Röntgenstr. 131 (1979) 249–255.
245. Naidich, T. P., Pudlowski, R. M., Leeds, N. E., Deck, M. D. F.: Hypoglossal palsy – Computed tomography demonstration of denervation hemiatrophy of the tongue associated with glomus jugulare tumor. J. Comput. Ass. Tomogr. 2 (1978) 630–632.
246. Osborn, A. G., Anderson, R. E.: Direct sagittal computed tomographic scans of the face and paranasal sinuses. Radiology 129 (1978) 81–87.
247. Pirschel, J., Hübener, K. H.: Computertomographische Differentialdiagnostik von Schilddrüsenerkrankungen unter besonderer Berücksichtigung des szintigraphisch kalten Knotens. Fortschr. Röntgenstr. 130 (1979) 175–179.
248. Sekiya, T., Tada, S., Kawakami, K., Kino, M. et al.: Clinical application of computed tomography to thyroid disease. Computerized Tomogr. 3 (1979) 185–193.
249. Shimshak, R. R., Schoenrock, G. J., Taekman, H. P. et al.: Preoperative localization of a parathyroid adenoma using computed tomography and thyroid scanning. J. Comput. Ass. Tomogr. 3 (1979) 117–119.
250. Som, P. M., Biller, H. F.: The combined CT-sialogram. Radiology 135 (1980) 387–390.
251. Som, P. M., Shugar, J. M. A.: The CT classification of ethmoid mucoceles. J. Comput. Ass. Tomogr. 4 (1980) 199–203.
252. Som, P. M., Shugar, J. M. A.: Antral mucoceles – a new look. J. Comput. Ass. Tomogr. 4 (1980) 484–488.
253. Takahashi, M., Tamakawa, Y., Shindo, M., Konno, A.: Computed tomography of the paranasal sinuses and their adjacent structures. Computerized Tomogr. 1 (1977) 295–311.
254. Thawley, S. E., Gado, M., Fuller, T. R.: Computerized tomography in the evaluation of head and neck lesions. Laryngoscope 88 (1978) 451–458.
255. Weber, A. L., Tadmor, R., Davis, R., Roberson, G.: Malignant tumors of the sinuses. Neuroradiology 16 (1978) 443–448.
256. Wegener, O. H., Balan, E. H., Bier, J.: Das Computertomogramm zur Beurteilung des Kiefergelenkes. Dtsch. Z. Mund-Kiefer-Gesichts-Chir. 2 (1978) 23 S–29 S.

Thorax
257. Adler, O., Rosenberger, A.: Computed tomography in guiding of fine needle aspiration biopsy of the lung and mediastinum. Fortschr. Röntgenstr. 133 (1980) 135–137.
258. Faer, M. J., Burnam, R. E., Beck, C.: Transmural thoracic lipoma – Demonstration by computed tomography. Am. J. Roentgenol. 130 (1978) 161–163.
259. Gouliamos, A. D., Carter, B. L., Emami, B.: Computed tomography of the chest wall. Radiology 134 (1980) 433–436.
260. Jost, R. G., Sagel, S. S., Stanley, R. J., Levitt, R. G.: Computed tomography of the thorax. Radiology 126 (1978) 125–136.
261. Lackner, K., Felix, R., Oeser, H., Wegener, O. H., Bücheler, E., Buurmann, R., Heuser, L., Mödder, U.: Erweiterung der Röntgendiagnostik im Thoraxbereich durch die Computer-Tomographie. Radiologe 19 (1979) 79.
262. Lloyd, T. V., Paul, D. J.: Erosion of the scapula by a benign lipoma – Computed tomography diagnosis. J. Comput. Ass. Tomogr. 3 (1979) 679–680.
263. Long, J. A., Doppman, J. L., Nienhuis, A. W.: Computed tomographic studies of thoracic extramedullary hematopoiesis. J. Comput. Ass. Tomogr. 4 (1980) 67–70.
264. McLoud, T. C., Wittenberg, J., Ferrucci, J. T.: Computed tomography of the thorax and standard radiographic evaluation of the chest – A comparative study. J. Comput. Ass. Tomogr. 3 (1979) 170–180.
265. Mendez, G., Isikoff, M. B., Isikoff, S. K., Sinner, W. N.: Fatty tumors of the thorax demonstrated by CT. AJR 133 (1979) 207–212.
266. Paling, M. R., Dwyer, A.: The first rib as the cause of a "pulmonary nodule" on chest computed tomography. J. Comput. Ass. Tomogr. 4 (1980) 847–848.

267. Rohlfing, B., Korobkin, M., Hall, A. D.: Computed tomography of intrathoracic omental herniation and other mediastinal fatty masses. J. Comput. Ass. Tomogr. 1 (1977) 181–183.
268. Rothman, S. L. G., Simeone, J. F., Allen, W. E. et al.: Computerized tomography in the assessment of diseases of the thorax. Computerized Tomogr. 1 (1977) 181–196.
269. Soteropoulos, G. C., Cigtay, O. S., Schellinger, D.: Pectus excavatum deformities simulating mediastinal masses. J. Comput. Ass. Tomogr. 3 (1979) 596–600.
270. Wegener, O. H., Gerstenberg, E., Oeser, H.: Die Computer-Tomographie der Thorax-Organe. Röntgen-Berichte 6 (1977) 294.

Mediastinum

271. Bein, M. E., Mancuso, A. A., Mink, J. H., Hansen, G. C.: Computed tomography in the evaluation of mediastinal lipomatosis. J. Comput. Ass. Tomogr. 2 (1978) 379–383.
272. Binder, R. E., Pugatch, R. D., Faling, L. J., Kanter, R. A. et al.: Diagnosis of posterior mediastinal goiter by computed tomography J. Comput. Ass. Tomogr. 4 (1980) 550–552.
273. Brown, L. R., Muhm, J. R., Gray, J. E.: Radiographic detection of thymoma. AJR 134 (1980) 1181–1188.
274. Carter, B. L., Stanley, B. I.: Neck and mediastinal angiography by computed tomography scan. Radiology 122 (1977) 515–516.
275. Crowe, J. K., Brown, L. R., Muhm, J. R.: Computed tomography of the mediastinum. Radiology 128 (1978) 75–87.
276. Daffner, R. H., Halber, M. D., Postlethwait, R. W., Korobkin, M., Thompson, W. M.: CT of the esophagus. II. Carcinoma. AJR 133 (1979) 1051–1055.
277. Doppman, J. L., Brennan, M. F., Koehler, J. O., Marx, S. J.: Computed tomography for parathyroid localization. J. Comput. Ass. Tomogr. 1,1 (1977) 30 ff.
278. Fagan, C. J., Schreiber, M. H., Amparo, E. G. et al.: Traumatic diaphragmatic hernia into the pericardium – Verification of diagnosis by computed tomography. J. Comput. Ass. Tomogr. 3 (1979) 405–408.
279. Goldwin, R. L., Heitzman, E. R., Proto, A. V.: Computed tomography of the mediastinum. Radiology 124 (1977) 235–241.
280. Halber, M. D., Daffner, R. H., Thompson, W. M.: CT of the esophagus. I. Normal appearance. AJR 133 (1979) 1047–1050.
281. Heitzman, E. R., Goldwin, R. L., Proto, A. V.: Radiological analysis of the mediastinum utilizing on computed tomography. Sem. Roentgenol. 13 (1978) 277–292.
282. Homer, M. J., Wechsler, R. J., Carter, B. L.: Mediastinal lipomatosis. Radiology 128 (1978) 657–661.
283. Komaiko, M. S., Lee, M. E., Birnberg, F. A.: The contrast enhanced paravascular neoplasm – A potential CT pitfall. J. Comput. Ass. Tomogr. 4 (1980) 516–520.
284. Kormano, M., Yrjana, J.: The posterior tracheal band – Correlation between computed tomography and chest radiography. Radiology 136 (1980) 689–694.
285. Machida, K., Yoshikawa, K.: Aberrant thyroid gland demonstrated by computed tomography. J. Comput. Ass. Tomogr. 3 (1979) 689–690.
286. Mink, J. H., Bein, M. E., Sukov, R., Herrmann, C. et al.: Computed tomography of the anterior mediastinum in patients with myasthenia gravis and suspected thymoma. Am. J. Roentgenol. 130 (1978) 239–246.
287. Modic, M. T., Janicki, P. C.: Computed tomography of mass lesions of the right cardiophrenic angle. J. Comput. Ass. Tomogr. 4 (1980) 521–526.
288. Onitsuka, H., Kuhns, L. R.: Dextroconvexity of the mediastinum in the azygoesophageal recess – A normal CT variant in young adults. Radiology 135 (1980) 126.
289. Owens, G. R., Arger, P. H., Mulhern, C. B., Coleman, B. G. et al.: CT evaluation of mediastinal pseudocyst. J. Comput. Ass. Tomogr. 4 (1980) 256–259.
290. Pugatch, R. D., Faling, L. J., Robbins, A. H., Spira, R.: CT diagnosis of benign mediastinal abnormalities. AJR 134 (1980) 685–694.
291. Sinner, W. N.: Zur computertomographischen Differentialdiagnostik von gut- und bösartigen lipoiden Raumforderungen des Mediastinums und deren Ausbreitung. Fortschr. Röntgenstr. 132 (1980) 613–621.
292. Stratt, B., Steiner, R. M.: The radiologic findings in posterior mediastinal chordoma. Skeletal Radiol. 5 (1980) 171–173.
293. Walter, E., Hübener, K. H.: Computertomographische Charakteristika raumfordernder Prozesse im vorderen Mediastinum und ihre Differentialdiagnose. Fortschr. Röntgenstr. 133 (1980) 391–400.
294. Wegener, O. H.: Die Computertomographie des Mediastinums. Fortschr. Röntgenstr. 129 (1978) 727–735.
295. Wolf, B. S., Nakagawa, H., Yeh, H. C.: Visualization of the thyroid gland with computed tomography. Radiology 123 (1977) 368.

Heart, pericardium

296. Baim, R. S., MacDonald, I. L., Wise, D. J., Lenkei, S. C.: Computed tomography of absent left pericardium. Radiology 135 (1980) 127–128.
297. Carlsson, E., Lipton, M. J., Skiöldebrand, C. G. et al.: Erfahrungen mit der Computer-Tomographie bei der in-vivo-Herzdiagnostik. Radiologe 20 (1980) 44–49.
298. Felix, R., Lackner, K., Simon, H., Grube, E., Thurn, P.: Das Herz im „schnellen" Computertomogramm „Computer-Kardio-Tomographie" (CKT). Methodik und erste Ergebnisse. Fortschr. Röntgenstr. 129 (1978) 401–409.
299. Felix, R., Lackner, K., Thurn, P.: Derzeitige und zukünftige Möglichkeiten des CT-Einsatzes am Herzen. Radiologe 20 (1980) 50–55.
300. Guthaner, D. F., Wexler, L., Harell, G.: CT demonstration of cardiac structures. AJR 133 (1979) 75–81.
301. Harell, G. S., Guthaner, D. F., Breiman, R. S. et al.: Stop-action cardiac computed tomography. Radiology 123 (1977) 515–517.
302. Hessel, S. J., Dougless, F. A., Judy, P. F. et al.: Detection of myocardial ischemia in vitro by computed tomography. Radiology 127 (1978) 413–418.
303. Houang, M. T. W., Arozena, X., Shaw, D. G.: Demonstration of the pericardium and pericardial effusion by computed tomography. J. Comput. Ass. Tomogr. 3 (1979) 601–603.
304. Huang, H. K., Mazziotta, J. C.: Heart imaging from computerized tomography. Computerized Tomogr. 2 (1978) 37–44.
305. Huggins, T. J., Huggins, M. J., Schnapf, D. J., Brott, W. H. et al.: Left atrial myxoma – Computed tomography as a diagnostic modality. J. Comput. Ass. Tomogr. 4 (1980) 253–255.
306. Janson, R., Lackner, K., Grube, E., Klehr, H. U., Thurn, P.: Computertomographische Diagnostik des Perikardergusses. Fortschr. Röntgenstr. 131 (1979) 173–179.
307. Janson, R., Lackner, K., Grube, E., Brecht, G., Thurn, P.: Computerkardiotomographie der idiopathischen hypertrophen subvalvulären Aortenstenose (IHSS) – Ein neuartiger Beitrag zur nicht-invasiven Diagnostik. Fortschr. Röntgenstr. 130 (1979) 536–542.
308. Jeffrey, R. B., Webb, W. R.: CT appearance of rheumatoid pericarditis. J. Comput. Ass. Tomogr. 4 (1980) 866–868.
309. Lackner, K., Heuser, L., Friedmann, G., Thurn, P.: Computerkardiotomographie bei Tumoren des linken Vorhofes. Fortschr. Röntgenstr. 129,6 (1979) 735–739.
310. Lackner, K., Simon, H., Thurn, P.: Kardio-Computertomographie – Neue Möglichkeiten in der radiologischen nicht-invasiven Herzdiagnostik. Z. Kardiol. 68 (1979) 667–675.
311. Lackner, K., Thurn, P.: EKG-gesteuerte Kardiocomputertomographie. Fortschr. Röntgenstr. 132 (1980) 164–169.
312. Lackner, K., Thurn, P., Orellano, L. et al.: Der aortokoronare Bypass im Computertomogramm. Fortschr. Röntgenstr. 133 (1980) 459–465.
313. Lipton, M. J., Hayashi, T. T., Boyd, D., Carlsson, E.: Measurement of left ventricular cast volume by computed tomography. Radiology 127 (1978) 419–423.
314. Rankin, R. N., Raval, B., Finley, R.: Primary chylopericardium – Combined lymphangiographic and CT diagnosis. J. Comput. Ass. Tomogr. 4 (1980) 869–870.
315. Rogers, C. I., Seymour, E. Q., Brock, J. G.: Atypical pericardial cyst location – The value of computed tomography. J. Comput. Ass. Tomogr. 4 (1980) 683–694.
316. Sagel, S. S., Weiss, E. S., Gillard, R. G., Hounsfield, G. N. et al.: Gated computed tomography of the human heart. Invest. Radiol. 12 (1977) 563–566.
317. Ter-Pogossian, M. M., Weiss, E. S., Coleman, R. E., Sobel, B. E.: Computed tomography of the heart. Am. J. Roentgenol. 127 (1976) 79–90.

Lung, pleura

318. Ayers, W. R., Huang, H. K.: The use of computerized tomography in the diagnosis of pulmonary nodules. Computerized Tomogr. 2 (1978) 55–62.
319. Baber, C. E., Hedlund, L. W., Oddson, T. A. et al.: Differentiating empyemas and peripheral pulmonary abscesses. Radiology 135 (1980) 755–758.
320. Berger, P. E., Kuhn, J. P., Kuhns, L. R.: Computed tomography and the occult tracheobronchial foreign body. Radiology. 134 (1980) 133–135.
321. Ekholm, S., Albrechtsson, U., Kugelberg, J. et al.: Computed tomography in preoperative staging of bronchogenic carcinoma. J. Comput. Ass. Tomogr. 4 (1980) 763–765.
322. Emami, B., Melo, A., Carter, B. L., Munzenrider, J. E., Piro, A. J.: Value of computed tomography in radiotherapy of lung cancer. Am. J. Roentgenol. 131 (1978) 63–67.
323. Godwin, J. D., Webb, W. R., Gamsu, G. et al.: Computed tomography of pulmonary embolism. AJR 135 (1980) 691–695.

324. Kreel, L.: Computer tomography in the evaluation of pulmonary asbestosis. Acta Radiol. Diagn. 17 (1976) 405–412.
325. Kreel, L.: Computed tomography of the lung and pleura. Sem. Roentgenol. 13 (1978) 213–225.
326. Mintzer, R. A., Malave, S. R., Neiman, H. L. et al.: Computed vs. conventional tomography in evaluation of primary and secondary pulmonary neoplasms. Radiology 132 (1979) 653–659.
327. Muhm, J. R., Brown, L. R., Crowe, L. K.: Detection of pulmonary nodules by computed tomography. Am. J. Roentgenol. 128 (1977) 267–270.
328. Naidich, D. P., Terry, P. B., Stitik, F. P. et al.: Computed tomography of the bronchi – 1. Normal anatomy. J. Comput. Ass. Tomogr. 4 (1980) 746–753.
329. Naidich, D. P., Stitik, F. P., Khouri, N. F. et al.: Computed tomography of the bronchi – 2. Pathology. J. Comput. Ass. Tomogr. 4 (1980) 754–762.
330. Pugatch, R. D., Faling, L. J., Robbins, A. H., Snider, G. L.: Differentiation of pleural and pulmonary lesions using computed tomography. J. Comput. Ass. Tomogr. 2 (1978) 601–606.
331. Putman, C. E., Rothman, S. L., Littner, M. R. et al.: Computerized tomography in pulmonary sarcoidosis. Computerized Tomogr. 1 (1977) 197–209.
332. Raptopoulos, V., Schellinger, D., Katz, S.: Computed tomography of solitary pulmonary nodules – Experience with scanning times longer than breath-holding. J. Comput. Ass. Tomogr. 4 (1980) 55–60.
333. Schaner, E. G., Chang, A. E., Doppman, J. L. et al.: Comparison of computed and conventional whole lung tomography in detecting pulmonar nodules – A prospective radiologic-pathologic study. Am. J. Roentgenol. 131 (1978) 51–54.
334. Siegelman, S. S., Zerhouni, E. A., Leo, F. P. et al.:CT of the solitary pulmonary nodule. AJR 135 (1980) 1–13.
335. Sinner, W. N.: Computed tomographic patterns of pulmonary thromboembolism and infarction. J. Comput. Ass. Tomogr. 2 (1978) 395–399.
336. Solomon, A., Kreel, L., McNicol, M., Johnson, N.: Computed tomography in pulmonary sarcoidosis. J. Comput. Ass. Tomogr. 3 (1979) 754–758.
337. Wegener, O.-H.: Die Dichtebestimmung des Lungengewebes mittels Computertomographie. Habilitationsschrift, Berlin 1979.

Abdomen

338. Aronberg, D. J., Stanley, R. J., Levitt, R. G., Sagel, S. S.: Evaluation of abdominal abscess with computed tomography. J. Comput. Ass. Tomogr. 2 (1978) 384–387.
339. Aspestrand, F.: Demonstration of thoracic and abdominal fistulas by computed tomography. J. Comput. Ass. Tomogr. 4 (1980) 536–537.
340. Bernardino, M. E., Jing, B. S., Wallace, S.: Computed tomography diagnosis of mesenteric masses. AJR 132 (1979) 33–36.
341. Boldt, D. W., Reilly, B.: Computed tomography of abdominal mass lesions in children. Radiology 124 (1977) 371–378.
342. Brasch, R. C., Abols, I. B., Gooding, C. A., Filly, R. A.: Abdominal disease in children. AJR 134 (1980) 153–158.
343. Bryan, P. J., Dinn, W. M.: Isodense masses on CT – Differentiation by gray scale ultrasonography. Am. J. Roentgenol. 129 (1977) 989–992.
344. Callen, P. W.: Computed tomographic evaluation of abdominal and pelvic abscesses. Radiology 131 (1979) 171–175.
345. Chuang, V. P., Fried, A. M., Oliff, M., Ellis, G. T., Sachatello, C. R.: Abdominal CSF pseudocyst secondary to ventriculoperitoneal shunt – Diagnosis by computed tomography in two cases. J. Comput. Ass. Tomogr. 2 (1978) 88 ff.
346. Daffner, R. H., Halber, M. D.: Pitfall in the CT diagnosis of abdominal abscess – The full stomach. Computerized Tomogr. 3 (1979) 33–36.
347. Druy, E. M., Rubin, B. E.: Computed tomography in the evaluation of abdominal trauma. J. Comput. Ass. Tomogr. 3 (1979) 40–44.
348. Dunnick, N. R., Ihde, D. C., Johnston-Early, A.: Abdominal CT in the evaluation of small cell carcinoma of the lung. AJR 133 (1979) 1085–1088.
349. Dwyer, A.: The displaced crus – A sign for distinguishing between pleural fluid and ascites on computed tomography. J. Comput. Ass. Tomogr. 2 (1978) 598–599.
350. Ferrucci, J. T., Wittenberg, J.: CT biopsy of abdominal tumors – Aids for lesion localization. Radiology 129 (1978) 739–744.
351. Feuerbach, S., Gullotta, U., Reiser, M., Ingianni, G.: Röntgensymptomatik intraabdomineller Abszesse im Computertomogramm. Fortschr. Röntgenstr. 133 (1980) 296–298.
352. Gerhardt, P., Kaick, G.: Indikation und Wertigkeit der Computertomographie in der Abdominaldiagnostik. Radiologe 18 (1978) 243–251.
353. Haertel, M., Fuchs, W. A.: Computertomographie nach stumpfem Abdominaltrauma. Fortschr. Röntgenstr. 131 (1979) 487–492.
354. Halber, M. D., Daffner, R. H., Morgan, C. L. et al.: Intraabdominal abscess – Current concepts in radiologic evaluation. AJR 133 (1979) 9–13.
355. Jeffrey, R. B.: CT demonstration of peritoneal implants. AJR 135 (1980) 323–326.
356. Jolles, H., Coulam, C. M.: CT of ascites – Differential diagnosis. AJR 135 (1980) 315–322.
357. Korobkin, M., Callen, P. W., Filly, R. A. et al.: Comparison of computed tomography, ultrasonography, and gallium–67 scanning in the evaluation of suspected abdominal abscess. Radiology 129 (1978) 89–93.
358. Lee, J. K. T., Levitt, R. G., Stanley, R. J., Sagel, S. S.: Utility of body computed tomography in the clinical follow-up of abdominal masses. J. Comput. Ass. Tomogr. 2 (1978) 607–611.
359. Levitt, R. G., Jost, R. G., Trachtman, J., Sagel, S. S., Stanley, R. J.: A computer-assisted method to determine the diagnostic efficacy of computed tomography of the body. Radiology 123 (1977) 97–101.
360. Levitt, R. G., Biello, D. R., Sagel, S. S., Stanley, R. J. et al.: Computed tomography and 67 – Ga citrate radionuclide imaging for evaluating suspected abdominal abscess. AJR 132 (1979) 529–534.
361. Mödder, U., Friedmann, G., Heuser, L., Buess, G.: Polyzystische Degeneration parenchymatöser Organe des Abdomens oder maligner Tumor – Computertomographische Abklärung. Fortschr. Röntgenstr. 127,5 (1977) 414–416.
362. Passariello, R., Simonetti, G., Rovighi, L., Ciolina, A.: Characteristic CT pattern of giant superior mesenteric artery aneurysms. J. Comput. Ass. Tomogr. 4 (1980) 621–626.
363. Pripstein, S., Cavoto, F. V., Gerritsen, R. W.: Spontaneous mycotic aneurysm of the abdominal aorta. J. Comput. Ass. Tomogr. 3 (1979) 681–683.
364. Quinn, M. J., Sheedy, P. F., Stephens, D. H. et al.: Computed tomography of the abdomen in evaluation of patients with fever of unknown origin. Radiology 136 (1980) 407–411.
365. Robbins, A. H., Pugatch, R. D., Gerzof, S. G. et al.: Observations on the medical efficacy of computed tomography of the chest and abdomen. Am. J. Roentgenol. 131 (1978) 15–19.
366. Robbins, A. H., Pugatch, R. D., Gerzof, S. G. et al.: Further observations on the medical efficacy of computed tomography of the chest and abdomen. Radiology 137 (1980) 719–725.
367. Sagel, S., Stanley, R. J., Evens, R. G.: Early clinical experience with motionless whole-body computed tomography. Radiology 119 (1976) 321–330.
368. Shin, M. S., Ferrucci, J. T., Wittenberg, J.: Computed tomographic diagnosis of pseudoascites (floating viscera syndrome). J. Comput. Ass. Tomogr. 2 (1978) 594–597.
369. Wegener, O. H., Hartmann, K.: Möglichkeiten und Grenzen der Computertomographie bei intraabdominellen Abszessen. In: Peritonitis (Ed.: Häring, R.). TM-Verlag, Bad Oeynhausen (1979).
370. Vujic, I., Rogers, C. I., Leveen, H. H.: Computed tomographic detection of portal vein thrombosis. Radiology 135 (1980) 697–698.
371. Wittenberg, J., Fineberg, H. V., Black, E. B., Kirkpatrick, R. H. et al.: Clinical efficacy of computed body tomography. Am. J. Roentgenol. 131 (1978) 5–14.
372. Wolverson, M. K., Jagannadharao, B., Sundaram, M. et al.: CT as a primary diagnostic method in evaluating intraabdominal abscess. AJR 133 (1979) 1089–1095.
373. Yeh, H. C., Chahinian, A. P.: Ultrasonography and computed tomography of peritoneal mesothelioma. Radiology 135 (1980) 705–712.

Liver

374. Alfidi, R. J., Haaga, J. R., Havrilla, T. R., Pepe, R. G., Cook, S. A.: Computed tomography of the liver. Am. J. Roentgenol. 127 (1976) 69–74.
375. Araki, T., Itai, Y., Furui, S. et al.: Dynamic CT densitometry of hepatic tumors. AJR 135 (1980) 1037–1043.
376. Barnett, P. H., Zerhouni, E. A., White, R. I. et al.: Computed tomography in the diagnosis of cavernous hemangioma of the liver. AJR 134 (1980) 439–447.
377. Bernardino, M. E.: Computed tomography of calcified liver metastases. J. Comput. Ass. Tomogr. 3 (1979) 32–35.
378. Biello, D. R., Levitt, R. G., Siegel, B. A., Sagel, S. S., Stanley, R. J.: Computed tomography and radionuclide imaging of the liver – A comparative evaluation. Radiology 127 (1978) 159–163.
379. Biondetti, P. R., Fiore, D., Muzzio, P. C.: Computed tomography of the liver in von Gierke's disease. J. Comput. Ass. Tomogr. 4 (1980) 685–686.

380. Bryan, P. J., Dinn, W. M., Grossman, Z. D., Wistow, B. W. et al.: Correlation of computed tomography, gray scale ultrasonography, and radionuclide imaging of the liver in detecting space-occupying processes. Radiology 124 (1977) 387–393.
381. Bücheler, E., Hagemann, J., Remmecke, J.: Postpartaler akuter Leberarterienverschluß. Fortschr. Röntgenstr. 133 (1980) 285–289.
382. Callen, P. W., Filly, R. A., Marcus, F. S.: Ultrasonography and computed tomography in the evaluation of hepatic microabscesses in the immunosuppressed patient. Radiology 136 (1980) 433–434.
383. Dunnick, N. R., Ihde, D. C., Doppman, J. L. et al.: Computed tomography in primary hepatocellular carcinoma. J. Comput. Ass. Tomogr. 4 (1980) 59–62.
384. Foley, W., Berland, L. L., Lawson, T. L. et al.: Computed tomography in the demonstration of hepatic pseudoaneurysm with hemobilia. J. Comput. Ass. Tomogr. 4 (1980) 863–865.
385. Freeny, P. C.: Portal vein tumor thrombus – Demonstration by computed tomographic arteriography. J. Comput. Ass. Tomogr. 4 (1980) 263–264.
386. Frick, M. P., Knight, L. C., Feinberg, S. B., Loken, M. K., Gedgaudas, E.: Computer tomography, radionuclide imaging and ultrasonography in hepatic mass lesions. Computerized Tomogr. 3 (1979) 49–55.
387. Haertel, M., Fretz, C., Fuchs, W. A.: Zur computertomographischen Diagnostik der Echinokokkose. Fortschr. Röntgenstr. 133 (1980) 164–170.
388. Haertel, M.: Das kavernöse Leberhämangiom im Computertomogramm. Fortschr. Röntgenstr. 133 (1980) 379–381.
389. Hübener, K. H., Hippeli, R.: Das Leberlipom. Fortschr. Röntgenstr. 133 (1980) 176–179.
390. Inamoto, K., Sugiki, K., Yamasaki, H. et al.: Computed tomography and angiography of hepatocellular carcinoma. J. Comput. Ass. Tomogr. 4 (1980) 832–839.
391. Ishikawa, T., Tsukune, Y., Ohyama, Y. et al.: Venous abnormalities in portal hypertension demonstrated by CT. AJR 134 (1980) 271–276.
392. Itai, Y., Nishikawa, J., Tasaka, A.: Computed tomography in the evaluation of hepatocellular carcinoma. Radiology 131 (1979) 165–170.
393. Itai, Y., Furui, S., Araki, T. et al.: Computed tomography of cavernous hemangioma of the liver. Radiology 137 (1980) 149–155.
394. Janson, R., Lackner, K., Paquet, K. J. et al.: Computertomographische und angiographische Synopsis histologisch gesicherter intrahepatischer Raumforderungen. Fortschr. Röntgenstr. 132 (1980) 658–665.
395. Kirschner, L. P., Ferris, R. A., Mero, J. H., Moss, M. L.: Hydatid disease of the liver evaluated by computed tomography. J. Comput. Ass. Tomogr. 2 (1978) 229–230.
396. Kolbenstvedt, A., Kjolseth, I., Klepp, O. et al.: Postirradiation changes of the liver demonstrated by computed tomography. Radiology 135 (1980) 391.
397. Kressel, H. Y., Korobkin, M., Goldberg, H. I., Moss, A. A.: The portal venous tree simulating dilated biliary ducts on computed tomography of the liver. J. Comput. Ass. Tomogr. 1 (1977) 169–175.
398. Kuhns, L. R., Borlaza, G. S., Seigel, R. et al.: Lack of visualization of the portal venous tree in cirrhosis of the liver – A computed tomography finding with possible diagnostic significance. J. Comput. Ass. Tomogr. 2 (1978) 400–403.
399. Kuhns, L. R., Borlaza, G.: Normal roentgen variant – Aberrant right hepatic artery on computed tomography. Radiology 135 (1980) 392.
400. Kunstlinger, F., Federle, M. P., Moss, A. A., Marks, W.: Computed tomography of hepatocellular carcinoma. AJR 134 (1980) 431–437.
401. Levitt, R. G., Sagel, S. S., Stanley, R. J., Jost, R. G.: Accuracy of computed tomography of the liver and biliary tract. Radiology 124 (1977) 123–128.
402. Marchal, G. J., Baert, A. L., Wilms, G. E.: CT of noncystic liver lesions – Bolus enhancement. AJR 135 (1980) 57–65.
403. Marks, W. M., Filly, R. A.: Computed tomographic demonstration of intraarterial air following hepatic artery ligation. Radiology 132 (1979) 665–666.
404. Mills, S. R., Doppman, J. L., Nienhuis, A. W.: Computed tomography in the diagnosis of disorders of excessive iron storage of the liver. J. Comput. Ass. Tomogr. 1,1 (1977) 101–104.
405. Morgan, C. L., Trought, W. S., Daffner, R. H.: The use of CT scanning in resolving "pseudo" lesions of the liver. Computerized Tomogr.2 (1978) 295–301.
406. Moss, A. A., Schrumpf, J., Schnyder, P. et al.: Computed tomography of focal hepatic lesions – A blind clinical evaluation of the effect of contrast enhancement. Radiology 131 (1979) 427–430.
407. Newmark, H., Smith, J. J., Burrows, R., Silberman, E. L.: Echinococcal cyst of the liver seen on computed tomography. J. Comput. Ass. Tomogr. 2 (1978) 231–232.
408. Noon, M. A., Young, S. W., Castellino, R. A.: Leiomyosarcoma metastatic to the liver – CT appearance. J. Comput. Ass. Tomogr. 4 (1980) 527–530.
409. Prando, A., Wallace, S., Bernardino, M. E., Lindell, M. M.: Computed tomographic arteriography of the liver. Radiology 130 (1979) 697–701.
410. Reh, T. E., Srivisal, S., Schmidt, E. H.: Portal venous thrombosis in ulcerative colitis – CT diagnosis with angiographic correlation. J. Comput. Ass. Tomogr. 4 (1980) 545–547.
411. Scherer, U., Lissner, J., Eisenburg, J., Zrenner, M., Schildberg, F. W.: Computertomographie der Leber. Fortschr. Röntgenstr. 130 (1979) 531–535.
412. Scherer, U., Rothe, R., Eisenburg, J., Schildberg, F. W. et al.: Diagnostic accuracy of CT in circumscript liver disease. Am. J. Roentgenol. 130 (1978) 711–714.
413. Scherer, U., Lissner, J.: CT of the liver. Intern. Symp. Heidelberg 1977. Eds.: Paul Gerhardt, Gerhard van Kaick. G. Thieme, Stuttgart (1979) 87–94.
414. Scherer, U., Buell, U., Rothe, R., Eisenburg, J. et al.: Computerized tomography and nuclear imaging of the liver. Eur. J. Nucl. Med. 3 (1978) 71–80.
415. Scherer, U., Santos, M., Lissner, J.: CT studies of the liver in vitro – A report on 82 cases with pathological correlation. J. Comput. Ass. Tomogr. 3 (1979) 589–595.
416. Scherer, U., Weinzierl, M., Sturm, R., Schildberg, F. W. et al.: Computed tomography in hydatid disease of the liver – A report on 13 cases. J. Comput. Ass. Tomogr. 2 (1978) 612–617.
417. Schnyder, P. A., Candardjis, G.: Extreme hydronephrosis versus echinococcal cyst of the liver – Computed tomography evaluation. J. Comput. Ass. Tomogr. 3 (1979) 126–127.
418. Scott, W. W., Sanders, R. C., Siegelman, S. S.: Irregular fatty infiltration of the liver – Diagnostic dilemmas. AJR 135 (1980) 67–71.
419. Snow, J. H., Goldstein, H. M., Wallace, S.: Comparison of scintigraphy, sonography, and computed tomography in the evaluation of hepatic neoplasms. AJR 132 (1979) 915–918.
420. Stephens, D. H., Sheedy, P. F., Hattery, R. R., MacCarty, R. L.: Computed tomography of the liver. Am. J. Roentgenol. 128 (1977) 579–590.
421. Tschakert, H.: Zeitlicher Ablauf des Dichteverhaltens von Lebermetastasen nach Kontrastmittelgabe. Fortschr. Röntgenstr. 133 (1980) 171–176.
422. Vigo, M., Faveri, D., Biondetti, P. R. et al.: CT demonstration of portal and superior mesenteric vein thrombosis in hepatocellular carcinoma. J. Comput. Ass. Tomogr. 4 (1980) 627–629.
423. Vogel, H., Schumpelick, V., Bücheler, E. et al.: Transkatheteraler Verschluß der A. hepatica. Fortschr. Röntgenstr. 133 (1980) 289–292.
424. Wenzel, E., Erbe, W.: Computertomographische Untersuchungen bei zystischen Leberveränderungen. Röntgen-Bl. 32 (1979) 401–407.
425. Zerhouni, E. A., Barth, K. H., Siegelman, S. S.: Computed tomographic demonstration of inferior vena cava invasion in a case of hepatocellular carcinoma. J. Comput. Ass. Tomogr. 2 (1978) 363–365.

Bile ducts

426. Araki, T., Itai, Y., Tasaka, A.: CT of choledochal cyst. AJR 135 (1980) 729–734.
427. Berland, L. L., Doust, B. D., Foley, W. D.: Acute hemorrhage into the gallbladder diagnosed by computed tomography and ultrasonography. J. Comput. Ass. Tomogr. 4 (1980) 260–262.
428. Buck, J., Bosnjakovic, S., Heuck, F., Schulze, R.: Ein Beitrag der Röntgen-Ganzkörper-Computer-Tomographie zur Diagnose und Differentialdiagnose des Ikterus. Radiologe 19 (1979) 353–360.
429. Ferris, R. A., Kirschner, L. P., Mero, J. H., Chung, D. H.: Increased attenuation value in a hydropic gallbladder. J. Comput. Ass. Tomogr. 3 (1979) 545–546.
430. Foley, W. D., Wilson, C. R., Quiroz, F. A. et al.: Demonstration of the normal extrahepatic biliary tract with computed tomography. J. Comput. Ass. Tomogr. 4 (1980) 48–52.
431. Goldberg, H. I., Filly, R. A., Korobkin, M., Moss, A. A., Kressel, H. Y., Callen, P. W.: Capability of CT body scanning and ultrasonography to demonstrate the status of the biliary ductal system in patients with jaundice. Radiology 129 (1978) 731–737.
432. Grant, E. G., Borts, F., Schellinger, D. et al.: Pneumobilia – A comparison of four imaging modalities. J. Comput. Ass. Tomogr. 4 (1980) 630–633.
433. Havrilla, T. R., Reich, N. E., Haaga, J. R., Seidelmann, F. E. et al.: Computed tomography of the gallbladder. Am. J. Roentgenol. 130 (1978) 1059–1067.
434. Havrilla, T. R., Haaga, J. R., Alfidi, R. J., Reich, N. E.: Computed tomography and obstructive biliary disease. AJR 128 (1977) 765–768.

435. Heuck, F., Buck, J.: Der Informationswert der Röntgen-Computer-Tomographie für die Beurteilung von Gallenwegen und Gallenblase. Radiologe 20 (1980) 6–15.
436. Itai, Y., Araki, T., Furui, S. et al.: Computerized tomography and ultrasound in the diagnosis of intrahepatic calculi. Radiology 136 (1980) 399–405.
437. Itai, Y., Araki, T., Yoshikawa, K. et al.: Computed tomography of gallbladder carcinoma. Radiology 137 (1980) 713–718.
438. Kaiser, J. A., Mall, J. C., Salmen, B. J. et al.: Diagnosis of Caroli disease by computed tomography – Report of two cases. Radiology 132 (1979) 661–664.
439. Moss, A. A., Filly, R. A., Way, L. W.: In vitro investigation of gallstones with computed tomography. J. Comput. Ass. Tomogr. 4 (1980) 827–831.
440. Nacianceno, S. E., Gross, S. C., Raju, J. S. et al.: Pancreatic pseudocyst simulating dilated biliary duct system on computed tomography. Radiology 134 (1980) 165–166.
441. Solomon, A., Kreel, L., Pinto, D.: Contrast computed tomography in the diagnosis of acute cholecystitis. J. Comput. Ass. Tomogr. 3 (1979) 585–588.
442. Thomas, J. L., Bernardino, M. E.: Segmental biliary obstruction – Its detection and significance. J. Comput. Ass. Tomogr. 4 (1980) 155–158.

Pancreas

443. Ariyama, J., Shirakabe, H., Shimaguchi, S. et al.: Kritischer Vergleich der Untersuchungsmethoden bei der Frage nach einem Pankreaskarzinom. Fortschr. Röntgenstr. 133 (1980) 6–9.
444. Baert, A. L., Ponette, E., Pringot, J., Marchal, G., Dardenne, A., Coenen, Y.: Axiale Computer-gesteuerte Tomometrie bei akuter und chronischer Pankreatitis. Radiologe 17 (1977) 181–188.
445. Borlaza, G. S., Kuhns, L. R., Seigel, R., Pozderac, R., Eckhauser, F.: Computed tomographic and angiographic demonstration of gastroduodenal artery pseudoaneurysm in a pancreatic pseudocyst. J. Comput. Ass. Tomogr. 3 (1979) 612–614.
446. Butzelaar, R. M. J. M., Mulder, G. L., Kuhler, W. J. et al.: Computer tomography in acute pancreatitis. Acta Radiol. Diagnosis 19 (1978) 417–422.
447. Callen, P. W., Breiman, R. S., Korobkin, M. et al.: Carcinoma of the tail of the pancreas – An unusual CT appearance. AJR 133 (1979) 135–137.
448. Charnsangavej, C., Elkin, M.: Displacement of the tail of the pancreas in the absence of the left kidney. Radiology 137 (1980) 156.
449. Dembner, A. G., Jaffe, C. C., Simeone, J., Walsh, J.: A new computed tomographic sign of pancreatitis. AJR 133 (1979) 477–479.
450. Dunnick, N. R., Doppman, J. L., Mills, S. R., McCarthy, D. M.: Computed tomographic detection of nonbeta pancreatic islet cell tumors. Radiology 135 (1980) 117–120.
451. Dunnick, N. R., Long, J. A., Krudy, A. et al.: Localizing insulinomas with combined radiographic methods. AJR 135 (1980) 747–752.
452. Fawcitt, R. A., Forbes, W., Isherwood, I., Braganza, J. M.: Computed tomography in pancreatic disease. Brit. J. Radiol. 51 (1978) 1–4.
453. Ferrucci, J. T., Wittenberg, J., Black, E. B. et al.: Computed body tomography in chronic pancreatitis. Radiology 130 (1979) 175–182.
454. Fishman, A., Isikoff, M. B., Barkin, J. S., Friedland, J. T.: Significance of a dilated pancreatic duct on CT examination. AJR 133 (1979) 225–227.
455. Foley, W. D., Lawson, T. L., Quiroz, F.: Sagittal and coronal image reconstruction – Application in pancreatic computed tomography. J. Comput. Ass. Tomogr. 3 (1979) 717–721.
456. Freeny, P. C., Ball, T. J., Ryan, J.: Impact of new diagnostic imaging methods on pancreatic angiography. AJR 133 (1979) 619–624.
457. Fricke, M., Zick, R., Mitzkat, H. J.: Das Insulinom im Computer-Tomogramm. Radiologe 18 (1978) 252–254.
458. Grabbe, E., Hagemann, V., Klapdor, R., Pfeiffer, M.: Sonographie und Computertomographie in der Verlaufskontrolle des Pankreaskarzinoms. Fortschr. Röntgenstr. 133 (1980) 149–154.
459. Haaga, J. R., Alfidi, R. J., Zeich, M. G., Meany, T. F. et al.: Computed tomography of the pancreas. Radiology 120 (1976) 589–595.
460. Haaga, J. R., Alfidi, R. J., Havrilla, T. R., Tubbs, R. et al.: Definitive role of CT scanning of the pancreas. Radiology 124 (1977) 723–730.
461. Haertel, M., Tillmann, U., Fuchs, W. A.: Die akute Pankreatitis im Computertomogramm. Fortschr. Röntgenstr. 130 (1979) 525–530.
462. Haertel, M., Kreel, L.: Das normale Pancreas im computerisierten Tomogramm. Fortschr. Röntgenstr. 128 (1978) 1–7.
463. Haertel, M., Zaunbauer, W., Fuchs, W. A.: Die computertomographische Morphologie des Pankreaskarzinoms. Fortschr. Röntgenstr. 133 (1980) 1–5.
464. Hauser, H., Battikha, J. G., Wettstein, P.: Computed tomography of the dilated main pancreatic duct. J. Comput. Ass. Tomogr. 4 (1980) 53–58.
465. Heller, A. H. J., Rupp, N., Weiss, H. D., Fuchs, H.: Die Computer-Tomographie des Pankreas. Dt. med. Wschr. 102 (1977) 3–5.
466. Husband, J. E., Meire, H. B., Kreel, L.: Comparison of ultrasound and computer-assisted tomography in pancreatic diagnosis. Brit. J. Radiol. 50 (1977) 855–862.
467. Kaplan, J. O., Isikoff, M. B., Barkin, J., Livingstone, A. S.: Necrotic carcinoma of the pancreas – The pseudo-pseudocyst. J. Comput. Ass. Tomogr. 4 (1980) 166–167.
468. Kivisaari, L., Kormano, M., Rantakokko, V.: Contrast enhancement of the pancreas in computed tomography. J. Comput. Ass. Tomogr. 3 (1979) 722–726.
469. Kreel, L., Haertel, M., Katz, D.: Computed tomography of the normal pancreas. J. Comput. Ass. Tomogr. 1 (1977) 290–299.
470. Kressel, H. Y., Margulis, A. R., Gooding, G. W., Filly, R. A. et al.: CT scanning and ultrasound in the evaluation of pancreatic pseudocysts – A preliminary comparison. Radiology 126 (1978) 153–157.
471. Kuhns, L. R., Borlaza, G. S., Seigel, R., Cho, K. J.: Localization of the head of the pancreas using the junction of the left renal vein and the inferior vena cava. J. Comput. Ass. Tomogr. 2 (1978) 170–172.
472. Lammer, J., Lepuschuetz, H., Sager, W. D., et al.: ERCP und CT in der Diagnostik von chronischen Pankreatitis, Pseudozysten und Pankreaskarzinom – ein Vergleich. Röntgen-Bl. 33 (1980) 602–611.
473. Levin, D. C., Wilson, R., Abrams, H. L.: The changing role of pancreatic arteriography in the era of computed tomography. Radiology 136 (1980) 245–249.
474. Maraist, D. V., Sibille, P. J.: Cystadenoma of the pancreas demonstrated by computed tomography with the ACTA-scanner – A case report. Comput. Tomogr. 1 (1977) 121–124.
475. Marchal, G., Baert, A. L., Wilms, G.: Intravenous pancreaticography in computed tomography. J. Comput. Ass. Tomogr. 3 (1979) 727–723.
476. Mendez, G., Isikoff, M. B.: Significance of intrapancreatic gas demonstrated by CT – A review of nine cases. AJR 132 (1979) 59–62.
477. Mödder, U., Friedmann, G., Bücheler, E., Baert, E., Lackner, C., Brecht, G. et al.: Wert und Ergebnisse der Computertomographie bei Pankreaserkrankungen. Fortschr. Röntgenstr. 130 (1979) 57–61.
478. Moss, A. A., Kressel, H. Y., Korobkin, M., Goldberg, H. I. et al.: The effects of Gastrografin and glucagon on CT scanning of the pancreas. Radiology 126 (1978) 711–714.
479. Moss, A. A., Kressel, H. Y.: Computed tomography of the pancreas. Digest. Diseases 22,11 (1977) 1018–1027.
480. Moss, A. A., Federle, M., Shapiro, H. A. et al.: The combined use of computed tomography and endoscopic retrograde cholangiopancreatography in the assessment of suspected pancreatic neoplasm – A blind clinical evaluation. Radiology 134 (1980) 159–163.
481. Neumann, C. H., Hessel, S. J.: CT of the pancreatic tail. AJR 135 (1980) 741–745.
482. Pistoletsi, G. F., Marzoli, G. P., Colosso, P. Q., Pederzoli, P., Procacci, C.: Computed tomography in surgical pancreatic emergencies. J. Comput. Ass. Tomogr. 2 (1978) 165–169.
483. Raptopoulos, V., Schellinger, D.: Imaging of the pancreas with computed tomography. Computerized Tomogr. 3 (1979) 37–47.
484. Santos, L. A., Bernardino, M. E., Paulus, D. D., Martin, R. E.: Computed tomography of cystadenoma of the pancreas. J. Comput. Ass. Tomogr. 2 (1978) 222–225.
485. Seidelmann, F. E., Cohen, W. N., Bryan, P. J., Brown, J.: CT demonstration of the splenic vein-pancreatic relationship: The pseudo-dilated pancreatic duct. Am. J. Roentgenol. 129 (1977) 17–21.
486. Sheedy, P. F., Stephens, D. H., Hattery, R. R., MacCarty, R. L.: Computed tomography in the evaluation of patients with suspected carcinoma of the pancreas. Radiology 124 (1977) 731–737.
487. Siegelman, S. S., Copeland, B. E., Saba, G. P. et al.: CT of fluid collections associated with pancreatitis. AJR 134 (1980) 1121–1132.
488. Stanley, R. J., Sagel, S. S., Levitt, R. G.: Computed tomographic evaluation of the pancreas. Radiology 124 (1977) 715–722.
489. Stanley, R. J., Sagel, S. S., Evens, R. G.: The impact of new imaging methods on pancreatic arteriography. Radiology 136 (1980) 251–253.
490. Steele, J. R., Sones, P. J.: Computed tomography of the pancreas – The use of intravenous contrast to define the dorsal surface of the pancreas. Computerized Tomogr. 2 (1978) 303–307.

Stomach, bowel

491. Douleday, L. C., Bernardino, M. E.: CT findings in the perirectal area following radiation therapy. J. Comput. Ass. Tomogr. 4 (1980) 634–638.
492. Grabbe, E., Buurmann, R., Winkler, R., Bücheler, R., Schreiber, H. W.: Computertomographische Befunde nach Rektumamputation. Fortschr. Röntgenstr. 131 (1979) 135–139.
493. Husband, J. E., Hodson, N. J., Parsons, C. A.: The use of comput-

ed tomography in recurrent rectal tumors. Radiology 134 (1980) 677–682.
494. Kaye, M. D., Young, S. W., Hayward, R. et al.: Gastric pseudotumor on CT scanning. AJR 135 (1980) 190–193.
495. Kressel, H. Y., Callen, P. W., Montagne, J. P., Korobkin, M., Goldberg, H. I. et al.: Computed tomographic evaluation of disorders affecting the alimentary tract. Radiology 129 (1978) 451–455.
496. Kuhns, L. R., Seigel, R., Borlaza, G., Rapp, R.: Visualization of the longitudinal fold of the duodenum by computed tomography. J. Comput. Ass. Tomogr. 3 (1979) 345–347.
497. Kuwabara, Y., Nishitani, H., Numaguchi, Y. et al.: Afferent loop syndrome. J. Comput. Ass. Tomogr. 4 (1980) 687–689.
498. Mayes, G. B., Zornoza, J.: Computed tomography of colon carcinoma. AJR 135 (1980) 43–46.
499. Megibow, A. J., Redmond, P. E., Bosniak, M. A., Horowitz, L.: Diagnosis of gastrointestinal lipomas by CT. AJR 133 (1979) 743–745.
500. Parienty, R. A., Smolarski, N., Pradel, J., Ducellier, R., Lubrano, J. M.: Computed tomography of the gastrointestinal tract – Lesion recognition and pitfalls. J. Comput. Ass. Tomogr. 3 (1979) 615–619.
501. Seigel, R. S., Kuhns, L. R., Borlaza, G. S. et al.: Computed tomography and angiography in ileal carcinoid tumor and retractile mesenteritis. Radiology 134 (1980) 437–440.
502. Steinbrich, W., Mödder, U., Rosenberger, J., Friedmann, G.: Computertomographische Diagnostik lokaler Rezidive von Rektumkarzinomen. Fortschr. Röntgenstr. 131 (1979) 499–503.

Urogenital tract
503. Ammon, J., Frik, W., Karstens, J. H., Rübben, H., Schoffers, J.: Ganzkörper-Computertomographie bei Erkrankungen des Urogenitalsystems. Urologe 18 (1979) 1–13.
504. Ammon, J., Karstens, J. H., Rübben, H.: Unterstützung einer am TNM-System orientierten Bestrahlungsplanung urologischer Tumoren durch die Computertomographie. Fortschr. Röntgenstr. 129 (1978) 253–259.
505. Apitzsch, D. E., Wegener, O. H., Khalil, M., Sörensen, R.: Advances in the diagnosis of renal angiomyolipoma. Acta Radiol. Diagn. 20 (1979) 105–110.
506. Baert, A. L., Marchal, G., Staelens, B., Coenen, Y.: C.T. evaluation of renal space occupying lesions. Fortschr. Röntgenstr. 126, 4 (1977) 285–291.
507. Baert, A. L., Marchal, G., Wilms, G., Dooren, W.: Vergleich Computertomographie und Ultraschall bei Nierenerkrankungen. Röntgen-Bl. 31 (1978) 641–645.
508. Baert, A. L., Marchal, G., Coenen, Y., Wilms, G. et al.: CT in diseases of the kidney and suprarenal glands. Intern. Symp. Heidelberg 1977. Eds.: Paul Gerhardt, Gerhard van Kaick. Georg Thieme, Stuttgart (1979) 124–134.
509. Baert, A. L., Wilms, G., Marchal, G. et al: Contrast enhancement by bolus technique in the CT examination. Radiologe 20 (1980) 279–287.
510. Bernardino, M. E., Santos, L. A., Johnson, D. E., Bracken, R. B.: Computed tomography in the evaluation of post-nephrectomy patients. Radiology 130 (1979) 183–187.
511. Braedel, H. U., Rzehak, L., Schindler, E. et al: Computertomographische Unterschungen bei Nierenverletzungen. Fortschr. Röntgenstr. 132 (1980) 49–54.
512. Breit, A., Rohde, U.: Computertomographie in der Gynäkologie. Med. Klin. 74 (1979) 1881–1893.
513. Buck, D. R., Dunnick, N. R., Doppman, J. L.: Retrorenal cysts. J. Comput. Ass. Tomogr. 3 (1979) 765–767.
514. Coleman, C. C., Saxena, K. M., Johnson, K. W.: Renal vein thrombosis in a child with the nephrotic syndrome – CT diagnosis. AJR 135 (1980) 1285–1286.
515. Colley, D. P., Clark, R. A.: The influence of computed tomography on clinical decision making in the evaluation of a nonvisualizing kidney. Computerized Tomogr. 2 (1978) 309–313.
516. Dailey, E. T., Rozanski, R. M., Kieffer, S. A., Dinn, W. M.: Computed tomography in genitourinary pathology. Urology 12, 1 (1978) 95–105.
517. Delmonico, F. L., McKusick, K. A., Cosimi, A. B., Russell, P. S.: Differentiation between renal allograft rejection and acute tubular necrosis by renal scan. Am. J. Roentgenol. 128 (1977) 625–628.
518. Dunnick, N. R., Long, J. A., Javadpour, N.: Perirenal extravasation of urographic contrast medium demonstrated by computed tomography. J. Comput. Ass. Tomogr. 4 (1980) 538–539.
519. Engelshoven, J. M. A., Kreel, L.: Computed tomography of the prostate. J. Comput. Ass. Tomogr. 3 (1979) 45–51.
520. Engelstad, B. L., McClennan, B. L., Levitt, R. G. et al.: The role of pre-contrast images in computed tomography of the kidney. Radiology 136 (1980) 153–155.
521. Epstein, L., Wacksman, J., Daughtry, J. et al.: Multilocular cysts of kidney – A diagnostic dilemma. Urology 11 (1978) 573–576.
522. Forbes, W. St., Isherwood, I., Fawcitt, R. A.: Computed tomography in the evaluation of the solitary or unilateral nonfunctioning kidney. J. Comput. Ass. Tomogr. 2 (1978) 389–394.
523. Frick, M. P., Feinberg, S. E., Knight, L. C.: Evaluation of retroperitoneum with computerized tomography and ultrasonography in patients with testicular tumors. Computerized Tomogr. 3 (1979) 181–184.
524. Friedman, G., Mödder, U., Tismer, R., Vlaho, M.: Lymphocele nach Nieren-Transplantation. Computer-tomographische und lymphographische Abklärung. Radiologe 17 (1977) 393–395.
525. Frija, J., Larde, D., Belloir, C. et al.: Computed tomography diagnosis of renal angiomyolipoma. J. Comput. Ass. Tomogr. 4 (1980) 843–846.
526. Gooding, G. A. W.: The ultrasonic and computed tomographic appearance of splenic lobulations – A consideration in the ultrasonic differential of masses adjacent to the left kidney. Radiology 126 (1978) 719–720.
527. Haaga, J. R., Zelch, M. G., Alfidi, R. J., Stewart, B. H., Daugherty, J. D.: CT-guided antegrade pyelography and percutaneous nephrostomy. Am. J. Roentgenol. 128 (1977) 621–624.
528. Haaga, J. R., Morrison, S. C.: CT appearance of renal infarct. J. Comput. Ass. Tomogr. 4 (1980) 246–247.
529. Haertel, M.: Zur Computertomographie gynäkologischer Karzinome. Fortschr. Röntgenstr. 132 (1980) 652–657.
530. Hattery, R. R., Williamson, B., Stephens, D. H. et al.: Computed tomography of renal abnormalities. Radiol. Clin. North Am. 15 (1977) 401–418.
531. Heinz, E. R., Dubois, P. J., Drayer, B. P. et al.: A preliminary investigation of the role of dynamic computed tomography in renovascular hypertension. J. Comput. Ass. Tomogr. 4 (1980) 63–66.
532. Heuser, L., Friedmann, G., Mödder, U., Bischofsberger, M., Heising, J.: Diagnose und Differentialdiagnose raumfordernder Prozesse der Nieren im Computer-Tomogramm. Röntgen-Blätter 30 (1977) 479–489.
533. Hoffman, E. P., Mindelzun, R. E., Anderson, R. U.: Computed tomography in acute pyelonephritis associated with diabetes. Radiology 135 (1980) 691–695.
534. Jaques, P. F., Staab, E., Richey, W., Photopulos, G., Swanton, M.: CT-assisted pelvic and abdominal aspiration biopsies in gynecological malignancy. Radiology 128 (1978) 651–655.
535. Jaschke, W., Kaick, G., Palmtag, H.: Vergleich der Wertigkeit von Echographie und Computertomographie bei der Diagnostik raumfordernder Prozesse der Nieren. Fortschr. Röntgenstr. 132 (1980) 145–151.
536. Javadpour, N., Doppman, J. L., Bergman, S. M., Anderson, T.: Correlation of computed tomography and serum tumor markers in metastatic retroperitoneal testicular tumor. J. Comput. Ass. Tomogr. 2 (1978) 176–180.
537. Jentsch, F., Stringaris, K., Kaiser, G., Kirschner, H.: Computertomographie des kleinen Beckens als Grundlage für strahlentherapeutische Vorgehen, Lokalisation und Bestrahlungsplanung beim Prostatakarzinom. Radiologe 17 (1977) 268–270.
538. Kim, D. S., Woesner, M. E., Howard, T. F., Olson, L. K.: Emphysematous pyelonephritis demonstrated by computed tomography. AJR 132 (1979) 287–288.
539. Kittredge, R. D., Brensilver, J., Pierce, J. C.: Computed tomography in renal transplant problems. Radiology 127 (1978) 165–169.
540. Küster, W., Imhof, H.: Die Bedeutung der Computertomographie für die Abklärung von Patienten mit Hodentumoren. Röntgen-Bl. 32 (1979) 526–532.
541. Kuhns, L. R., Thornbury, J., Seigel, R.: Variation of position of the kidneys and diaphragm in patients undergoing repeated suspension of respiration. J. Comput. Ass. Tomogr. 3 (1979) 620–621.
542. Lee, J. K. T., McClennan, B. L., Stanley, R. J., Sagel, S. S.: Computed tomography in the staging of testicular neoplasms. Radiology 130 (1979) 387–390.
543. Lee, J. K. T., McClennan, B. L., Stanley, R. J., Sagel, S. S.: Utility of computed tomography in the localization of the undescended testis. Radiology 135 (1980) 121–125.
544. Lee, J. K. T., McClennan, B. L., Melson, G. L., Stanley, R. J.: Acute focal bacterial nephritis – Emphasis on gray scale sonography and computed tomography. AJR 135 (1980) 87–92.
545. Love, L., Reynes, C. J., Churchill, R., Moncada, R.: Third generation CT scanning in renal disease. Radiol. Clin. North Am. 17 (1979) 77–90.
546. Magilner, A. D., Ostrum, B. J.: Computed tomography in the diagnosis of renal masses. Radiology 126 (1978) 715–718.

547. Marchal, G., Coenen, Y., Wilms, G., Baert, A. L.: The accuracy of CT-scan in the diagnosis of retroperitoneal metastases of malignant testicular tumours. Fortschr. Röntgenstr. 128 (1978) 746–753.
548. McClennan, B. L., Stanley, R. J., Melson, G. L., Levitt, R. G., Sagel, S. S.: CT of the renal cyst – Is cyst aspiration necessary? AJR 133 (1979) 671–675.
549. Panigel, M., Leo, F. P., Donner, M. W.: In vitro computed tomography of the human placenta. J. Comput. Ass. Tomogr. 3 (1979) 181–183.
550. Petersen, R. W.: A computerized tomographic evaluation of malignancies of the bladder and prostate. Computerized Tomogr. 1 (1977) 283–293.
551. Probst, P., Fischedick, A. R., Haertel, M.: Computertomographie nach Nierentumorembolisation. Fortschr. Röntgenstr. 133 (1980) 633–636.
552. Riehle, R. A., McCarron, J. P., Kazam, E., Muecke, E.: Computed tomography in urologic patients. Urology 10 (1977) 529–535.
553. Rohde, U., Spechter, H. J., Breit, A.: Computed tomography in gynecology. Intern. Symp. Heidelberg 1977. Eds.: Paul Gerhardt, Gerhard van Kaick. Georg Thieme, Stuttgart (1979) 183–188.
554. Rubin, B. E.: Computed tomography in the evaluation of renal lymphoma. J. Comput. Ass. Tomogr. 3 (1979) 759–764.
555. Ryan, K. G., Hoch, W. H., Craven, R. M.: Intraureteral tumor demonstrated by computed tomography. J. Comput. Ass. Tomogr. 3 (1979) 474–477.
556. Sagel, S. S., Stanley, R. J., Levitt, R. G., Geisse, G.: Computed tomography of the kidney. Radiology 124 (1977) 359–370.
557. Sandler, C. M., Conley, S. B., Fogel, S. R., Brewer, E. D.: Splenic compression of the left kidney simulating pathologic unilateral renal enlargement. J. Comput. Ass. Tomogr. 4 (1980) 248–250.
558. Schaner, E. G., Balow, J. W., Doppman, J. L.: Computed tomography in the diagnosis of subcapsular and perirenal hematoma. AJR 129 (1977) 83–88.
559. Segal, A. J., Spitzer, R. M.: Pseudo thick-walled renal cyst by CT. AJR 132 (1979) 827–828.
560. Segal, A. J., Spataro, R. F., Linke, C. A., Frank, I. et al.: Diagnosis of nonopaque calculi by computed tomography. Radiology 129 (1978) 447–450.
561. Seidelmann, F. E., Cohen, W. N., Bryan, P. J., Temes, S. P. et al.: Accuracy of CT staging of bladder neoplasms using the gas-filled method – Report of 21 patients with surgical confirmation. AJR 130 (1978) 735–739.
562. Smith, W. P., Levine, E.: Sagittal and coronal CT image reconstruction – Application in assessing the inferior vena cava in renal cancer. J. Comput. Ass. Tomogr. 4 (1980) 531–535.
563. Steele, J. R., Sones, P. J., Heffner, L. T.: The detection of inferior vena caval thrombosis with computed tomography. Radiology 128 (1978) 385–386.
564. Sukov, R. J., Scardino, P. T., Sample, W. F. et al.: Computed tomography and transabdominal ultrasound in the evaluation of the prostate. J. Comput. Ass. Tomogr. 1 (1977) 281–289.
565. Takahashi, M., Tamakawa, Y., Shibata, A., Fukushima, Y.: Computed tomography of 'page' kidney. J. Comput. Ass. Tomogr. 1 (1977) 344–348.
566. Takao, R., Amamoto, Y., Matsunaga, N. et al.: Computed tomography of multicystic kidney. J. Comput. Ass. Tomogr. 4 (1980) 548–549.
567. Turner, R. J., Young, S. W., Castellino, R. A.: Dynamic continuous computed tomography – Study of retroaortic left renal vein. J. Comput. Ass. Tomogr. 4 (1980) 109–111.
568. Wegener, O. H., Rost, A., Souchon, R., Fiedler, M.: Erste Ergebnisse der Computer-Tomographie bei der Klassifikation von Harnblasentumoren. Verh. Ber. d. Dtsch. Ges. f. Urol. 29 (1977) 76–80.
569. Wenzel, E., Scherer, K., Vogel, H. M.: Sonographie, Computertomographie und Angiographie bei Nierenbeckenhämangiom. Fortschr. Röntgenstr. 130, 5 (1979) 583–586.
570. Williamson, B., Hattery, R. R., Stephens, D. H. et al.: Computed tomography of the kidneys. Sem. Roentgenol. 13 (1978) 249–255.
571. Wilms, G., Baert, A. L., Marchal, G., Bruneel, M.: CT demonstration of gas formation after renal tumor embolization. J. Comput. Ass. Tomogr. 3 (1979) 838–839.
572. Wolverson, M. K., Jagannadharao, B., Sundaram, M. et al.: CT in localization of impalpable cryptorchid testes. AJR 134 (1980) 725–729.

Adrenals

573. Behan, M., Martin, E. C., Muecke, E. C., Kazam, E.: Myelolipoma of the adrenal – Two cases with ultrasound and CT findings. Am. J. Roentgenol. 129 (1977) 993–996.
574. Berger, P. E., Kuhn, J. P., Munschauer, R. W.: Computed tomography and ultrasound in the diagnosis and management of neuroblastoma. Radiology 128 (1978) 663–667.
575. Brownlie, K., Kreel, L.: Computer assisted tomography of normal suprarenal glands. J. Comput. Ass. Tomogr. 2 (1978) 1–10.
576. Dunnick, N. R., Schaner, E. G., Doppman, J. L., Strott, C. A. et al.: Computed tomography in adrenal tumors. AJR 132 (1979) 43–46.
577. Eghrari, M., McLoughlin, M. J., Rosen, I. E. et al.: The role of computed tomography in assessment of tumoral pathology of the adrenal glands. J. Comput. Ass. Tomogr. 4 (1980) 71–77.
578. Falappa, P., Mirk, P., Rossi, M. et al.: Bilateral pseudocystic pheochromocytoma. J. Comput. Ass. Tomogr. 4 (1980) 860–862.
579. Galanski, M., Friemann, J., Thiede, G. et al.: Computertomographische Diagnostik von Nebennierenerkrankungen. Röntgen-Bl. 33 (1980) 272–278.
580. Galanski, M., Fischer, M., Cramer, B. M. et al.: Computertomographische Lokalisationsdiagnostik beim primären Aldosteronismus. Fortschr. Röntgenstr. 133 (1980) 629–633.
581. Georgi, M., Jaschke, W., Trede, M. et al.: Erfahrungen mit der Computertomographie und der Nebennierenphlebographie in der Diagnostik hormonaktiver Nebennierenprozesse. Radiologe 20 (1980) 172–180.
582. Haertel, M., Probst, P., Bollmann, J. et al.: Computertomographische Nebennierendiagnostik. Fortschr. Röntgenstr. 132 (1980) 31–36.
583. Heuck, F., Buck, J., Reiser, U.: Die gesunde und kranke Nebenniere im Röntgen-Computer-Tomogramm. Radiologe 20 (1980) 158–171.
584. Hübener, K. H., Grehn, S., Schulze, K.: Indikationen zur computertomographischen Nebennierenuntersuchung – Leistungsfähigkeit, Stellenwert und Differentialdiagnostik. Fortschr. Röntgenstr. 132 (1980) 37–44.
585. Karstaedt, N., Sagel, S. S., Stanley, R. J. et al.: Computed tomography of the adrenal gland. Radiology 129 (1978) 723–730.
586. Korobkin, M., White, E. A., Kressel, H. Y. et al.: Computed tomography in the diagnosis of adrenal disease. AJR 132 (1979) 231–238.
587. Laursen, K., Damgaard-Pedersen, K.: CT for pheochromocytoma diagnosis. AJR 134 (1980) 277–280.
588. Long, J. A., Dunnick, N. R., Doppman, J. L.: Noninflammatory gas formation following embolization of adrenal carcinoma. J. Comput. Ass. Tomogr. 3 (1979) 840–841.
589. Montagne, J. P., Kressel, H. Y., Korobkin, M., Moss, A. A.: Computed tomography of the normal adrenal glands. Am. J. Roentgenol. 130 (1978) 963–966.
590. Sample, W. F., Sarti, D. A.: Computed tomography and gray scale ultrasonography of the adrenal gland – A comparative study. Radiology 128 (1978) 377–383.
591. Schaner, E. G., Dunnick, N. R., Doppman, J. L., Strott, C. A. et al.: Adrenal cortical tumors with low attenuation coefficients – A pitfall in computed tomography diagnosis. J. Comput. Ass. Tomogr. 2 (1978) 11–15.
592. Stadler, H. W., Grabner, W., Fuchs, H. F.: Computertomographische Untersuchung der Nebennieren. Klinikarzt 8 (1979) 399–406.
593. Stewart, B. H., Straffon, R. A., Haaga, J., Seidelmann, F. E.: Urological applications of computerized axial tomography. Transactions Am. Assoc. Genito-Urinary Surgeons 70 (1979) 117–130.
594. Stiris, M. G.: Accessory spleen versus left adrenal tumor – Computed tomographic and abdominal angiographic evaluation. J. Comput. Ass. Tomogr. 4 (1980) 543–544.
595. Tisnado, J., Amendola, M. A., Konerding, K. F. et al.: Computed tomography versus angiography in the localization of pheochromocytoma. J. Comput. Ass. Tomogr. 4 (1980) 853–859.
596. Wilms, G., Baert, A., Marchal, G., Goddeeris, P.: Computed tomography of the normal adrenal glands – Correlative study with autopsy specimens. J. Comput. Ass. Tomogr. 3 (1979) 467–469.

Retroperitoneum, pelvis

597. Borlaza, G. S., Kuhns. L. R., Seigel, R. S., Rapp, R.: The posterior pararenal space – An escape route for retrocrural masses. J. Comput. Ass. Tomogr. 3 (1979) 470–473.
598. Brun, B., Kristensen, J. K.: Computed tomography in the evaluation of a pelvic tumor. J. Comput. Ass. Tomogr. 3 (1979) 547–549.
599. Carter, B. L., Kahn, P. C., Wolpert, S. M. et al.: Unusual pelvic masses – A comparison of computed tomographic scanning and ultrasonography. Radiology 121 (1976) 383–390.
600. Gerson, E. S., Gerzof, S. G., Robbins, A. H.: CT confirmation of pelvic lipomatosis – Two cases. Am. J. Roentgenol. 129 (1977) 338–340.
601. Gilula, L. A., Murphy, W. A., Tailor, C. C., Patel, R. B.: Computed tomography of the osseous pelvis. Radiology 132 (1979) 107–114.
602. Grauthoff, H., Hofmann, P., Lackner, K., Brackmann, H. H.: Hä-

mophiler Pseudotumor und Iliacushämatom; radiologische und klinische Befunde. Fortschr. Röntgenstr. 129 (1978) 614–620.
603. Guilford, W. B., Mintz, P. D., Blatt, P. M. et al.: CT of hemophilic pseudotumors of the pelvis. AJR 135 (1980) 167–169.
604. Haertel, M., Bollmann, J., Vock, P., Zingg, E.: Computertomographie und retroperitoneale Fibrose (Morbus Ormond). Fortschr. Röntgenstr. 131 (1979) 504–507.
605. Heller, M., Kötter, D., Wenzel, E.: Computertomographische Diagnostik des traumatisierten Beckens. Fortschr. Röntgenstr. 132 (1980) 386–391.
606. Jeffrey, R. B., Callen, P. W., Federle, M. P.: Computed tomography of psoas abscesses. J. Comput. Ass. Tomogr. 4 (1980) 639–641.
607. Kalman, M. A.: Radiologic soft tissue shadows in the pelvis – Another look. AJR 130 (1978) 493–498.
608. Korobkin, M., Callen, P. W., Fisch, A. E.: Computed tomography of the pelvis and retroperitoneum. Radiol. Clin. North Am. 17 (1979) 301–319.
609. Lange, T. A., Alter, A. J.: Evaluation of complex acetabular fractures by computed tomography. J. Comput. Ass. Tomogr. 4 (1980) 849–852.
610. Levine, E., Farber, B., Lee, K. R.: Computed tomography in diagnosis of pelvic lipomatosis. Urology 12 (1978) 606–608.
611. Levitt, R. G., Sagel, S. S., Stanley, R. J. et al.: Computed tomography of the pelvis. Sem. Roentgenol. 13 (1978) 193–200.
612. Mannes, E. J., Walsh, J. W., Simeone, J. F., Putnam, S. L.: Computer assisted tomographic evaluation of a ganglioneuroblastoma in an adult. J. Comput. Ass. Tomogr. 3 (1979) 120–123.
613. Mendez, G., Isikoff, M. B., Hill, M. C.: Retroperitoneal processes involving the psoas demonstrated by computed tomography. J. Comput. Ass. Tomogr. 4 (1980) 78–82.
614. Mitty, H. A.: CT for diagnosis and management of urinary extravasation. AJR 134 (1980) 497–501.
615. Musumeci, R., Palo, G., Kenda, R. et al.: Retroperitoneal metastases from ovarian carcinoma. AJR 134 (1980) 449–452.
616. Ralls, P. W., Boswell, W., Henderson, R., Rogers, W. et al.: CT of inflammatory disease of the psoas muscle. AJR 134 (1980) 767–770.
617. Reich, N.: Computed tomography of the retroperitoneum – Anatomic and pathologic considerations. Intern. Symp. Heidelberg 1977. Eds.: Paul Gerhardt, Gerhard van Kaick. Georg Thieme, Stuttgart (1979) 135–142.
618. Sagel, S. S., Siegel, M. J., Stanley, R. J., Jost, R. G.: Detection of retroperitoneal hemorrhage by computed tomography. Am. J. Roentgenol. 129 (1977) 403–407.
619. Sauser, D. D., Billimoria, P. E., Rouse, G. A. et al.: CT evaluation of hip trauma. AJR 135 (1980) 269–274.
620. Shirkhoda, A., Johnston, R. E., Staab, E. V. et al.: Optimal computed tomography technique for bone evaluation. J. Comput. Ass. Tomogr. 3 (1979) 134–139.
621. Shirkhoda, A., Brashear, H. R., Staab, E. V.: Computed tomography of acetabular fractures. Radiology 134 (1980) 683–688.
622. Simeone, J. F., Robinson, F., Rothman, S. L., Jaffe, C. C.: Computerized tomographic demonstration of a retroperitoneal hematoma causing femoral neuropathy. J. Neurosurg. 47 (1977) 946–948.
623. Somogyi, J., Cohen, W. N., Omar, M. M., Makhuli, Z.: Communication of right and left perirenal spaces demonstrated by computed tomography. J. Comput. Ass. Tomogr. 3 (1979) 270–273.
624. Steinbrich, W., Friedmann, G.: Computertomographische Untersuchung der Organe des kleinen Beckens (Untersuchungstechnik und normale Anatomie). Röntgen-Bl. 33 (1980) 595–601.
625. Stephens, D. H., Sheedy, P. F., Hattery, R. R., Williamson, B.: Diagnosis and evaluation of retroperitoneal tumors by computed tomography. Am. J. Roentgenol. 129 (1977) 395–402.
626. Vint, V. C., Usselman, J. A., Warmath, M. A. et al.: Aortic perianeurysmal fibrosis – CT density enhancement and ureteral obstruction. AJR 134 (1980) 577–580.
627. Walsh, J. W., Amendola, M. A., Konerding, K. F.: Computed tomographic detection of pelvic and inguinal lymph-node metastases from primary and recurrent pelvic malignant disease. Radiology 137 (1980) 157–166.

Vertebral column
628. Aaro, S., Dahlborn, M., Svensson, L.: Estimation of vertebral rotation in structural scoliosis by computer tomography. Acta Radiol. Diagnosis 19 (1978) 990–992.
629. Arredondo, F., Haughton, V. M., Hemmy, D. C. et al.: The computed tomographic appearance of the spinal cord in diastematomyelia. Radiology 136 (1980) 685–688.
630. Banzer, D., Risch, M. W., Wegener, O. H.: Eine neue Methode zur Messung des Rotationswinkels der Wirbelskoliose. Fortschr. Röntgenstr. 132 (1980) 403–405.
631. Bonafé, A., Ethier, R., Melançon, D. et al.: High resolution computed tomography in cervical syringomyelia. J. Comput. Ass. Tomogr. 4 (1980) 42–47.
632. Carrera, G. F., Haughton, V. M., Syvertsen, A., Williams, A. L.: Computed tomography of the lumbar facet joints. Radiology 134 (1980) 145–148.
633. Claussen, C. D., Lohkamp, F. W., Bazan, U.: The diagnosis of congenital spinal disorders in computed tomography (CT). Neuropädiatrie 8, 4 (1977) 405–417.
634. Claussen, C., Banniza, U., Jaschke, W. et al.: Die Bedeutung der Computertomographie in der Diagnostik kongenitaler spinaler Mißbildungen, insbesondere der Diastematomyelie. Fortschr. Röntgenstr. 133 (1980) 520–527.
635. Coin, C. G., Chan, Y. S., Keranen, V., Pennink, M.: Computer assisted myelography in disk disease. J. Comput. Ass. Tomogr. 1 (1977) 398.
636. Coin, C. G., Pennink, M., Ahmad, W. D., Keranen, V. J.: Diving-type injury of the cervical spine – Contribution of computed tomography to management. J. Comput. Ass. Tomogr. 3 (1979) 362–372.
637. Coin, C. G., Hucks-Folliss, A.: Cervical computed tomography in multiple sclerosis with spinal cord involvement. J. Comput. Ass. Tomogr. 3 (1979) 421–422.
638. Colley, D. P., Dunsker, S. B.: Traumatic narrowing of the dorsolumbar spinal canal demonstrated by computed tomography. Radiology 129 (1978) 95–98.
639. Faerber, E. N., Wolpert, S. M., Scott, R. M., Belkin, S. C., Carter, B. L.: Computed tomography of spinal fractures. J. Comput. Ass. Tomogr. 3 (1979) 657–661.
640. Geehr, R. B., Rothman, S. L. G., Kier, E. L.: The role of computed tomography in the evaluation of upper cervical spine pathology. Computerized Tomogr. 2 (1978) 79–97.
641. Gonsalves, C. G., Hudson, A. R., Horsey, W. J., Tucker, W. S.: Computed tomography of the cervical spine and spinal cord. Computerized Tomogr. 2 (1978) 279–293.
642. Haughton, V. M., Williams, A. L.: CT anatomy of the spine. Eds.: Caillé, J. M., Salamon, G.: Springer-Verlag Berlin – Heidelberg – New York 1980.
643. Haughton, V. M., Syvertsen, A., Williams, A. L.: Soft-tissue anatomy within the spinal canal as seen on computed tomography. Radiology 134 (1980) 649–655.
644. Heller, M., Ringe, J. D., Bücheler, E., Kuhlencordt, F.: Morbus Paget – Manifestationen an der Wirbelsäule. Fortschr. Röntgenstr. 130, 6 (1979) 652–658.
645. Herman, G. T., Coin, C. G.: The use of three-dimensional computer display in the study of disk disease. J. Comput. Ass. Tomogr. 4 (1980) 564–567.
646. James, H. E., Oliff, M.: Computed tomography in spinal dysraphism. J. Comput. Ass. Tomogr. 1 (1977) 391–397.
647. Lackner, K., Schroeder, S.: Computertomographie der Lendenwirbelsäule. Fortschr. Röntgenstr. 133 (1980) 124–131.
648. Lamarque, J. L., Ginestie, J. F., Dondelinger, R., Bruel, J. M. et al.: Initial experience with computerized tomography in osteoarticular and muscular pathologic conditions. Intern. Symp. Heidelberg 1977. Eds.: Paul Gerhardt, Gerhard van Kaick. Georg Thieme, Stuttgart (1979) 221–225.
649. Ledley, R. S., Park, C. M., Ray, R. D.: Application of the ACTA-scanner to visualization of the spine. Computerized Tomogr. 3 (1979) 57–69.
650. Lee, B. C. P., Kazam, E., Newman, A. D.: Computed tomography of the spine and spinal cord. Radiology 128 (1978) 95–102.
651. Naidich, T. P., King, D. G., Moran, C. J. et al.: Computed tomography of the lumbar thecal sac. J. Comput. Ass. Tomogr. 4 (1980) 37–41.
652. Naidich, T. P., Pudlowski, R. M.: High resolution CT of the cervical spinal cord. Eds.: Caillé, J. M., Salamon, G. Springer-Verlag Berlin – Heidelberg – New York 1980.
653. Nakagawa, H., Huang, Y. P., Malis, L. I., Wolf, B. S.: Computed tomography of intraspinal and paraspinal neoplasms. J. Comput. Ass. Tomogr. 1 (1977) 377–390.
654. O'Callaghan, J. P., Ullrich, C. G., Yuan, H. A. et al.: CT of facet distraction in flexion injuries of the thoracolumbar spine. AJR 134 (1980) 563–568.
655. Oon, C. L.: A method of locating the plane of CT scans of the abdomen. J. Comput. Ass. Tomogr. 4 (1980) 268–277.
656. Post, M. J. D., Gargano, F. P., Vining, D. Q. et al.: A comparison of radiographic methods of diagnosing constrictive lesions of the spinal canal. J. Neurosurg. 48 (1978) 360–368.
657. Resjoe, I. M., Harwood-Nash, D. C., Fitz, C. R., Chuang, S.: Normal cord in infants and children examined with computed tomographic metrizamide myelography. Radiology 130 (1979) 691–696.
658. Resjoe, I. M., Harwood-Nash, D. C., Fitz, C. R., Chuang, S.: CT metrizamide myelography for intraspinal and paraspinal neoplasms in infants and children. AJR 132 (1979) 367–372.

659. Resjoe, I. M., Harwood-Nash, D. C., Fitz, C. R., Chuang, S.: Computed tomographic metrizamide myelography in spinal dysraphism in infants and children. J. Comput. Ass. Tomogr. 2 (1978) 549–558.
660. Roub, L. W., Drayer, B. P.: Spinal computed tomography – Limitations and applications. AJR 133 (1979) 267–273.
661. Sartor, K., Richert, S.: Computertomographie des zervikalen Spinalkanals nach intrathekalem Enhancement – Zervikale CT-Myelographie. Fortschr. Röntgenstr. 130, 3 (1979) 261–269.
662. Sartor, K.: Computertomographie bei spinalen Tumoren. Fortschr. Röntgenstr. 132 (1980) 391–398.
663. Sartor, K.: Computertomographie bei Verletzungen der Halswirbelsäule und der oberen Brustwirbelsäule. Fortschr. Röntgenstr. 132 (1980) 132–138.
664. Sartor, K.: Spinale Computertomographie. Radiologe 20 (1980) 485–493.
665. Schöter, I., Wappenschmidt, J.: Die intraspinale Raumforderung im computerassistierten Myelogramm (CAM). Fortschr. Röntgenstr. 133 (1980) 527–530.
666. Scotti, L. N., Marasco, J. A., Pittman, T. A., Feczko, W. A. et al.: Computed tomography of the spinal canal and cord. Computerized Tomogr. 1 (1977) 229–234.
667. Scotti, G., Harwood-Nash, D. C., Hoffman, H. J.: Congenital thoracic dermal sinus – Diagnosis by computer assisted metrizamide myelography. J. Comput. Ass. Tomogr. 4 (1980) 675–677.
668. Sheldon, J. J., Sersland, T., Leborgne, J.: Computed tomography of the lower lumbar vertebral column. Radiology 124 (1977) 113–118.
669. Tadmor, R., Davis, K. R., Roberson, G. H., New, P. F., Taveras, J. M.: Computed tomographic evaluation of traumatic spinal injuries. Radiology 127 (1978) 825–827.
670. Taylor, A. J., Haughton, V. M., Doust, B. D.: CT imaging of the thoracic spinal cord without intrathecal contrast medium. J. Comput. Ass. Tomogr. 4 (1980) 223–224.
671. Ullrich, C. G., Binet, E. F., Sanecki, M. G., Kieffer, S. A.: Quantitative assessment of the lumbar spinal canal by computed tomography. Radiology 134 (1980) 137–143.
672. Wackenheim, A., Vallier, D., Babin, E.: Die konstitutionelle Stenose des Lumbalkanals. Radiologe 20 (1980) 470–477.
673. Williams, A. L., Haughton, V. M., Syvertsen, A.: Computed tomography in the diagnosis of herniated nucleus pulposus. Radiology 135 (1980) 95–99.

Lymphatic system (spleen)

674. Alcorn, F. S., Mategrano, V. C., Petasnick, J. P., Clark, J. W.: Contributions of computed tomography in the staging and management of malignant lymphoma. Radiology 125 (1977) 717–723.
675. Böttger, E., Semerak, M., Jaschke, W.: Computertomographische Befunde bei Milzruptur, subkapsulärem Milzhämatom und perisplenitischem Abszeß. Fortschr. Röntgenstr. 132 (1980) 282–286.
676. Brasch, R. C., Royal, S., Ammann, A. J., Crowe, J.: Pseudolymphoma in two immunodeficient children. AJR 132 (1979) 844–847.
677. Breiman, R. S., Castellino, R. A., Harell, G. S., Marshall, W. H. et al.: CT-pathologic correlations in Hodgkin's disease and non-Hodgkin's lymphoma. Radiology 126 (1978) 159–166.
678. Dossetor, R. S., Winter, J.: Computerized tomography, lymphangiography, and ultrasound in the diagnosis of lymph node enlargement – A comparison. Intern. Symp. Heidelberg 1977. Eds.: Paul Gerhardt, Gerhard van Kaick. Georg Thieme, Stuttgart (1979) 170–173.
679. Federle, M. P., Callen, P. W.: Cystic Hodgkin's lymphoma of the thymus – Computed tomography appearance. J. Comput. Ass. Tomogr. 3 (1979) 542–544.
680. Feuerbach, S., Gullotta, U., Rupp, N. et al.: Lymphknotenmetastasen maligner Hodentumoren in Lymphographie und Computertomographie – eine vergleichende Studie. Röntgen-Bl. 33 (1980) 267–271.
681. Feuerbach, S., Reiser, M., Gullotta, U. et al.: Die Bedeutung der CT für die Stadieneinteilung lymphatischer Systemerkrankungen. Fortschr. Röntgenstr. 133 (1980) 182–184.
682. Goodman, P. C., Federle, M. P.: Splenorrhaphy – CT appearance. J. Comput. Ass. Tomogr. 4 (1980) 251–252.
683. Harell, G. S., Breiman, R. S., Glatstein, E. J., Marshall, W. H., Castellino, R. A.: Computed tomography of the abdomen in the malignant lymphomas. Radiol. Clin. N. Amer. 3 (1977) 391–400.
684. Koehler, P. R., Jones, R.: Association of left-sided pleural effusions and splenic hematomas. AJR 135 (1980) 851–853.
685. Lackner, K., Weissbach, L., Boldt, I., Scherholz, K., Brecht, G.: Computertomographischer Nachweis von Lymphknotenmetastasen bei malignen Hodentumoren. Fortschr. Röntgenstr. 130, 6 (1979) 636–643.
686. Lackner, K., Brecht, G., Janson, R. et al.: Wertigkeit der Computertomographie bei der Stadieneinteilung primärer Lymphknotenneoplasien. Fortschr. Röntgenstr. 132 (1980) 21–30.
687. Lee, J. K. T., Stanley, R. J., Sagel, S. S., Melson, G. L. et al.: Limitations of the post-lymphangiogram plain abdominal radiograph as an indicator of recurrent lymphoma – Comparison to computed tomography. Radiology 134 (1980) 155–158.
688. Leonidas, J. C., Carter, B. L., Leape, L. L. et al.: Computed tomography in diagnosis of abdominal masses in infancy and childhood. Arch. Dis. Child. 53 (1978) 120–125.
689. Lissner, J., Scherer, U.: Der Wert der Computertomographie bei Leber- und Milzerkrankungen. Röntgen-Bl. 32 (1979) 1–14.
690. Mall, J. C., Kaiser, J. A.: CT diagnosis of splenic laceration. AJR 134 (1980) 265–269.
691. Marshall, W. H., Breiman, R. S., Harell, G. S. et al.: Computed tomography of abdominal paraaortic lymph node disease – Preliminary observations with a 6 second scanner. AJR 128 (1977) 759–764.
692. Moss, M. L., Kirschner, L. P., Peereboom, G., Ferris, R. A.: CT demonstration of a splenic abscess not evident at surgery. AJR 135 (1980) 159–160. G. Thieme, Stuttgart.
693. Piekarski, J., Federle, M. P., Moss, A. A. et al.: Computed tomography of the spleen. Radiology 135 (1980) 683–689.
694. Pilepich, M. V., Rene, J. B., Munzenrider, J. E., Carter, B. L.: Contribution of computed tomography to the treatment of lymphomas. Am. J. Roentgenol. 131 (1978) 69–73.
695. Redman, H. C., Glatstein, E., Castellino, R., Federal, W. A.: Computed tomography as an adjunct in the staging of Hodgkin's disease and non-Hodgkin's lymphomas. Radiology 124 (1977) 381–385.
696. Schaner, E. G., Head, G. L., Doppman, J. L., Young, R. C.: Computed tomography in the diagnosis, staging, and management of abdominal lymphoma. J. Comput. Ass. Tomogr. 1 (1977) 176–180.
697. Schertel, L.: Computertomographie der Milz. Röntgen-Bl. 33 (1980) 91–99.

Large vessels

698. Aiello, M. R., Cohen, W. N.: Inflammatory aneurysm of the abdominal aorta. J. Comput. Ass. Tomogr. 4 (1980) 265–267.
699. Alder, W., Zwicker, H.: Computertomographischer Nachweis eines Entrapment-Syndroms der Arteria poplitea. Fortschr. Röntgenstr. 130,5 (1979) 543–545.
700. Axelbaum, S. P., Schellinger, D., Gomes, M. N., Ferris, R. A., Hakkal, H. G.: Computed tomographic evaluation of aortic aneurysms. Am. J. Roentgenol. 127 (1976) 75–78.
701. Bergström, M., Riding, M., Greitz, T.: The limitations of definition of blood vessels with computer intravenous angiography. Neuroradiology 11 (1976) 35–40.
702. Brecht, G., Lackner, K., Brecht, Th., Thurn, P.: Das Aortenaneurysma im Computertomogramm. Fortschr. Röntgenstr. 130,2 (1979) 162–171.
703. Breda, A., Rubin, B. E., Druy, E. M.: Detection of inferior vena cava abnormalities by computed tomography. J. Comput. Ass. Tomogr. 3 (1979) 164–169.
704. Chuang, V. P., Fried, A. M., Chen, Ch.: Computed tomographic evaluation of para-aortic hematoma following translumbar aortography. Radiology 130 (1979) 711–712.
705. Clark, K. E., Foley, W. D., Lawson, T. L. et al.: CT evaluation of esophageal and upper abdominal varices. J. Comput. Ass. Tomogr. 4 (1980) 510–515.
706. Egan, T. J., Neiman, H. L., Herman, R. J. et al.: Computed tomography in the diagnosis of aortic aneurysm dissection or traumatic injury. Radiology 136 (1980) 141–146.
707. Faer, M. J., Lynch, R. D., Evans, H. O., Chin, F. K.: Inferior vena cava duplication – Demonstration by computed tomography. Radiology 130 (1979) 707–709.
708. Ferris, R. A., Kirschner, L. P., Mero, J. H., McCabe, D. J. et al.: Computed tomography in the evaluation of inferior vena cava obstruction. Radiology 130 (1979) 710.
709. Ginaldi, S., Chuang, V. P., Wallace, S.: Absence of hepatic segment of the inferior vena cava with azygous continuation. J. Comput. Ass. Tomogr. 4 (1980) 112–114.
710. Godwin, J. D., Herfkens, R. L., Skiöldebrand, C. G. et al.: Evaluation of dissections and aneurysms of the thoracic aorta by conventional and dynamic CT scanning. Radiology 136 (1980) 125–133.
711. Goldberg, R. P., Carter, B. L.: Absence of thoracic osteophytosis in the area adjacent to the aorta – Computed tomography demonstration. J. Comput. Ass. Tomogr. 2 (1978) 173–175.
712. Gomes, M. N.: ACTA scanning in the diagnosis of abdominal aortic aneurysms. Computerized Tomogr. 1 (1977) 51–61.
713. Gomes, M. N., Hakkal, H. G., Schellinger, D.: Ultrasonography and CT scanning – A comparative study of abdominal aortic aneurysms. Computerized Tomogr. 2 (1978) 99–110.
714. Gross, S. C., Barr, I., Eyler, W. R. et al.: Computed tomography in dissection of the thoracic aorta. Radiology 136 (1980) 135–139.

715. Harris, R. D., Usselman, J. A., Vint, V. C., Warmath, M. A.: Computerized tomographic diagnosis of aneurysms of the thoracic aorta. Computerized Tomogr. 3 (1979) 81–91.
716. Heuser, L., Friedmann, G., Mödder, U.: Computer-tomographischer Nachweis der Aorten-Aneurysmen. Radiologe 18 (1978) 482–486.
717. Lackner, K., Frommhold, H., Thurn, P.: Vergleich der Gefäßdarstellungen im Abdomen und Retroperitonealraum mit Computertomographie und Ultraschall. Fortschr. Röntgenstr. 131 (1979) 479–486.
718. Larde, D., Belloir, C., Vasile, N. et al.: Computed tomography of aortic dissection. Radiology 136 (1980) 147–151.
719. Machida, K., Tasaka, A.: CT patterns of mural thrombus in aortic aneurysm. J. Comput. Ass. Tomogr. 4 (1980) 840–842.
720. Marchal, G., Wilms, G., Baert, A., Ponette, E.: Applications of specific vascular opacification in CT of the upper abdomen. Fortschr. Röntgenstr. 132 (1980) 45–48.
721. Moncada, R., Reynes, C., Churchill, R., Love, L.: Normal vascular anatomy of the abdomen on computed tomography. Radiol. Clin. North Am. 17 (1979) 25–37.
721a. Royal, S. A., Callen, P. W.: CT evaluation of anomalies of the inferior vena cava and left renal vein. AJR 132 (1979) 759–763.
722. Taber, P., Chang, L. W. M., Campion, G. M.: Diagnosis of retro-esophageal right aortic arch by computed tomography. J. Comput. Ass. Tomogr. 3 (1979) 684–685.
723. Taber, P., Chang, L. W. M., Campion, G. M.: The left brachiocephalic vein simulating aortic dissection on computed tomography. J. Comput. Ass. Tomogr. 3 (1979) 360–361.
724. Tisnado, J., Amendola, M. A., Vines, F. S., Beachley, M. C.: Computed tomography of a double inferior vena cava – the 'double cava' sign. Computerized Tomogr. 3 (1979) 195–199.
725. Usselman, J. A., Vint, V. C., Kleiman, S. A.: CT diagnosis of aortic pseudoaneurysm causing vertebral erosion. AJR 133 (1979) 1177–1179.
726. Weiand, G., Lackner, K., Koischwitz, D.: CT-Nachweis des venösen Umgehungskreislaufs bei Verschluß oder Agenesie der Vena cava. Fortschr. Röntgenstr. 133 (1980) 250–258.
727. Zerhouni, E. A., Barth, K. H., Siegelman, S. S.: Demonstration of venous thrombosis by computed tomography. AJR 134 (1980) 753–758.

Muscles, skeleton
728. Archer, C. R., Yeager, V.: Internal structures of the knee visualized by computed tomography. J. Comput. Ass. Tomogr. 2 (1978) 181–183.
729. Barlow, R. E., Goldman, M. L.: Computed tomography of the skeletal system. Computerized Tomogr. 2 (1978) 27–35.
730. Berger, P. E., Kuhn, J. P.: Computed tomography of tumors of the musculoskeletal system in children. Radiology 127 (1978) 171–175.
731. Chew, F. S., Hudson, T. M., Hawkins, I. F.: Radiology of infiltrating angiolipoma. AJR 135 (1980) 781–787.
732. Dihlmann, W., Gürtler, K. F., Heller, M.: Sakroiliakale Computertomographie. Fortschr. Röntgenstr. 130,6 (1979) 659–665.
733. Dunnick, N. R., Schaner, E. G., Doppman, J. L.: Detection of subcutaneous metastases by computed tomography. J. Comput. Ass. Tomogr. 2 (1978) 275–279.
734. Gerhardt, P., Kaick, G., Puhl, W., Prawitz, R., Jaschke, W.: Die Computertomographie des Hüftgelenks. Röntgenpraxis 32 (1979) 42–50.
735. Grabbe, E., Heller, M., Böcker, W.: Computertomographie bei Weichteilsarkomen. Fortschr. Röntgenstr. 131 (1979) 372–378.
736. Grote, R., Elgeti, H., Saure, D.: Bestimmung des Antetorsionswinkels am Femur mit der axialen Computertomographie. Röntgen-Bl. 33 (1980) 31–42.
737. Hermann, G., Rose, J. S.: Computed tomography in bone and soft tissue pathology of the extremities. J. Comput. Ass. Tomogr. 3 (1979) 58–66.
738. Hinderling, Th., Rüegsegger, P., Anliker, M., Dietschi, C.: Computed tomography reconstruction from hollow projections – An application to in vivo evaluation of artificial hip joints. J. Comput. Ass. Tomogr. 3 (1979) 52–57.
739. Jend, H. H., Heller, M., Schöntag, H. et al.: Eine computertomographische Methode zur Bestimmung der Tibiatorsion. Fortschr. Röntgenstr. 133 (1980) 22–25.
740. Lackner, K., Hofmann, P., Grauthoff, H., Brecht, G., Thurn, P.: Computertomographischer Nachweis von Muskelhämatomen bei Hämophilie. Fortschr. Röntgenstr. 129,3 (1978) 298–302.
741. Levine, E., Lee, K. R., Neff, J. R., Maklad, N. F. et al.: Comparison of computed tomography and other imaging modalities in the evaluation of musculoskeletal tumors. Radiology 131 (1979) 431–437.
742. Levinsohn, E. M., Bryan, P. J.: Computed tomography in unilateral extremity swelling of unusual cause. J. Comput. Ass. Tomogr. 3 (1979) 67–70.
743. McLeod, R. A., Stephens, D. H., Beabout, J. W., Sheedy, P. F., Hattery, R. R.: Computed tomography of the skeletal system. Sem. Roentgenol. 13 (1978) 235–247.
744. McLoughlin, M. J.: CT and percutaneous fine-needle aspiration biopsy in tropical myositis. AJR 134 (1980) 167–168.
745. O'Connor, J. F., Cohen, J.: Computerized tomography in orthopedic surgery. AJR 132 (1979) 1037.
746. O'Doherty, D. S., Schellinger, D., Raptopoulos, V.: Computed tomographic patterns of pseudohypertrophic muscular dystrophy – Preliminary results. J. Comput. Ass. Tomogr. 1 (1977) 482–486.
747. Pavlov, H., Freiberger, R. H., Deck, M. F. et al.: Computer-assisted tomography of the knee. Invest. Radiol. 13 (1978) 57–61.
748. Penkava, R. R.: Iliopsoas bursitis demonstrated by computed tomography. AJR 135 (1980) 175–176.
749. Reiser, M., Gullotta, U., Feuerbach, S. et al.: Die computertomographische Diagnostik des Meniskusganglion. Fortschr. Röntgenstr. 133 (1980) 671–672.
750. Santos, L. A., Goldstein, H. M., Murray, J. A., Wallace, S.: Computed tomography in the evaluation of musculoskeletal neoplasms. Radiology 128 (1978) 89–94.
751. Weinberger, G., Levinsohn, E. M.: Computed tomography in the evaluation of sarcomatous tumors of the thigh. Am. J. Roentgenol. 130 (1978) 115–118.
752. Wilson, J. S., Korobkin, M., Genant, H. K., Bovill, E. G.: Computed tomography of musculoskeletal disorders. Am. J. Roentgenol. 131 (1978) 55–61.

Technique
753. Bassano, D. A., Chamberlain, C. C., Corry, J. M., Robinson, S., Getz, S.: Physical performance and dosimetric characteristics of the △-scan 50 whole-body/brain scanner. Radiology 123 (1977) 455–462.
754. Ewen, K., Fischer, P. G., Fiebach, B. J. O.: Die Strahlenexposition durch Nutz- und Störstrahlung bei der Computertomographie. Electromedica 1 (1977) 7.
755. Ewen, K., Steiner, H., Jungblut, R. et al.: Die Bestimmung von Organdosen bei Röntgenaufnahmen und computertomographischen Untersuchungen sowie die Berechnung der somatisch signifikanten Dosisindizes. Fortschr. Röntgenstr. 133 (1980) 425–429.
756. Hounsfield, G. N.: Picture quality of computed tomography. Am. J. Roentgenol. 127 (1976) 3–9.
757. Hounsfield, G. N.: Computerized transverse axial scanning (tomography). Part I. Description of system. Brit. J. Radiol. 46 (1973) 1016–1022.
758. McCullough, E. C., Payne, J. T.: Patient dosage in computed tomography. Radiology 129 (1978) 457–463.
759. Schittenhelm, R., Schwierz, G.: Das Computertomogramm – Seine Erzeugung und sein Bildcharakter. Medizintechnik 98 (1978) 87–94.
760. Schneider, G., Sager, W. D., Spreizer, H.: Strahlenbelastung der Orbita bei der Computertomographie mit dem EMI-Scanner CT 1010. Fortschr. Röntgenstr. 128,6 (1978) 687–690.
761. Wall, B. F., Green, D. A. C., Veerappan, R.: The radiation dose to patients from EMI brain and body scanners. Brit. J. Radiol. 52 (1979) 189–196.
762. Wegener, O. H.: Artefakte in der Computertomographie. Fortschr. Röntgenstr. 132 (1980) 643–651.

Index (99-00)

A

Abdominal wall
-- abscess 72-43, 81-51
-- hernia 74-30
Abscess 3-53
- abdominal wall 92-40, 72-43, 81-51
- cystic transformation 3-53
- density 3-53
- Douglas' abscess 85-52
- fresh abscess 3-53
- granulation tissue 3-53
- hypostatic
-- pyogenic 86-37, 86-32
-- tuberculous 93-58
- intraperitoneal 75-50
- kidney 81-51
- liver 71-55
-- for monitoring the course of therapy 71-55
-- necrotic metastases 71-55
-- vs. solid lesions 71-55
- mediastinal 61-81
- membrane 3-53
-- contrast enhancement 71-55
- muscle 92-40
- pancreas 73-53, 73-51, 73-32
- paracolic 86-35
- pararenal 86-35, 86-36
- paravertebral 93-58
- pelvic 86-38, 85-53
- perirenal 86-31
- peritoneal cavity 75-10
- prostate 84-40
- psoas muscle 86-37
- pyogenic, hepatic 71-55
- radiodensity 3-53
- retroperitoneal 86-31, 86-35, 86-38
- spleen 76-50
- stages 3-53
- subhepatic 75-50
- subphrenic 75-50
- thoracic wall 64-40
- tuberculous 93-58, 71-50, 71-55
- tuboovarian 85-52
- uterine myoma 85-31
Absorption
- coefficient, linear 1-40
- of X-rays 97-00
- physiology and contrast media 4-22
- resolution 97-00
Addition of image slices 97-00
Adenocarcinoma
- biliary tract 72-70
- gallbladder 72-50
- ovarian 85-43
- pancreas 73-42
Adenoma
- adrenals 82-32
- gallbladder 72-50
- kidney 81-42
-- degree of vascularity 81-42
- lacrimal gland 51-52
- liver 71-41
-- degree of vascularity 71-41
- pleomorphic 51-52
- prostate 84-30
- thyroid 53-40
Adenomyomatosis
- gallbladder 72-50
- of the uterus 85-41
Adenopathy cf. lymph nodes
Adnexae 85-10
Adnexitis 55-52
Adrenal 82-00
- adenoma 82-32
-- vascularity 82-32
- atrophy 82-72
-- idiopathic 82-71
-- sequela 82-72
- carcinoma 82-33
- cysts 82-50
- haemorrhage 82-60
- hyperplasia 82-31
- hypoplasia 82-70
- inflammation 82-70
- metastases 82-45
- size 82-10
- tumours 82-30, 82-40
- weight 82-10
Adrenogenital syndrome 82-30
Agenesis
- kidney 81-90
Algorithm 97-00
Alveolitis 63-52, 63-53
Amoebic abscess
-- liver 71-55
Amyloidosis 3-55
- spleen 76-21
Anatomy
- adrenals 82-10
- biliary system 72-10
- colon 74-10
- female genital organs 85-10
- gastrointestinal tract 74-10
- heart 62-10
- in the computed tomogram (arteries, veins, muscles, bone) 2-00
- kidney 81-10
- lung 63-10
- mediastinum 61-10

- orbit   51-10
- osseous pelvis   93-61
- pancreas   73-10
- parapharyngeal space   52-10
- pararenal space   86-15
- pericardium   62-81
- perirenal space   86-14
- pleura   64-10
- prostate   84-10
- retroperitonal space   86-10
- skeleton   93-10
- spinal canal   93-51
- spleen   76-10
- thoracic wall   64-10
- urinary bladder   83-10
- vertebral canal   93-51
- vertebral column   93-51
- visceral cranium   52-10

Aneurysms
- abdominal   86-71
- abdominal aorta, forms   86-72
- aortic dissection   61-72, 86-72
- arteriovenous, pulmonary   63-40
- brachiocephalic trunk   61-73
- cardiac wall   62-50
- etiology   61-72, 86-72
- haemorrhage   86-72, 86-73
- myocardium   62-50
- spurious   61-92
- thoracic aorta, forms   61-72
---- delineation from paraaortic lesions   61-72

Angle measurement   97-00
Angio-computerized tomography (angio-CT)   4-31
Angiofibroma, juvenile
-- nasopharynx   52-51
-- paranasal sinuses   52-31

Angiomyolipoma
- kidney   81-43

Aorta
- abdominal   86-11
- diameter   86-11
- mural thrombus   86-72
- rupture   61-92
- stenosis, idiopathic, hypertrophic subvalvular   62-32
- thoracic   61-12
- valvular stenosis   62-32

Aortic arch
-- malformations   61-71

Aortic trauma
-- after translumbar puncture   86-73

Aplasia
- kidney   81-90

Area measurement   97-00

Arrhenoblastoma
- ovary   85-43

Artery
- coronary   62-10
- hepatic   71-10, 86-11
- pulmonary   61-12
- splenic   73-10
- superior mesenteric   86-11
--- relationship to the pancreas   73-10

Arthritis, iliosacral   93-64
Arthrosis, intervertebral   93-53
Artifacts   97-00, 3-20
- visceral cranium   52-20
Asbestosis   63-85
- pleural changes   63-85
- pulmonary manifestation   63-85

Ascites
- and cirrhosis of the liver   71-53
- and ovarian tumour   85-40
- and uterine myoma   85-31
- as a secondary sign   75-30
- etiology   75-30

Asplenia   76-80

Atrophy, pancreas
-- lipomatous   73-70
-- partial   73-52

B

Back-projection   97-00
Bechterev's disease cf. arthritis, sacroiliac   93-64
Biliary system   72-00
Biliary tract
-- dilation cf. cholestasis
--- cystic   72-72
-- intrahepatic
--- air-containing   72-60
--- contrast enhancement   72-10
--- demonstration   72-10
-- tumours   72-70

Bladder, trabeculated   83-40
Bladder, urinary   83-00
-- CT imaging conditions   83-10
-- lumen
--- administration of contrast medium   4-21
-- opacification   4-21
-- position   83-30
-- tumours   83-50
--- diagnosis of expansion   83-51
--- staging   83-51
-- wall   83-10
--- calcification   83-40
--- thickness   83-40
-- substratification   4-35
-- trabeculated   83-40

Blastoma, teratoid
— mediastinal   61-43
Blood
- coagulated, density value   3-52
- liquid, density value   3-52
- plasma
—— density value   3-52
Blood-fluid barrier   4-10, 4-50
Bolus injection cf. also use of contrast media   4-30
—— arteriovenous transit time   4-32
—— circulation time   4-32
—— controlled   4-33
——— conditions   4-33
—— guided   4-32
——— administration technique   4-32
——— with long scan times   4-32
—— lead time   4-32
—— multiple bolus technique   4-32
—— reduced   4-35
—— start of scanning   4-31
—— transit time   4-32
Bolus length   4-32
Bone
- medullary invasion   93-40
- mineralization   93-30
—— densitometry   93-30, 3-54
- skeleton   93-00
- tissue, radiodensity   3-54
- tumours
—— administration of contrast medium   93-40
—— soft tissue infiltration   93-40
Bowel, opacification
—— for organ delineation   4-22
—— oral   4-22
——— artifacts   4-22
——— diagnosis of abscess   75-50
——— diagnosis of biliary system   72-20
——— diagnosis of kidney   81-20
——— diagnosis of lymphoma   86-15, 86-51
——— diagnosis of ovarian lesion   85-10
——— diagnosis of pancreas   73-20, 73-10
——— diagnosis of peritoneal cavity   75-20
——— diagnosis of spleen   76-20
——— diagnosis of uterine lesion   85-20
—— partial   4-23
—— total   4-23
Bronchial carcinoma
—— central
——— conventional tomography   63-62
——— hilar lymph node enlargement   63-62
——— mediastinal lymph node enlargement   63-62
——— obstructive syndrome   63-62
——— radiation planning   63-62

——— subpleural metastases   63-62
—— chest wall metastasis   64-30
—— hilar visualization   63-62
—— lymph node metastases, mediastinal   61-32
—— paratracheal   63-62, 61-15
—— peripheral
——— vs. tuberculoma   63-62
Bronchiectasis   63-40
Bronchiectatic deformation   63-30
Bypass, aorto-coronary   62-50

C
Calcification   3-55
- adenoma, parathyroid   61-45
- adrenal cyst   82-50
- adrenal inflammation   82-71
- aneurysm, abdominal   86-71
—— thoracic   61-72
- dermoid cyst, mediastinal   61-43
——— ovarian   85-42
- echinococcus alveolaris   71-34
- echinococcus granulosus   71-33
- ganglioneurinoma, mediastinal   61-61
- histoplasmoma, pulmonary   63-54
- liver   71-7a
- lymphoma, malignant   61-31
- mediastinitis, chronic   61-82
- nephroblastoma   81-45
- neuroblastoma, mediastinal   61-61
—— adrenal   82-44
- ovarian cyst   85-41
- ovarian tumour   85-43
- pancreatitis, chronic   73-52
- pleura
—— asbestosis   63-85
—— hyaloserositis   63-86
—— trauma   63-84
—— tuberculosis   63-64
- prostate   84-40
- pulmonary tuberculoma   63-54
- renal tumour   81-41
- spleen   76-9a
- splenic cyst   76-30
- teratoma, mediastinal   61-43
- tuberculoma, pulmonary   63-54
- urinary bladder   83-40
- uterine myoma   85-31
- Wilms' tumour   81-45
Carbuncle, renal   81-51
Carcinoma
- adrenal   82-33
- bronchial   63-62
- cervical   85-32
—— parametrane expansion   85-32
—— recurrence   85-34

-- staging 85-32
- cholangiocellular 71-46
- gallbladder 72-50
-- contrast enhancement 72-50
- gastrointestinal tract 74-30
- hepatocellular 71-45
-- categories 71-45
-- incidence 71-45
- hypernephroid 81-41
-- criteria of malignancy 81-41
-- differential diagnosis 81-41
-- local recurrence 81-41
-- staging 81-41
-- vascularity 81-41
- lacrimal gland 51-52
- mammary
-- retrobulbar metastases 51-45
- oesophagus 61-63
- ovaries 85-43
- pancreas 73-42
-- cholestasis 73-42
-- direct CT signs 73-42
-- indirect CT signs 73-42
-- infiltration 73-42
-- metastases 73-45
-- types 73-42, 73-43, 73-44
- paranasal sinuses 52-33
- prostate 84-30
- tongue 52-60
- tonsils 52-60
- urinary bladder 83-51
- uterus
-- body 85-33
-- cervical carcinoma 85-32
-- expansion 85-33
-- recurrence 85-34
-- staging 85-33
-- vs. other malignant uterine growth 85-33
Cardio-computerized tomography (CCT) 62-00
Cardiomyopathy 62-40
Caroli syndrome 72-72
Cava cf. vena cava
Cava-gallbladder line 71-10
Cholangitis 72-60
Cholecystitis 72-41
- acute
-- bolus injection 72-41
-- floridity 72-41
-- vs. gallbladder carcinoma 72-41
- chronic 72-41
- emphysematous 72-41
Cholecystolithiasis
- gallbladder tumour 72-50
Cholecystomegaly 72-30

- negative cholecystogram 72-30
Cholecystoses, hyperplastic 72-50
Cholelithiasis 72-42
- calcareous gallstones 72-42
- CT indication 72-42
- oral cholegraphy vs. CT 72-42
- sonography vs. CT 72-42
Cholestasis, obstructive
-- cholelithiasis 72-42
-- inflammation of the biliary tract 72-60
-- lymph node enlargement 86-50
-- tumours of the biliary tract 72-70
-- tumours of the gallbladder 72-50
Cholesterol stones 72-42
Cholesterolosis 72-50
Chondroma 93-40
Chondromatosis, pelvic 93-62
Chondromyxoid fibroma 93-40
Chondrosarcoma 93-40, 93-55, 93-62
Chordoma
- nasopharynx 52-51
- sacral 93-62
- spinal 93-55
Choriocarcinoma 61-43
Chorioepithelioma
- uterus 85-33
Chylothorax 63-83
Circular foci, pulmonary
--- inflammatory 63-60
--- neoplastic 63-60
Circulation time 4-32
Cirrhosis, hepatic 71-53
Coagulation (of blood) 3-52
Coccyx cf. pelvis, osseous 93-60
Common bile duct
--- after opacification of the pancreas 72-10
--- cysts 72-71
--- dilation
---- inflammations 72-60
---- lithiasis 72-42
---- tumours 72-70, 73-42
--- lithiasis 72-42
--- tumours 72-70
--- visualization 72-10
Computed tomogram 1-10
Computer cf. equipment, computerized tomographic 97-00
Computerized tomographic system
--- multidetector rotation-translation scanners 1-20
--- rotation scanners with movable detector system 1-20
--- rotation system with stationary detectors 1-20

--- single-detector rotation-translation scanners 1-20
Computerized tomographic terminology 97-00
Computerized tomography
-- historical development 1-00
-- sequential 4-32
-- spatial resolution 1-10
-- technical realization 1-20
Concha nasalis 52-10
Congestion, pulmonary 63-70
Conn's syndrome 82-30
Contraindication
- oral contrast media 4-22
Contrast enhancement
-- abscesses 3-53
-- administration technique 4-31
-- cysts 3-51
-- distribution volume 4-10
-- injection time 4-31
-- maintenance dose 4-35
-- vascularity 4-50
Contrast gradient
-- bolus vs. infusion 4-31
Contrast media
-- accumulation, renal 4-35
-- administration
--- bolus injection 4-32
--- infusion
---- bolus infusion 4-35
---- high-dosed 4-35
---- mode of administration 4-36
---- normal dose 4-35
--- intracavitary vs. intravascular 4-10
-- biliary 4-40
--- biligraphic effect 4-10
--- maximum enhancement 4-40
--- mode of administration 4-40
-- distribution spaces 4-31
-- intravascular use
---- abscesses 3-53
---- biliary system 4-10, 72-20, 72-50
---- carcinoma of the liver 71-45
---- cerebral diagnosis 4-10
---- heart 4-33, 62-20, 62-50
---- kidney 81-20
---- liver haematoma 71-60
---- liver parenchyma 4-10, 71-20, 71-40
---- lung 63-20
---- mediastinum 61-20, 61-30, 61-42, 61-81, 61-92
---- orbit 51-20, 51-65
---- pancreas 73-20, 73-32, 73-42
---- pancreatic parenchyma 73-10
---- parenchyma, general 4-31
---- pericardium 62-82
---- peritoneal cavity 75-20
---- pleura 63-82, 63-86
---- prostate 84-20
---- pulmonary diagnosis 63-20
---- renal parenchyma 4-10
---- spleen 76-20, 76-61
---- thoracic wall 64-20, 64-30
---- thyroid 53-30
---- visceral cranium 52-20
-- pharmacokinetics 4-31
-- protein binding 4-10
-- redistribution 4-10
-- renal 4-30
-- transit time, arteriovenous
----- brain 4-32
----- definition 4-32
----- kidney 4-32
----- liver 4-32
Contrast reversal 71-10
Control console 97-00
Convolution core 97-00
Convolution function 97-00
Coordinates 97-00
Coronal slice technique 97-00, 51-10, 52-10
CT cf. computerized tomography
- indication 5-00
Cushing's syndrome 82-30
Cyst(s)
- administration of contrast medium 3-51, 3-53
- adrenal 82-50
- bronchogenic 61-52
- chocolate, ovarian 85-41
- common bile duct 72-71
- corpus luteum, ovarian 85-41
- dermoid
-- mediastinal 61-43
-- orbital 51-54
-- ovarian 85-42
- dysontogenetic 71-31, 73-31
- follicular, lutein, ovarian 85-41
- gastroenteral 61-62
- kidney
-- multilocular 81-33
-- parenchymal 81-31
- liver
-- dysontogenetic 71-31
-- solitary 71-32
- mediastinal, neuroenteric 61-61
- neurogenic 52-31
- odontogenic 52-31
- oesophageal 61-62
- ovarian 85-41
-- dermoid 85-42
- pancreas, dysontogenetic 73-31

- paranasal sinuses 52-31
- pharyngeal bursa 52-51
- pleuropericardial 61-53
- post-inflammatory 3-53
- post-traumatic 3-52
- protein-rich 3-53
- radiodensity 3-51, 3-53
- spleen 76-30
- teratoid, mediastinal 61-43
- thoracic duct 61-62
- thyroid 53-40
Cystadenocarcinoma
- ovary 85-43
- pancreas 73-43
- vs. cystadenoma 73-43
Cystadenoma
- kidney 81-42
- lacrimal gland 51-52
- ovary 85-41
- pancreas 73-41
Cystic cystitis 83-40
Cystic degeneration 3-55
-- of the kidneys 81-32
--- complication 81-32
Cystic disease of the pancreas 73-30
Cystic duct, occlusion
--- gall bladder 72-43
Cystic echinococcosis, hepatic 71-33
Cystic hepatopathy 71-30
Cystic kidneys 81-32
-- dysgenetic 81-33
Cystography, retrograde 4-21
Cystoma pseudomucinosum
  glandulare 85-41
Cystoma serosum glandulare
  cillatum 85-41
Cystoma serosum simplex 85-41

D

Dacryoadenitis 51-63
- bilateral 51-63
- enhancement 51-63
- Mikulicz syndrome 51-63
- Sjögren syndrome 51-63
- unilateral 51-63
Dacryocystitis 51-61
Densitometry, bone
  mineralization 93-30, 3-54
Density cf. radiodensity
Density measurement 3-10
-- at boundaries of a structure 3-20
Density profile 97-00
Density resolution cf. absorption resolution
Density scale (Hounsfield scale) 3-30
Density-time curve (diagram) 4-30
---- hepatic tumour 71-40

Density unit cf. density value
Density value 1-40
-- accuracy 3-10
-- analysis 3-00
-- falsification 3-20, 1-50
Dentigerous cysts 52-31
Dermoid
- cysts
-- mediastinal 61-43
-- orbital 51-54
-- ovarian 85-42
- intraspinal 92-55
Detector 97-00, 1-20
Diaphragm 86-13
- crura 86-13
- hernia 61-40
Diastematomyelia 93-55
Digital X-ray 97-00
Directory 97-00
Disk, intervertebral
-- herniation 93-54
-- imaging conditions 93-50
-- prolapse 93-54
Display 97-00
Dissection, aortic 61-72
Distance measurement 97-00
Dose 97-00
Douglas' abscess 75-50
Douglas' pouch 75-10
Duct, pancreatic cf. pancreatic duct
Duodenal infiltration
-- pancreatic carcinoma 73-42
Dysgerminoma, ovarian 85-43
Dysmorphism, renal lobar 81-50
Dysplasia
- cystic, of the lung 63-40
- fibrous 52-31

E

ECG triggering 62-10
Echinococcosis 71-33
Echinococcus alveolaris 71-34
-- differential diagnosis 71-34
-- kidney 71-34
Echinococcus granulosus 71-33
-- adrenal 82-50
-- liver 71-33
-- spleen 76-30
Ectopia of the kidney 81-90
Edge enhancement 97-00
Effusion
- pericardial 62-83
- peritoneal 75-10, 75-30
- pleural 63-83
Electrolytes, density value 3-51
Element volume 1-50

Emphysema
– lung   63-30
– mediastinal   61-91
– pulmonary density value   63-30
Empyema
– gallbladder   72-43
– pleura   63-51, 63-83
Encephalocele   52-31
Enema, colonic   4-22
Enhancement cf. contrast enhancement
– edge   97-00
Ependymoma   93-55
Epidermoid
– intraspinal   93-55
– paranasal   52-31
Epipharynx
– anatomy   52-10
– tumours   52-50
Equidense cf. isodensity
Equipment, computerized
   tomographic   97-00
Ethmoid bone   52-10
−− mucocele   52-41
−− tumours   52-30
Ethmoiditis   51-61
Examination technique
−− adrenals   82-20
−− biliary system   72-20
−− cholelithiasis   72-42
−− fascial spaces, retroperitoneal   86-20
−− female genital organs   85-20
−− gastrointestinal tract   4-20
−− heart   61-20
−− kidneys   81-20
−− liver   71-20
−− lung   63-20
−− mediastinum   61-20
−− muscle   92-10
−− orbit   51-20
−− pancreas   73-20
−− pericardium   62-82
−− peritoneal cavity   75-20
−− pleura   63-82
−− prostate   84-20
−− skeleton   93-20
−− soft tissues   91-20
−− spleen   76-20
−− thoracic wall   64-20
−− thyroid   53-20
−− urinary bladder   83-20
−− vertebral canal   93-52
−− vertebral column   93-52
−− visceral cranium   52-20
Exophthalmos
– dacryoadenitis   51-63
– due to tumour   51-40, 51-50

– granulomatous inflammation   51-62
– inflammatory   52-40
– malignant (endocrine) 51-65
– pseudotumours   51-64
– pulsatile   51-72
Exposure time cf. scan time
Exudate, density value   3-51

F
Fan beam   1-20, 97-00
Fascia
– anterior renal   86-14
– Gerota's   61-14
– mediastinal   61-14
– perivisceral   61-14
– pharyngeal   52-10
– posterior renal   86-14
– prevertebral   61-14
Fascial spaces, retroperitoneal   86-14
Fat-containing tumours
−−− abdominal wall   74-30
−−− adrenal   82-41
−−− kidney   81-43
−−− mediastinum   61-40
−−− ovary   85-42
−−− peritoneum   74-30
−−− retroperitoneum   86-60
Fatty degeneration, liver
−−− degree   71-51
−−− vs. neoplasias   71-51
Fatty tissue, retrobulbar   51-10
Fibrin bodies, pleural   63-86
Fibrolipomatosis
– pelvic   86-42
– renal   81-56
Fibroma
– mediastinal   61-41
– orbit   51-55
– soft tissues   91-40
Fibrosarcoma
– mediastinal   61-41
– retroperitoneal   86-60
– soft tissues   91-10
Fibrosis
– perirectal   86-40, 83-40
– perirenal   86-34
– perivesicular   83-40
– pulmonary   83-53
– retroperitoneal, idiopathic   86-40
−− secondary   86-40
File   97-00
Fistula, carotid cavernous sinus   51-72
Floppy disc   97-00
Fluid, accumulation of
−− pericardial   62-83
−− peritoneal 75-10, 75-30

-- pleural 63-83
Foramina, intervertebral 61-61
Foreign bodies
-- artifacts 97-00
-- intra- and extraocular 51-73
Fossa, infratemporal 52-10
- lacrimal 51-10
-- infiltration 51-52
- pterygopalatine 52-10

G

Gallbladder
- carcinoma 72-50
- density 72-10
- empyema 72-43
- examination technique 72-20
- hydrops 72-43
- imaging conditions 72-10
- localization 72-10
- position 71-10
- thickening of the wall 72-41
- tumours 72-50, 72-30
Gallstones
- demonstrability 72-42
- vacuum phenomenon 72-42
Gantry 97-00
Gastrinoma 73-44
Gastrografin®, use of
--- in bowel opacification 4-22
--- in oesophageal diagnosis 61-12, 61-63
Gastrointestinal tract 74-00, 4-22
-- conventional X-ray examination 74-30
-- CT indication 74-30
Genital organs, female 85-00
-- male 84-00
Gland, parotid 52-10
- submandibular 52-10
Glioblastoma multiforme 93-55
Glioma of the optic nerve 51-42
--- enhancement after contrast medium 51-42
--- intracranial expansion 51-42
Goitre cf. struma
Gonadal dose 97-00
Gonadoblastoma 85-43
Granuloma, pulmonary 63-54
Granulosa cell tumour 85-43
Grey shade 97-00
-- display 1-00

H

Haemangioblastoma 93-55
Haemangioendothelioma
- liver 71-43
- mediastinal 61-41

Haemangioma
- extremities 93-54
- liver 71-43
- mediastinum 61-41
- orbit 51-41
- soft tissue 91-10
- spleen 76-40
- vertebra 93-54
Haemangiosarcoma, mediastinal 61-41
Haematocrit
- radiodensity of the blood 3-52
Haematoma
- cystic transformation 3-52
- fresh 3-52
- intraperitoneal haemorrhage 75-60
- kidneys 81-61
- liver 71-60
-- subcapsular vs. intraperitoneal fluid 71-60
- mediastinal 61-92
- muscle 92-50
- pancreas 73-60
- pararenal 86-35, 86-36
- perirenal 86-33
-- etiology 81-61
- perisplenic 76-61
- psoas muscle 86-37
- retrobulbar 51-72
- retroperitoneal 86-30
- spleen 76-61
- thoracic wall 64-50
Haemochromatosis
- liver 71-54
- secondary 71-54
Haemoglobin content
- blood 3-52
Haemorrhage cf. haematoma
- adrenal 82-60
-- etiology 82-60
- intraabdominal 75-60
Haemosiderosis of the liver 71-54
Haemothorax 63-83
Hamartoma
- gallbladder cf. adenomyomatosis
- liver, mesenchymal 71-42
- lung 63-61
Heart 62-00
- aneurysms of the wall 62-50
--- apical thrombus 62-50
- atrial myxoma 62-70
- atrial thrombus 62-60, 62-70
- CT diagnosis 62-10
- functional states 62-30
- infarct 62-50
- pressure load 62-32
- pressure stress 62-32

- ventricles, demonstration of 62-10
- volume load 62-31
- volume stress 62-31

Heart disease, coronary 62-50

Hepatitis
- calcification 71-52
- CT indication 71-52
- purulent (bacterial) 71-52
- non-purulent (granulomatous) 71-52

Hepatomegaly
- cirrhosis 71-53
- fatty degeneration of liver 71-51
- hepatitis 51-52
- hepatocellular carcinoma 71-45

Hernia, abdominal 74-30

Highlighting 97-00
- resolution, CT 97-00

Histiocytosis, intraorbital 51-62

Histogram analysis 97-00

Histoplasmoma of the lung 63-54

Hodgkin's disease 61-31, 86-51
-- hepatic involvement 86-51
-- lymph node involvement 61-31, 86-51
-- mesenteric involvement 86-51
-- morbidity 61-31, 86-51
-- pulmonary involvement 61-31
-- splenic involvement 86-51
-- thoracic wall involvement 64-30

Honeycombing 63-53

Horseshoe kidney 81-90

Hounsfield scale 1-40
- units 3-30

HR/CT (high resolution) 97-00

Hyalinization 3-55

Hyaloserositis, pleural 63-86

Hydroma cf. lymphangioma

Hydromyelia 93-55

Hydronephrosis
- acute 81-71
- cause 81-71
- chronic 81-71

Hydrosalpinx 85-52

Hydroureter 81-70

Hyperaemia, local 3-53

Hyperaldosteronism 82-30

Hyperdensity 3-40
- granulation tissue 4-50
- hypervascularized regions 4-50

Hypernephroma 81-41
- calcification 81-41
- intravascular expansion 86-41
- perirenal expansion 86-34
- recurrence 81-41
- staging 81-41

Hyperplasia, adenomatous
-- liver 71-41

--- vs. hepatoadenoma 71-41

Hyperplasia, adrenal 82-31
-- vs. adrenal adenoma 82-30

Hyperplasia, focal nodular (FNH)
--- liver 71-41
---- vs. hepatoadenoma 71-41

Hypertension
- portal 71-53, 71-54, 72-72
-- Caroli syndrome 72-72

Hypertrophy, cardial 62-32

Hypervascularization
- absorptive processes 4-50
- inflammatory processes 4-50
- neoplasias 4-50

Hypodensity 3-40
- hypovascularized tissue 4-50

Hypoplasia, renal 81-90

I

Image
- evaluation 97-00
- filing 97-00
- filtration 97-00
- matrix 97-00, 1-20
- noise 97-00, 3-10
- reconstruction 97-00
- reproduction 97-00
- store 97-00
- window 97-00

Indications for computerized tomography 5-00

Infarct
- kidneys 81-81
- lung 63-70
- myocardium 62-50
- spleen 76-71

Infiltration, leukaemic
-- orbit 51-44

Inflammation 3-53
- abdominal cavity 75-50
- adnexae 85-52
- adrenals 82-70
- biliary tract 72-60
- gallbladder 72-41
- general 3-53
- iliosacral joints 93-64
- intraorbital 51-60
- kidneys 81-50
- liver 71-50
- lung 63-50
- mediastinum 61-80
- muscle 92-40
- ocular muscle 51-64, 51-65
- pancreas 73-50
- parametrium 85-53
- paranasal sinuses 52-40

- pericardium 62-83
- pleura 63-83
- prostate 84-40
- retrobulbar space 51-61
- retroperitoneal space 86-30
- spleen 76-50
- thoracic wall 64-40
- urinary bladder 83-40
- uterus 85-51
- vertebral column 93-58

Infraorbitomeatal line (OML) 51-10
Insulinoma cf. tumour, islet cell
Interactive display 97-00
Intestinal gas, reduction
--- renal diagnosis 81-20
Isodensity 3-40

J

Jaundice cf. cholestasis, cf. hepatitis
Joints
- sacroiliac 93-64
-- inflammation 93-64
-- luxation 93-64
- sternoclavicular 65-10
Joystick 97-00

K

Kidney 81-00
- abscess 81-51
- agenesis 81-90
- angiomyolipoma 81-43
- anomaly 81-90
- aplasia 81-90
- arteries 86-11
- atrophy 81-53, 81-51
- carcinoma 81-41
- concrements 81-73
- cyst 81-30
- degeneration, polycystic 81-32
- dysmorphism, lobar 81-90
- dystrophy 81-90
- embolism 81-81
- hilar region 86-15
- lesion, vascular 81-80
- main arteries 81-10
- medullary pyramids 81-10
- metastases 81-47
- pelvis
-- dilation 81-70
-- tumours 81-46
- reniculus 81-90
- rudimentary 81-90
- sacciform 81-71, 81-72
- silent 81-70
- stones 81-73
- transplantation 81-55

- tuberculosis 81-54
- veins 86-11

L

Lacrimal gland 51-10
-- inflammation 51-63
-- tumours 51-52
Large bowel cf. opacification of the colon
Lead time 4-32
Leiomyoma
- soft tissue 91-10
- urinary bladder 83-52
- uterine 85-31
Leiomyosarcoma
- soft tissue 91-10
- urinary bladder 83-52
- uterine 85-33
Lesion
- space occupying cf. tumour
- vascular
-- orbit 51-71
- vertebragenic, tumour-like 93-55
Lesser sac 75-10
Ligament, falciform 71-10
Ligamentum teres hepatis 71-10
Light pencil 97-00
Linear attenuation coefficient 97-00
Lipoid tumours cf. fat-containing tumours
Lipoma
- abdominal wall 74-30
- intraspinal 93-56
- liver 71-44
- mediastinal 61-41
- pleural 63-86
- retroperitoneal 86-60
- soft tissue 91-10, 91-30
- thoracic wall 64-30
Lipomatosis
- mediastinal 61-41
- pancreas 73-70
- pelvic 86-42
Liponecrosis, pericardial 61-53
Liposarcoma
- mediastinal 61-41
- retroperitoneal 86-60
- soft tissue 91-30
Liver 71-00
- abscess 71-55
- adenoma 71-41
- adjacent structures 71-10, 75-10
- carcinoma 71-45
- cava-gallbladder line 71-10
- cirrhosis 71-53
- cysts 71-30
- degree of fatty degeneration 3-54, 71-51
- echinococcosis 71-33, 71-34

- haemangioma 71-43
- haematoma 71-60
- injury 71-60
- lobes 71-10
- metastases
-- administration of contrast medium 71-47
-- regressive changes 71-47
-- solitary focus 71-47
-- vascularity 71-40
-- vs. abscess 71-47
- porta hepatis 71-10
- portal structures 71-10
- rupture 71-60
- size 71-10
- tumours 71-40
- veins 71-10
- vessels 71-10
Lobe, caudate of the liver 71-10
- quadrate of the liver 71-10
Lung 63-00
- abscess 63-51
- boundaries of lobes 63-10
- circular focus 63-12, 63-60
- coin lesion 63-12, 63-60
- cysts 63-40
- degeneration, cystic 63-40
- density 63-13
- disease
-- inflammatory 63-50
-- inflammatory exudative 63-51
-- inflammatory granulomatous 63-52
-- neoplastic 63-60
- fibrosis 63-53
- hilum 61-12
- infarct 63-70
- infiltration
-- in effusion 63-51
- metastasis
-- CT vs. conventional tomography 63-63
-- intrapulmonary distribution 63-63
- structure 63-11
-- honeycombing 63-53
-- reticulation 63-53
- tissue
-- density range 3-54
-- fine structure 63-11
Lymph node metastases (cf. also under the individual organ tumours)
--- mediastinal 61-32
--- mediastinal, extrathoracic tumour 61-32
--- retroperitoneal 86-52
---- cervical carcinoma 85-32
---- primary tumour 86-52
---- vascularity 86-52

Lymph nodes (groups)
--- bifurcation (mediastinal) 61-15
--- bronchopulmonary 61-15
--- bronchopulmonary, bolus injection 61-15
--- iliac groups 86-15
--- intercostal 61-15
--- mediastinal, posterior 61-15, 86-15
--- mesenteric 86-15
--- obturator groups 86-15
--- paratracheal 61-15
--- periaortic 86-15
--- peripancreatic 86-15
--- porta hepatis 86-15
--- prevascular (mediastinal) 61-15
--- renal hilum 86-15
--- splenic hilum 86-15
--- sternal (mediastinal) 61-15
--- subclavicular 61-15
--- tracheobronchial 61-15
Lymph nodes (main groups) 61-15
---- mediastinum 61-15
---- retroperitoneal space 86-15
Lymphadenopathy, benign 86-53
Lymphangioma
- mediastinal 61-41
- retroperitoneal 86-36
Lymphangiosis, carcinomatous
-- lung 61-32
Lymphogranulomatosis cf. Hodgkin's disease
Lymphography
- prostatic carcinoma 84-30
- vs. computerized tomography 86-15
Lymphoma, malignant 61-31, 86-51
-- epipharynx 52-52
-- general characterstics
---- contrast enhancement 61-31
---- expansion 61-31, 86-51
---- Hodgkin's vs. non-Hodgkin's 86-51, 61-31
---- liver involvement 86-51
---- mesenteric involvement 86-51
---- morbidity 61-31
---- splenic involvement 86-51
-- lacrimal gland 51-52
-- mediastinum 61-31
-- mesenterium 74-30
-- orbit 51-44
-- paranasal sinuses 52-33
-- retroperitoneal space 86-51
-- thoracic wall 64-30

M

Magnetic disc 97-00
Magnetic tape 97-00
Malformation
- bronchopulmonary 63-40
Malformations, vascular, arteriovenous
--- orbital 51-71
Malignant tumour cf. also tumour, carcinoma, sarcoma, cystadenocarcinoma
-- ethmoid bone 52-33
-- frontal sinus 52-33
-- maxillary sinus 52-33
-- paranasal sinuses 52-33
-- periorbital 51-33
-- recurrence 85-34
-- sphenoid bone 52-33
-- thyroid 53-40
-- uterus 85-34
Mass cf. tumour
Mean value, statistical 3-10
Measuring accuracy, statistical 3-10
Measuring errors, systematic 3-20
Measuring time cf. scan time
Mediastinal spaces 61-11
Mediastinitis
- acute 61-81
- chronic 61-82
-- idiopathic 61-82
-- sclerotic 61-82
-- tuberculous 61-82
Mediastinum 61-00
- division according to Fraser-Paré 61-11
- lymph node groups 61-15
- tumours 61-40, 61-50, 61-60
- vascular lesions 61-70
Medullary sponge kidney 81-33
Melanoma, malignant
-- metastases 86-52
-- ocular bulb 51-46
Meningeoma, orbital
-- extraconal 51-51
-- optic nerve 51-42
Meningocele
- intraspinal 93-56
- mediastinal 61-62
- sacral 93-56
Mesopharynx
- anatomy 52-10
- tumours 52-60
Mesothelioma
- asbestosis 63-85
- pleural, diffuse 63-87
-- local 63-86
Metastases
- adrenal 82-45
- kidney 81-47
- liver 71-40, 71-47
- lung 63-63
- orbit 51-45
- peritoneal 75-40
-- CT demonstrability 75-40
-- localization 75-40
- spleen 76-40
- vertebral canal 93-56
- vertebral column 93-55
Monitor 97-00
Mouth, floor of 52-10
Movement artifacts cf. artifacts 97-00
Mucocele
- paranasal sinuses 52-41, 51-67
- vs. tumour 52-42
Multiplanar reconstruction cf. secondary slices 97-00
Muscle
- atrophy 92-20
- calcifications 92-43, 92-50
- dystrophy
-- progressive 92-30
-- pseudohypertrophy 92-30
- haematoma 92-50, 86-37
- iliopsoas 86-37
- psoas 86-37
- tissue 92-00
-- radiodensity 3-30
-- reduction of density 3-54
Musculature, retroocular 51-10
Musculi recti oculi 51-10
Musculus levator palpebrae 51-10
Musculus obliquus superior 51-10
Myasthenia gravis 61-42
Myelography 93-56
Myelolipoma, adrenal 82-40
Myocardium 62-10
Myoma 92-10
- uterus 85-31
Myomatosis
- gallbladder 72-50
Myosarcoma
- uterus 85-33
Myositis purulent 92-41
Myxoma 92-10
- heart 62-70
- retroperitoneal space 86-6a
Myxosarcoma 92-10, 86-6a

N

Necrosis 3-55
- density range 3-55
- hypernephroma 81-41
- liver metastases 71-47
- phaeochromocytoma 82-42

Neoplasia cf. tumour,
  adenoma, cyst,
  carcinoma, sarcoma etc.
- ovarian   85-42, 85-43
Nephrectomy   81-41
Nephritis, local, bacterial   81-51
Nephroblastoma   81-45
Nephrographic effect   4-10
Nerve
- optic   51-10
- phrenic   61-12
- vagus   61-12, 53-10
- visceral cranium   52-10
Neurinoma, orbital   51-43
Neuritis, retrobulbar   51-66
Neuroblastoma, adrenal   82-44
Neurofibroma
- orbit   51-56
- retroperitoneal space   86-60
Neuroocular plane   51-10
Non-Hodgkin's lymphoma
- mediastinal   61-31
- retroperitoneal   86-51

O
Ocular bulb   51-10
Oedema   3-54
Oesophagus   61-13
- administration of Gastrografin®   61-13
- carcinoma   61-63
-- expansion   61-63
-- signs of infiltration   61-63
- tumours   61-63
Omental bursa   75-10
Opacification
- colon   4-22
-- oral   4-23
-- rectal   4-23
- intravascular   4-31
- parenchymal   4-31
Ophthalmopathy, endocrine   51-65
Orbit   51-00
- anatomy   51-10
- frontal computed tomogram   51-10
- intermuscular membrane   51-10
- lacrimal gland   51-10
- multiplanar reconstruction   51-10
- phlegmon   51-61
- slice thickness   51-10
- tumour   51-30, 51-40, 51-50
Orbitomeatal line   51-10
Organ size cf. anatomy
Osteoblastoma   93-40
Osteochondroma   93-40
Osteoidosteoma   93-40
Osteoma
- paranasal sinuses   51-67

- skeleton   93-40
Osteomalacia   93-30
Osteoporosis   93-30
Osteosarcoma   93-40
Ovaries   85-00
- CT demonstrability   85-10
Over-hydration, haemodialysis   63-70

P
Paget's disease   52-32
Pancreas   73-00
- anatomy   73-10
- calcifications   73-32, 73-52
- carcinoma cf. carcinoma of the pancreas
- contours, obliterated   73-51
- enlargement of the head   73-10
- examination technique   73-20
- haematoma   73-60, 73-51
- inflammation cf. pancreatitis
- lipomatosis   73-70
- main duct cf. pancreatic duct
- organ boundary   73-10
- organ size   73-10
--- estimation of   73-10
- pseudocyst cf. pseudocyst   73-32, 73-51
- radiodensity   3-30
-- inhomogeneity of density   73-32, 73-42, 73-45
- retention cyst   73-32
- secondary tumour   73-45
--- malignant lymphomas   73-45
--- remote metastasis   73-45
- shape   73-10
-- abrupt alteration of width   73-42
- tail   73-10
-- delineation from the jejunum   73-10
- topography   73-10
- trauma   73-60
- tumour cf. carcinoma   73-40
- uncinate process   73-10
Pancreatic duct   73-10
-- dilation due to carcinoma   73-42
-- dilation due to chronic pancreatitis   73-42
-- normal diameter   73-10
Pancreatitis, acute   73-51
-- abscess formation   73-51
-- carcinoma of the pancreas   73-42
-- etiology   73-51
-- haemorrhagic necrotic   73-51
-- incidence   73-51
-- oedematous   73-51
-- pancreatic pseudocyst   73-32
-- suppurative   73-51
Pancreatitis, chronic   73-52
-- atrophy   73-52

-- calcifying 73-52
-- clinical forms 73-52
-- dilation of the duct 73-52
-- etiology 73-52
-- fibrosis, perilobular 73-52
-- incidence 73-52
-- lithiasis 73-52
-- pseudocyst 73-52
-- retention cyst 73-32
-- shrinkage of the pancreas 73-52
Papillitis, stenosing 72-60
Papilloma
- gallbladder 72-50
- urinary bladder 83-51
Parametritis 85-53
Paranephritis 86-35, 86-36
Parapharyngeal space 52-10
Pararenal space 86-15
-- anterior 86-15
---- exudations, genesis 86-35
-- exudative haemorrhagic lesions 86-35
-- posterior 86-15
---- exudations, genesis 86-36
Parathyroid 53-10
- anatomy 53-10
- ectopic 61-45
Parenchyma, focal lesions 4-31
--- contrast enhancement 4-31
Partial volume effect 1-50, 3-20
--- orbital diagnosis 51-10
--- prostatic diagnosis 84-10
Pelvis
- bone tumours 93-62
- mural abscess 86-38
- osseous
-- anatomy 93-60
- sacrolisthesis 93-64
- trauma 93-63
- vessels 86-11
- wall, recurrent tumours 85-34
Pericarditis 62-83
- bacterial 62-83
- chronic constrictive 62-84
- cyst 61-52
- differential diagnosis 62-83
- etiology 62-83
- non-infectious 62-83
Pericardium 62-80
- effusion cf. pericarditis 62-83
Perinephritis 86-31
Perirenal space 86-15
-- exudative haemorrhagic lesions 86-31
Peritoneal cavity 75-00
-- fluid collections 75-10
-- inframesocolic spaces 75-10
-- omental bursa 75-10

-- subhepatic space 75-10
-- subphrenic space 75-10
-- supramesocolic spaces 75-10
Peritoneography 4-24
- contrast enhancement 4-24
Peritonitis, carcinomatous 75-30
Phaeochromoblastoma 82-43
- hormonal activity 82-43
- metastatic disease 82-43
Phaeochromocytoma
- adrenal 82-42
-- contrast enhancement 82-42
- mediastinal 61-61
Pharmacokinetics
- biliary contrast media 4-40
- bolus injection 4-31
- contrast medium infusion 4-31
Phlegmon
- mediastinal 61-81
- retrobulbar 51-61
- retroperitoneal 86-35, 86-36, 85-53
Photon flow 3-10
Picture element 97-00
Pixel 97-00
Plane, ethmoidal 52-10
- frontal cf. slice, plane 97-00
Pleura 63-80
- calcification 63-84, 63-85, 63-86
- demonstrability 63-81
- effusion
-- etiology 63-83
-- exudative 63-83
-- transudative 63-83
- thickening 63-84
- vs. artifact 63-81
Pleuritis 63-83
- fibrous 63-84
-- uraemia 63-84
Plexus, prostatic 84-10
Plexus, uterovaginal 85-10
Plexus, vertebral, venous 93-51
Pneumectomy 63-84
- status after 63-62
Pneumomediastinum cf. emphysema,
   mediastinal 61-91
Polymyositis 92-43
Polysplenia 76-80
Pre-oedema, pulmonary 73-70
Pressure load, cardiac 62-32
Pressure stress, cardiac 62-32
Process, pterygoid 52-10
Proctectomy 74-31
- late abscess formation 74-31
- recurrence 74-31
- secondary retroperitoneal fibrosis 74-31
Prolapse, nucleus pulposus 93-54

Prostate 84-00
- abscess 84-40
- adenoma 84-30
- calcifications 84-10
- carcinoma 84-30
- position of seminal vesicles 84-10
- size 84-10
- stones
-- primary 84-40
-- secondary 84-40
Protein content of fluids 3-51
Protrusion of the bulb 51-40, 51-50, 51-60
Pseudocyst
- adrenal 82-50
- pancreatic 73-32
-- etiology 73-32
-- incidence 73-32
-- localization 73-32
-- necrotic zones 73-51
---- inflammatory vs. neoplastic 73-32
-- pancreatitis, acute 73-51
--- chronic 73-52
-- traumatic 73-32
- perirenal 86-32
- splenic 76-30
Pseudomyxoma peritonaei 85-41
Pseudotumour
- lacrimal gland 51-52
- orbital 51-64
-- etiology 51-64
-- histology 51-52
-- in idiopathic mediastinitis 61-82
Psoas cf. muscle, psoas
Puncture, translumbar 86-73
-- indication for CT-guided 5-00
Pyelonephritis
- chronic 81-53
- xanthogranulomatous 81-52
Pyocele, paranasal 52-41
-- contrast enhancement 52-41
-- localization 51-67
Pyonephrosis
- chronic course 81-72
- pathogenesis 81-72
Pyosalpinx 85-52

R
Radiation dose 97-00
Radiodensity
- accumulation of fluid
--- pericardial 62-83
--- pleural 63-83
- adnexitis 85-52
- adrenal adenoma 82-32
- adrenal carcinoma 82-33
- adrenal haemangioma 82-60

- adrenal myelolipoma 82-40
- ascites 75-30
- blood 3-52
- bronchogenic cyst 61-52
- cystic tumours of the paranasal sinuses 52-31
- dysontogenetic cyst of the liver 71-31
- echinococcus alveolaris 71-34
- echinococcus granulosus 71-33
- empyema of the gallbladder 72-43
- exudate 3-51
- exudative haemorrhagic pararenal lesions 86-35
- exudative haemorrhagic perirenal lesions 86-31
- fatty degeneration of the liver 3-54, 71-51
- fatty tissue 3-54
- foreign bodies, ocular 51-73
- gallbladder 72-42
-- hydrops 72-43
- gallstones 72-42
- goitre, endothoracic 61-44
- Hodgkin's disease 86-51
- hydronephrosis 81-71
- hypernephroma 81-41
- islet cell tumour 73-44
- lipoma, mediastinal 61-41
-- paranasal 52-32
- lipomatosis, mediastinal 61-41
- liposarcoma 91-30
- liver 3-54
-- abscess 71-55
-- haemochromatosis 71-54
- lymph node metastasis 86-52
- lymphoma 61-31
- mediastinal fibroma 61-41
- mediastinal haematoma 61-92
- mediastinal lipoma 61-41
- mediastinal teratoid blastoma 61-43
- mesopharyngeal tumour 52-60
- mixed tissue 3-54
- mucocele 52-41, 51-67
- myxoma 91-30
- orbit 51-10
- orbital dermoid cyst 51-54
- ovarian cystadenoma 85-41
- ovarian retention cyst 85-34
- pancreatic cystadenoma 73-41
- pancreatic haematoma 73-60
- pancreatic pseudocyst 73-32
- pancreatitis, acute 73-51
- perirenal haematoma 86-33
- perirenal pseudocyst 86-32
- pleural empyema 63-51
- pleural fluid 63-83
- pyocele, paranasal 52-41

- pyonephrosis 81-72
- renal abscess 81-51
- renal cyst 81-31
- renal fibrolipomatosis 81-56
- renal haematoma 81-61
- renal parenchyma 81-10
- soft tissue tumour 91-30
- spleen, accessory 76-80
- splenic abscess 76-50
- splenic cyst 76-30
- splenic haematoma 76-61
- splenic parenchyma 76-10
- thymic cyst 61-42
- thymolipoma 61-42
- thymoma 61-42
- thyroid 53-10
-- adenoma 53-40
-- cyst 53-40
- transudate 3-51
- tumour
-- oropharynx 52-60
-- renal pelvis 81-46
-- thyroid 53-40
- uterine myoma 85-31
- Wilms' tumour 81-45
Recess, alveolar
-- maxilla 52-10
Recklinghausen's disease 51-42
Rectum, tumours 74-30
Region of interest 97-00
Reid's line 51-10
Retention cyst
-- ovarian 85-41
-- pancreatic 73-32
Retinoblastoma 51-46
Retrocrural space 86-12
Retromaxillary space 52-10
Retroperitoneal space 86-00
Retropharyngeal space 52-10
Rhabdomyoma
- heart 62-70
- soft tissue 91-10
- urinary bladder 83-52
Rhabdomyosarcoma
- orbit 51-45
- soft tissue 91-10
- urinary bladder 83-52
Ring artifacts cf. artifacts 97-00

S

Sacrum cf. pelvis, osseous
Sarcoidosis
- intraorbital 51-62
- muscular 92-42
- pulmonary 63-52
Sarcoma

- mediastinal 61-41
- orbital 51-45
- osteogenic 93-40
- paranasal 52-33
- reticulum cell 86-60, 93-40
- retroperitoneal 86-60
- soft tissue 91-10
- thoracic wall 64-30
- uterine 85-33
Scan 97-00
- field 97-00
- time 97-00, 1-20
-- heart 62-10
Scanner 1-20
- generation 1-20
Scanning 97-00
- area 97-00
-- biliary diagnosis 72-20
-- cardiac diagnosis 62-20
-- liver diagnosis 71-20
-- mediastinum 61-20
-- pancreatic diagnosis 73-20
-- pericardium 82-82
-- peritoneal cavity 75-20
-- pleura 64-20
-- prostatic diagnosis 84-20
-- pulmonary diagnosis 62-20
-- thyroid diagnosis 53-20
-- visceral cranium 52-20
- principles 1-20
- series time 4-32
--- definition 4-32
--- dimensioning 4-32
- technique
-- coronal slices 97-00, 51-10, 52-10
-- foreign bodies, ocular 51-73
-- orbital fibroma 51-55
-- orbital pseudotumours 51-64
- unit 97-00
Scattering of X-rays 97-00
Schwannoma 86-60
Schwan's cell, proliferation 51-43
Scout view 97-00
-- vertebral column 93-10
SD = standard deviation 3-10
Secondary slices 97-00
Sector scan 97-00
Seminal vesicles 84-10
Seminoma
- mediastinal 61-43
- metastases 86-52
- ovarian 85-43
- retroperitoneal 86-60
Septum, nasal 52-10
Septum, orbital 51-10
Serial computerized tomography

cf. computerized tomography, sequential
Sheehan's syndrome 82-72
Sinus
- frontal 52-10
-- tumours 52-30
- maxillary
-- inflammation 52-40
-- tumours 52-30
- paranasal 52-00
-- bone sclerosis 52-33
- renal 81-10
Sjögren syndrome 51-63
Skeleton 93-00
- imaging criteria 93-10
Slice 97-00
- geometry 97-00
- plane 97-00
- thickness 97-00
Soft tissue
-- definition 3-54
-- tumours 91-00
Sonography
- cholelithiasis 72-42
- pericardial effusion 62-83
Spasmolytics cf. examination technique
Spinal canal 93-51
-- narrow 93-53
Spinal cord 93-51
Spinal nerves 93-51
Spleen 76-00
- abscess 76-50
- accessory 76-80
- amyloidosis 76-20
- anomaly 76-80
- artery 86-11
-- aneurysm 86-70
- cyst 76-30
- echinococcosis 76-30
- enlargement 76-2a
- estimation of size 76-10
- hilum 76-30
- index 76-10
- infarct 76-71
- injury 76-60
- parenchyma 76-10
- pseudocyst 76-30
- rupture 76-61
- tumour
-- cystic 76-30
-- solid 76-40
- vein 86-11
-- thrombosis 76-72
Splenomegaly 86-2a
Spondylitis 93-58
Standard deviation 3-10, 97-00
Stenosis

- spinal 93-53
-- morphometric data 93-53
Sternum 65-10
Streak artifacts cf. artifacts 97-00
Struma
- endothoracic 61-44
- mediastinal, dystopic 61-44
- ovarian 85-43
- Riedel's 61-82
Subperitoneal space
-- exudative haemorrhagic lesions 86-38
Substratification, urinary bladder 4-35
Subtraction of computed
 tomograms 97-00
Syndrome
- Pancoast 63-62, 64-40
- superior orbital fissure 52-41
- vena cava superior occlusion
Syringomyelia 93-56

T
Table advance 97-00
Talcosis 63-85
Technique of computerized
 tomography 1-00, 97-00
Teratoma
- intraspinal 93-56
- malignant
-- ovarian 85-43
- mediastinal 61-43
Thoracic duct 86-12, 61-12
Thoracic wall 64-00
-- anatomy 64-10
-- inflammation 63-40
-- metastases 63-30
-- trauma 63-50
-- tumours 63-30
Thrombophlebitis
- liver abscess 71-55
- orbital 51-71
Thymoma 61-42
- criteria of malignancy 61-42
- forms 61-42
Thymus
- carcinoma 61-42
- Hodgkin's disease 61-42
- hyperplasia 61-42
- persistence 61-42
Thyroid 53-00
- adenoma 53-40
- anatomy 53-10
- carcinoma 53-40
- cyst 52-40
- mediastinal 61-44
- retrotracheal 61-44
- tissue density 53-10

Tissue density cf. radiodensity
-- relative 3-40
Tissue, solid 3-54
Topogram 97-00
Topography cf. anatomy
- female pelvis 85-10
- male pelvis 84-10
- pancreas 73-10
- parapharyngeal space 52-10
- pararenal space 86-15
- pericardium 62-81
- perirenal space 86-14
- peritoneal cavity 75-10
- porta hepatis 71-10, 75-10
- pulmonary hilum 61-10
- retroperitoneal space 86-10
- thoracic wall 64-00
- vertebral canal 93-51
- visceral cranium 52-10
Trachea 61-12
- displacement 61-44
- tumours 61-51
Transit time cf. contrast media, transit time
Trauma
- kidney 81-56
- liver 71-60
- oesophagus 61-91
- orbit 51-72
- pancreas 73-60
- pelvis, osseous 93-63
- spleen 76-60
- thoracic wall 64-50
- thorax 64-50
- vertebral column 93-57
--- vs. conventional X-ray examination 93-57
Trunk, brachiocephalic 61-10
-- compression 61-73
Trunk, coeliac 86-11
Tube voltage 97-00
Tuberculoma, pulmonary 63-54
Tuberculosis
- kidney 81-54
- liver 71-55
- lung 63-51
- miliary 63-50
- prostate 84-40
- vertebral column 93-58
Tumor
- calcification 3-55
- necrosis 3-55
- vascularization 4-50
Tumour, cystic cf. cyst, cystadenoma, cystadenocarcinoma
Tumour, solid
-- adrenal cortex 82-30
-- adrenal medulla 82-40
-- anterior mediastinum 61-40
-- biliary tract 72-70
-- bone 93-40
-- epipharynx 52-52
-- gallbladder 72-50
-- giant cell 91-10
---- orbit 51-45
-- islet cell
---- hormone activity 73-44
---- localization 73-44
---- malignancy 73-44
---- types 73-44
---- vascularity 73-44
-- lacrimal gland 51-52
-- liver 71-40
-- lung 63-60
-- mediastinal mestastases 61-32
-- mediastinal, neurogenic 61-61
-- mediastinum
--- anterior 61-40
--- middle 61-50
--- posterior 61-60
-- mesopharynx 52-60
-- nasopharynx 52-50
-- ontogenic 52-32
-- optic nerve 51-42
-- orbit 51-30
--- extraconal 51-50
--- intraconal 51-40
-- oropharynx 52-60
-- osseous pelvis 93-62
-- osteogenic 93-40
-- ovaries 85-40
--- hormone-producing 85-43
-- Pancoast 63-62, 64-40
-- paranasal sinuses 72-30
-- parathyroid 61-45
-- pelvic, osseous 93-62
-- pericardium 62-85
-- perirenal space 86-34
-- pleura
--- primary 64-31
--- secondary 64-63
-- renal parenchyma 81-44
-- renal pelvis 81-46
-- retroperitoneal, primary 86-60
-- soft tissue 91-30
-- spinal 93-56
-- testicular
--- retroperitoneal metastases 86-52
-- theca cell, ovarian 85-43
-- thoracic wall 64-30
-- trachea 61-51
-- urinary bladder 83-50
-- uterus 85-30

– – vertebragenic   93-55

U

Ureter
– dilation   81-71
– tumour   81-71
Urine, extravasation
– – perirenal pseudocyst   86-32
Urinoma   86-32
Urographic agents
– – intravascular opacification   4-31
– – parenchymal opacification   4-31
– – pathophysiological correlate of enhancement   4-50
Urography
– retroperitoneal fibrosis   86-40
– tumours of the renal pelvis   81-46
Urolithiasis   81-73
– plain urographic diagnosis   81-73
– renal sinus   81-73
– vs. blood clot   81-73
Uropathy, obstructive   81-70
Uterus
– carcinoma   85-32, 85-33
– inflammation   85-51
– muscles   85-10
– myoma   85-31

V

Vacuum phenomenon
– – gallstones   72-42
Vagina   85-10
– marking   85-10
Valvular defects
– – CT follow-up   62-60
Varicosis, orbital   51-71
Vascularity   4-50
– avascular lesion   4-50
– hypervascular lesion   4-50
– hypovascular lesion   4-50
Vein
– azygos   86-11, 61-12
– – dilation   61-74
– – occlusion   61-74
– brachiocephalic   61-12
– – trauma   61-92
– – vs. dissecting aneurysm   61-72
– external jugular   61-12
– hemiazygos   86-11
– internal jugular   61-12
– pelvic   86-11
– portal   71-10, 73-10
– splenic
– – displacement   73-10
– – relationship to the pancreas   73-10
– subclavian   61-12
– superior mesenteric   73-10
– superior ophthalmic   51-10, 51-72
– umbilical, reopened   71-53
Vena cava inferior   86-11
– – – agenesis   86-74
– – – anomaly   86-74
– – – occlusion   61-74
– – – thrombosis   86-75
– – – vs. lymph node enlargement   86-74
Vena cava superior   61-12
– – – compression   61-43
– – – occlusion   61-74
– – – occlusion syndrome   61-82
Ventricles, enlargement, enddiastolic   62-31
Vertebral body   93-51
– – destruction   93-55
– – mineralization   93-30
– – osteoporosis   93-30
– – tumours   93-55
Vertebral column   93-50
Vertebral fracture   93-57
Vessels
– cervical   53-10
– lumbar   86-11
– mediastinal   61-12
– retroperitoneal   86-11
– visceral cranium   52-10
Visceral cranium   52-00
– – examination technique   52-20
– – muscular structures   52-10
– – osseous structures   53-10
Volume element   1-30
Volume measurement   97-00
Voxel   97-00

W

Waterhouse-Friderichsen syndrome   82-60
Wegener's granulomatosis
– intraorbital   51-62
– pulmonary   63-54
Wilms' tumour   81-45
– incidence   81-45
Window   97-00
– level   97-00
– width   97-00

X

X-, Y-coordinates   97-00
X-ray generator cf. equipment, computerized tomographic   97-00

Z

Z-axis   97-00